About the Authors

An anthropologist and cultural theorist, T. S. Wiley is a member of the New York Academy of Sciences and has been a guest investigator at Sansum Medical Research Institute. She lives in Santa Barbara, California.

Julie Taguchi, M.D., an oncologist, is a staff physician at Sansum Medical Clinic in Santa Barbara. She joined the team for Cancer Protocol to clinically test their progesterone theories at Cottage Hospital in 1999.

Bent Formby, Ph.D., holds doctorates in biochemistry, biophysics, and molecular biology from the University of Copenhagen in Denmark. He has pursued research projects in California for the last two decades with the University of California, Sansum Medical Research Institute, and now with the Rasmus Institute for Medical Research in Santa Barbara.

T. S. Wiley, Dr. Julie Taguchi, and Dr. Bent Formby are conducting cancer research in Santa Barbara, California, where they have partnered on numerous studies and published papers. At present they have two more papers out on the role of the newly discovered gene Survivin, and on the roles of natural progesterone and the gene P21. Their most recent publication is the textbook *Breast Cancer: Prognosis, Treatment, and Prevention.*

T.S. WILEY,
with Julie Taguchi, M.D.,
and Bent Formby, Ph.D.

The Shocking Truth About

SYNTHETIC HORMONES AND THE BENEFITS OF NATURAL ALTERNATIVES

SEX,

LIES,

and

MENOPAUSE

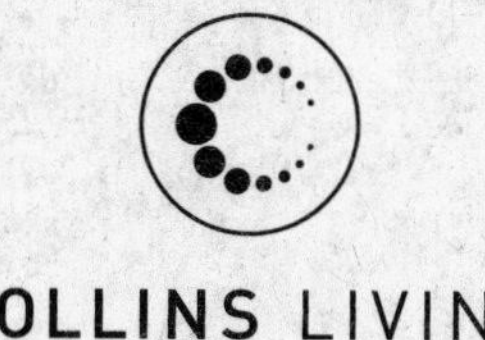

COLLINS LIVING

An Imprint of HarperCollins*Publishers*

This book contains advice and information relating to health care. It is not intended to replace medical advice and should be used to supplement rather than replace regular care by your doctor. It is recommended that you seek your physician's advice before embarking on any medical program or treatment. All efforts have been made to assure the accuracy of the information contained in this book as of the date of publication. The publisher and the author disclaim liability for any medical outcomes that may occur as a result of applying the methods suggested in this book.

Grateful acknowledgment is made to reprint the following excerpt from *Rosencrantz and Guildenstern Are Dead*, Act II, by Tom Stoppard. Copyright © 1966 by Tom Stoppard. Reprinted by permission of Grove Press and Faber and Faber.

A hardcover edition of this book was published in 2003 by William Morrow, an imprint of HarperCollins Publishers.

First Perennial Currents edition published 2004.

Designed by Adrian Leichter

The Library of Congress has catalogued the hardcover edition as follows:
Wiley, T. S.
Sex, lies, and menopause: the shocking truth about hormone replacement therapy / T. S. Wiley, Julie Taguchi, and Bent Formby.
p. cm.
ISBN 0-06-054233-0
1. Menopause—Hormone therapy—Complications.
2. Oral contraceptives.
3. Middle-aged women—Health and hygiene.
4. Menopause. I. Taguchi, Julie.
II. Formby, Bent. III. Title.
RG186.W49 2003
618.1'75061—dc21 2003050126

ISBN 0-06-054234-9 (pbk.)

08 ❖/RRD 10 9 8 7 6

The work in this book is dedicated to

ROSE KUSHNER

and

LINDA DONOFRIO

PLAYER: We only know what we're told, and that's little enough.
And for all we know, that isn't even true.
For all anyone knows, nothing is.
Everything has to be taken on trust;
truth is only that which is taken to be true.
It's the currency of living.
There may be nothing behind it, but it doesn't
make any difference so long as it is honored.
One acts on assumptions.
What do you assume?

—TOM STOPPARD,
Rosencrantz and Guildenstern Are Dead,
Act II

Contents

PART THREE | MENOPAUSE

Acknowledgments

The learning curve and research process for this book have taken over seven years. In the ensuing time, at least a hundred people all over America have, in part, collaborated with me to make this book possible.

Bent, Julie, and I are grateful to the cancer patients who courageously listened to their survival instincts and volunteered to try the principles of treatment that we've discovered. The volunteers include, but are not limited to, the women in Irvine, California, like Joanie Scott and Sandy Gardner, and Aileen Mostel in Florida. We also thank women, old and young, without cancer, who know that they must have hormone replacement to feel well, like Sofia and Erica Koltavary.

We've appreciated working with curious, open-minded doctors here in Santa Barbara, California, like David Laub, Ed Wroblewski, Alison Mayer-Oaks, Alex Depaoli, and Luc Maes, and in New York, the always-ahead-of-his-time Dr. Robert Atkins. As always, the ongoing dialogue and debate with Dr. John Lee is a sounding board for my own ideas.

The nurse practitioners like Barbara Winter on the East Coast and Anna Bunting and Alice Levine here in Santa Barbara, who provide the best care for women possible, gave us insights and practical advice all along the way. Barbara, in particular, has provided research and guidance with regard to the prescriptive needs of women in her practice and how to communicate the principles of self-managed menopause to the public. Dana Nelson at Health Plus Pharmacy, our friend and patron, was instrumental in determining the best-quality, safest transdermal hormone preparations and delivery system.

Perhaps the biggest thanks of all goes to my friend of thirty years and agent, Deborah Schneider. Deborah's enthusiasm and intelligence has made this project her first priority from the beginning. Without Deborah representation, we got the opportunity to work with Claire Wachtel.

I personally want to thank all of the people at William Morrow, but especially my editor Claire Wachtel. Claire gave us the chance to air this revolutionary new approach to women's health and breast cancer. She brought a new depth to my work with her incisive and probing questions. She has worked tirelessly, and I thank her for her commitment to safeguarding the evidence and helping us to bring the truth to women everywhere.

Bent and I have collaborated on two books, and both times Jane Cavolina did a wonderful job editing the original drafts. She's always been there for us. Her comments, suggestions, and support mean the world to me.

There is no greater intellectual pleasure that I know than to sit and debate scientific truths and mysteries with my partner, Bent Formby. I always feel that there's nothing I can't figure out with Bent's enormous wealth of knowledge.

Dr. Julie Taguchi is exactly what all doctors should aspire to be. She's willing to risk everything to understand what good health is and bring it to her patients. She's capable of evolving and moving in new directions to save lives and give comfort, even when her life and practice of medicine might be much easier if she'd stuck with the status quo. Julie understands that the practice of medicine is a "holy" ordinance of trust that requires the same devotion and vigilance that mothering does.

Maybe the best always does come last. Thanks to my mother, who at eighty-eight is of sound body and mind thanks to natural rhythmic HRT, and all of the mothers who stood in for me with my children while I worked—Mara Raden, Robin Bisio, Jenny Teton, Mary Turley, Liz Bosscocci, and Amy Sachs. I include my executive assistant and researcher, Chelsey Fink, as part of my family because her devotion to this project has, at this point, spanned a fourth of her life. And to Carol Wiley-Lorente who has my gratitude for years of research and support for this endeavor.

My treasured son-in-law, Ian McGuinness, did dishes and footnotes with charm, grace, and good humor and gave us our grandson, Harvey. All my children, Mara, Aja, Jake, Max, and Zoe, give me feedback and are the real reason I go on at all. I thank Aja, particularly, for the concepts of evolutionary biology in Chapter Four. They belong to her. My precious husband, Neil Raden, has listened in the dark to me about endocrinology for more hours than anyone could ever stay interested, and always encouraged me to write it down. As Deborah once said, "You can't tell everyone, one at a time." I love you, Neil. Thank you.

—T.S. Wiley

SEX, LIES, AND MENOPAUSE

part one

SEX

one

IT'S ONLY ROCK AND ROLL

The drums were pounding. The beat, getting louder and louder, was on the upswing. The sun made its mark for noon in the sky, and well-worn trails were lined with throngs of worshipers who would snake toward the flat open spaces where a festival would take place. Hundreds would gather near gigantic structures built for the occasion. Those who weren't engaged in work were engaged in play.

The ground was littered with small naked running children, mothers and babies nursing on blankets, and yapping dogs festooned with red strips of cloth. In an adjacent field, men naked to the waist except for the beads around their necks passed around a bamboo smoking tube and danced and laughed and shouted. Men and women, their long hair decorated with flowers and rawhide bands, started swaying in unison, and some seemed to be hallucinating. The drums were inside them now, in their brains and bones.

The lone drums and flutes were drowned out by instruments with strings; bigger, louder drums; and singing that would go on night and day for three days. The physicality of union on many levels, from eating to bathing and mating,[1] may have been the true purpose of the gathering.

Some of the fervid splashed naked in the small pond. Others, in pairs or groups, copulated openly. They stroked and petted each other and continuously displayed grooming behavior like combing hair, rubbing backs, and stroking one another's arms and feet. Finally, on the third day, the gods hosed them down. The skies cracked wide open, and a flood of near-biblical proportions ensued, the ultimate cosmic release at the end of the frenzy, an orgasm of nature. The place: Upstate New York. The tribe described is us, and the scene is from a documentary called *Woodstock*. We *thought* we invented music, love, and sex.

We were so young.

Since time began, men and women have heard music and been driven to sexual ecstasy. It's common knowledge that listening to music can be a religious experience—especially loud music. For many in Western culture, until the Renaissance, God was actually conceived of as only sound or a vibration. The scientific reason for this is that in the software controlling hearing and balance in your brain, a small organ called the *sacculus,* part of the balance-regulating system in the inner ear, is "tickled" at certain decibel levels.

Loud music can activate the sacculus and create the feeling of movement or floating. That's why listening to music above 70 decibels sends a pleasurable buzz through the sacculus that ends up at the hypothalamus, a buzz that thrills the listener in the way bungee jumping or swinging very high does, a simultaneous flying and falling feeling.[2-6] It's no coincidence that the distribution of frequencies typical of rock concerts and dance clubs is at exactly the right decibel level to make listeners feel as if they're floating. Your sacculus also speaks to the part of your brain that controls drives like hunger, sex, and more than a few other hedonistic responses—the hypothalamus.[7-13]

That's part of the reason sex, drugs, and rock and roll go so well together. Of course, the drugs we take now—Prozac, Paxil, Klonopin, Ambien, Tamoxifen, Vioxx, Claritin, or Lipitor, Beta-blockers or ACE Inhibitors, not to mention Advil and Tylenol PM, just aren't as much fun.

Talkin' About My Generation

Only about thirty-five of the seventy-five million of us born between 1948 and 1952 made it to college, where most of us were introduced to the principles of self-medication. By 1969, according to a Gallup survey of fifty-seven college campuses, 31 percent of students had smoked pot and between 10 and 15 percent admitted to using LSD. To clarify: At least ten to twelve million of us smoked marijuana and between three and five million of us dropped acid. Today we get a kick out of loading up on nutritional supplements at the health food store.

It's just not the same.

We're just not radical anymore. But we should be. Our very lives are at stake, because half of all of the women today have already been on synthetic *hormone replacement therapy* (HRT), and we're not even sure of the damage it's done. And on the opposite side of the coin, most of us aren't really sure that we want to give up our drugs (HRT).

Is living without hormones really living?

We need to find out how much harm has been done and whether or not we should ever put our hormones back at all. Most of us would admit that without them we don't really feel good—no matter how many supplements we buy or how many miles we jog or how little fat we eat. But, at the same time, we're all scared of heart disease, strokes, and cancer. We face the same inevitable health condition that made our parents obstinate, obdurate, and obsolete—a condition called *aging,* characterized by being stubborn, hardened, and out of date. None of us want to look and feel "old," but most of us are in menopause.

In 2002, forty-six million women will reach the age of menopause.[14]

Menopause is the hallmark of aging in women.

There exists today more than a few of us who once fought the good fight for personal freedom, but now sit back and spout the party line of our generation about menopause being *natural.* Of course it's "natural."

So is pregnancy in the wake of free love, but that didn't stop us from taking hormones to avoid it in our youth. Those miracle drugs—contraceptives—were the hormones that kept us in school or going to work every day while having all the sex we wanted, without the natural consequence of childbirth and breast-feeding.

It's a painful irony that when we were young and had everything to lose (our fertility and potential for genetic immortality), many of us eagerly tossed back hormones made out of mutated synthetic estrogens, fake progesterone, and even, sometimes, testosterone. In effect, a good many of us have been on synthetic HRT most of our adult lives. We may have taken them for a different purpose, but the drugs in contraceptives were basically the same synthetic hormones that are in HRT.

The doctors who prescribed them had no idea they might impact our future fertility or what those hormones might be doing to us physically by *preventing* pregnancy. And now the very same authorities who wrote those prescriptions without a thought are warning us every day against taking the very *same* hormones. Doctors and researchers are in a panic because medicine is just starting to figure out exactly how toxic the synthetic hormone "drugs" like PremPro can really be.

PremPro is a combination pill containing two synthetic (invented in a lab) *hormonelike* drugs. PremPro actually contains fake progesterone or progestin, called medroxyprogesterone (MPA), or Provera in combination with a metabolite of horse estrogen, equinol, which is *not* like human estrogen, called Premarin.

Back in the 1970s, when Provera was invented, Premarin, the "Prem" in PremPro, was prescribed alone. The low-dose chronic horse estrogen caused uterine cancer by fostering an *overgrowth* of the lining of the uterus. Originally, a doctor aiming to replace hormones only prescribed estrogen replacement therapy (ERT). But once the epidemic increase of uterine cancer was identified,[15-17] instead of pulling Premarin from the shelves, Upjohn, the original maker of MPA, invented another drug out of natural progesterone. The molecule of natural progesterone found in a compound called *genistein* in plants[18] was chemically altered into a patentable drug that has been proven to have life-threatening side effects like heart disease, breast cancer, stroke, and dementia.[19-23] The two drugs were eventually packaged together and remarketed as PremPro to prevent the horse estrogen from causing uterine cancer, and increase the market share to women with uteruses.

However, unlike real progesterone, which has a rhythmic, cyclical presence in your body two weeks out of every month, if you take PremPro, you receive Provera every day. In actuality, this combination of horse estrogen and fake progesterone[24] can't ever re-create a normal cycle, so although it's marketed as HRT, *it's not*. It's not really hormone *replacement* for two reasons: (1) because it's a drug, and (2) because it's prescribed in a static dose, which has no resemblance to what used to go on hormonally in your body when you were young.

In the end, the static, chronic dose of a progestin like Provera in a combination dose with an animal-source estrogen like Premarin blocks the horse estrogen's effect *every day*. So any benefits known to result in heart, brain, and breast from estrogen are lost or diminished. Even though this combination drug can cause breast cancer, heart disease, and dementia,[25-28] it's still widely available to women all over the world.

There's no question, in fact, that Wyeth-Ayerst knows this and still does not withdraw it voluntarily from the marketplace. There is no question because the side effects are published in the package inserts written by the company[29-30] and many of the studies reporting toxicity[31-34] were funded by Wyeth-Ayerst themselves, or they at the very least donated their product for testing. There's no question because they provided free drugs for the recent Women's Health Initiative study that said so.

Now, according to the news, hormone replacement not only increases your risk of cancer, but also causes heart disease and stroke.[35] Conventional HRT invented by Wyeth-Ayerst really *does* cause these side effects. The hormones made in your body really *don't*.

The Age of Aquarius

There is an alternative to hormonelike drugs available. The real bioidentical hormones (that Wyeth-Ayerst altered in the lab to create the unnatural HRT drugs) can be had *in their pure form* by prescription. More than likely your doctor has never heard of Natural Hormones. But getting your hands on the real McCoy isn't the only problem. Getting *enough* hormones to make yourself a real, normal, *physiologically rhythmic* cycle just like when you were young—that's the problem.

It wasn't just the chemical composition of the drugs in PremPro that made us sick. It was the dosage, too. Real hormones in your body pulse in waves of seconds, minutes, hours, days, weeks, and seasons because we have evolved as an integral part of nature and the cosmos, not in opposition to it. The rhythm of the planet we live on is in us, literally. Hormonal rhythms echo the pulse of life, of hearts beating, of lungs expanding and contracting, even of the gait of our walk. The hormones give us menstrual periods that count the beat of time for women month after month, year after year. Men, too, have rhythm. Young males peak hormonally in the fall and drop low in the spring after their testosterone kicks in.[36] Everything on Earth does. Birds sing and bees dance because of their respective testosterone levels.[37-38] There's the music again.

The only primate besides us that sings is the gibbon. Gibbons are monogamous because resources are scarce and a pair bond does a better job of defending a territory, ensuring the survival of offspring. As it is in all venues, female selection is the rule. The female chooses a territory, maybe one with a great fruit tree, and then invites a male to join her. She does this by rising at first light and singing a very, very complicated song. A cacophony of males try to return her call. The male who is smart enough to sing her song back note for note wins himself a life—children, a home, and a wife.[39]

Take a moment to remember. Before puberty, music was nice. But after your hormones kicked in, music was everything. Life, surely, still has a beat, but we aren't dancing to it. The big question is: How come no one's talking about the fact that we've lost our rhythm? When our menstrual cycles dwindle and cease, the hormones that kept us in step with each other to mate and survive are gone.

The Beat Goes On

The world as we know it, from bacteria to blue whales, the whole universe, in fact, is all about timing, within each of us and in relation to everything outside us. The individual rhythms overlap into larger patterns that then again weave in and out of each other. Human beings swim in this sea of rhythms; the examples are myriad.

The moon provides more light with its full face and sure enough, as the new moon ends, every twenty-eight days females bleed.[40] Babies in utero synchronize their movements to the sound of their mothers' voices. This sets up a pattern of emotional response to mom calling you for dinner as your very brain architecture is being laid down.[41] More babies are born between midnight and 6:00 A.M. than any other time period, thanks to our circadian clock.[42-60] The circadian clock in every cell measures one spin of the planet, or twenty-four hours.

Instrumental music is just an expression of those rhythms, ineffable to some, but quite tangible to others. Because there is a beat to it, it is generally accepted that the rhythm originates in the music, but more likely music is a highly specialized releaser of the rhythms already inherent in the listener. We, and all life on Earth, are dancers to a tune we've heard so long that we've forgotten we're dancing.[61]

A scientist named Hans Selye asserted that it's only when we *can't* dance that we get sick. He called it "perennial adaptation."[62] His hypothesis was that illness only occurs when an organism is stuck in a constant effort to adapt to the next level of existence, when it is no longer living in rhythm. When our menstrual cycles stop, it's evident that we won't make it to the next level—reproduction—ever again. Nature hates that.

Although we live unaware of it, consciousness itself is a manifestation of hormonal cues, and hormonal cues are the rhythmic regulators inside us.[63] Our desires for food, love, sex, and shelter are hormonal interfaces between our bodies and the world around us. The sun, the stars, and our own planet tick off the passing hours and seasons. This ticking is referred to as "time."

When life appeared on Earth, the light and dark cycles occasioned by the revolving of our planet as it exposed first one, then the other side to the Sun made up the environmental cues by which *human* life evolved. The roll of the tides caused by the forces of the moon and the seasonal rhythms that change as the planet travels in its orbit around our sun became the basis for yet another subset of clocks. So day/night, hot/cold, wet/dry, and the moon's gravitational effect are the clocks that strike the beat to which all life, including *our personal* life, keeps time.

It is not a coincidence that women menstruate in tandem with the lunar cycle.

We adapted to the rhythm of the planet and internalized it in our *hormonal* rhythms. Our hormones designed the rhythms of our sleep, our appetite for sex and food, and our menstrual, birth, and nursing cycles in tandem with the weather and food supply. In order to survive, all things alive had to integrate life-sustaining activities in rhythm with the planet's offerings. Sleeping, eating, mating, playing, learning, giving birth, and even dying are set to internal clocks.

When things cease to beat, they cease to be.

Do You Wanna Dance?

Living in Earth time means that when the warm sun shines, it's time to look for food and to mate, and when it's dark and cold, it's time to sleep and hide. We humans lived according to this rhythm for most of our history on this planet. All of us who share this planet know these calls for survival in our bones and soul. Fiddler crabs know the twelve-hour tidal clock and forage on the beach at low tide. Oysters know to feed at high tide, and human males know it's fall when the freshman girls appear on campus. Our internal clocks, regulated by hormones, keep all living things in step, not only with each other in our individual species, but with the rest of the universe. Staying "in phase" with all other life and bodies in motion creates biological *harmony*. Science calls this *homeostasis*.

In a healthy organism, the internal environment remains constant or self-maintaining, even when the external environment fluctuates wildly. Having the ability to translate an environmental cue like light, for example, gives all creatures great and small the capability to predict weather and food supply—because light means food grows, and food means survival.[64-68]

The rhythm of nature is so internalized that every molecular action of every hormone to its receptor, on every gene in every cell, functioning in every organ of your body, hears the cosmic tune.[69-71] It's called *entrainment*.[72-73] The internalization of planetary cues by hormone actions assures survival. Entrainment means that the environment sings the song and your hormones hum along. Cortisol, insulin, melatonin, prolactin, progesterone, estrogen, testosterone, and growth hormone all play like the keys of a grand piano in response to environmental sheet music.[74-75]

The spontaneity and ephemeral nature of hormonal response is how we are entrained to the rhythm of life. *The system is programmed to last as long as we remain reproductive*. We have just enough hormones on board to last at most fifty years in reasonably good health. Then, as we literally run out of hormones, we lose the ability to use the raw materials of life to create new life, and as far as nature is concerned, we're finished.

Riders on the Storm

Picture life as a Slinky lying on its side: circles connected in a spiral. Now picture the one-way arrow of time traveling the circles of loops that seem to go on forever. If we follow the arrow of time as it carries information and energy through the organism (us)—in the form of food and light—coming in from the outside, traveling through us and out again on the other end, it becomes obvious that all organisms are *dissipative* structures—that is, structures that lose energy just living.

We use up resources over time and literally wear ourselves out doing it. The Second Law of Classical Thermodynamics describes the process of the dissipation of energy as the movement of energy away from the point of equilibrium, which in humans is about the age of twenty-six years, when human growth hormone and estrogen start to decline.[76] In our individual lives, the circles or loops carrying information begin to narrow as we age and run out of hormones. We literally start to run down like an old record player unwinding, in terms of physical function. This dissipation of energy is called *entropy*.

Entropy is essentially an organism moving away from order to disorder.[77] Any closed system, like the human body or a cell, will spontaneously move in the direction of ever-increasing entropy or disregulation as the arrow of time moves away from equilibrium. With fewer hormones in place to regulate and mandate order, ever-increasing disorder ensues.

Aging is our personal experience of *cellular entropy*.[78-83]

The loops in the spiral of eternity get smaller and smaller as we age. Just as a dying heart slows its beat in old age, your menstrual periods get shorter and shorter and farther apart as you approach menopause because our ovaries are running out of eggs.

That's why we run out of estrogen and are no longer fertile. The eggs were the source. Without an estrogen peak in a woman's blood every month, her brain stops sending the monthly signal to ovulate, or release the egg the next month. The absence of a released or "popped" egg leaves her without the progesterone that would be secreted by the egg "shell," or degrading egg sac.

It is progesterone's major job to regulate the genes that cause all of a woman's cells all over her brain and body to grow, to differentiate, or to die.[84-94] Progesterone is one of the premier regulatory hormones. Without it rising cyclically, the woman becomes, literally and figuratively, on the cellular level, out of control. This is the beginning of aging and, ultimately, the onset of the death of the organism that is you.

Sex hormones register directly to genes[95] that flip on and off according to hormonal directives, elicited by environmental cues. Sex hormones determine which genes are expressed (turned on) or silenced (turned off) in the nucleus of every cell in the body. Estrogen, progesterone, cortisol, testosterone, insulin, prolactin, and melatonin reach all the way down into the nucleus of every cell in every organ in your body to hit "promoter regions" and "response elements" on genes that literally control the stuff of life.

Hormones not only cause you to think, behave, and react in ways that enhance your chances for survival, but they also cause you to go forth and multiply.[96-99]

Without *regular* ovulation, which must be stimulated by high enough levels of estrogen, and without the progesterone that follows ovulation, the regulatory genes involved in cancer, heart disease, diabetes, Alzheimer's, and autoimmunity are left "deranged," or uncontrolled.[100-107] Your particular experience of this disregulation will take whatever form your inherited genetics dictate. In other words, when your sex hormones fall off and you start to die, the disease that gets you will depend on your family's personal threshold of entropy.

Will your heart or breast or blood sugar go first?

When You're Strange

In a *natural* environment, not the one we live in today, with electricity and antibiotics, a woman's fertility would start to fall off in her late twenties, after she had given birth to and breast-fed four or five children. If she actually made it to the ripe old age of thirty-five—and she hadn't already died in childbirth, been eaten by a tiger, drowned in a flood, or pricked her finger gathering berries and died of an infection—she would be a grandmother.

In our world, a world that has encouraged us to postpone childbearing, fertility still drops off in our late twenties. Today, by thirty-five a woman who is finally financially and emotionally ready to have a child may have to spend a lot of money on fertility treatments or surrogates because inside, her reproductive machinery is still that of a grandmother. Electricity and antibiotics haven't made delaying childbearing any more physically possible at thirty-five than it was thirty thousand years ago.

We're in even more trouble *now*.

In most of us now, our biological age doesn't really match our chronological age anymore. When we lived outside most of the time and slept when it got dark and ate what the season offered us, we were as old, in years, as the number of trips we'd taken around the sun or how many "moons" or months we had lived. But now, at thirty-five, many of us are years older *inside*.

Now we live in a world where it seems as if the sun never sets and we never run out of fruit (sugar). Although we have evolved to experience one mating season a year, which is one summer, our lives in the modern world are all sex all the time. When the light is long—that is, in summer—we are programmed to feel sexy because the sunlight and plentiful carbohydrates of summer increase our insulin, which provides us with extra circulating estrogen and testosterone to let us appreciate it *hormonally*. That's why the beach seems so sexy—it's the light, not just the bikinis.

Conversely, when the days are short and dark outside, even though we may be sitting in front of a blinking computer screen under fluorescent lights, rising melatonin lowers our body temperature a few tenths of a degree,[108] which is enough to cause a shiver and yawn. Your body is trying to remind you that it's winter outside and should be winter inside—of you, too. In nature, before now, we went dormant (more sleep, no sugar, very little sex) when the temperature dropped in winter, just like the other animals and plants. That's all different now. Now we turn up the heat and get a cup of coffee.

By creating endless summer, we have changed the rules of life. Since the light is long all the time in our world, it has put us—our bodies—out of rhythm with the earth, on which we evolved to survive. Everything in this life is all about timing, and we've altered what had to be a rhythm, to be a constant. There is no tempo without variation. That's why it is as much of a physical and mental problem when your menstrual periods stop as it is when your heart starts skipping beats.

It's a physical impossibility to be part of life and not be able to keep time.

This fundamental change in our environmental cues for mating and aging began in the mid-1860s. Then, in the mid-1960s, after about ten decades of altered light and food in exaggerated rhythms, birth control pills were invented and took us even farther away from the beat of nature and our own bodies.

When Proud Mary Keeps on Burnin'

In the world we live in today, the extended periods of artificial heat, light at night, and year-round carbohydrates out of season create a condition of endless summer that is read loud and clear by the systems' response-clocking mechanisms imbedded in us all. The artificial triggers of man-made light and food not only fool your insulin, cortisol, and melatonin systems—which wreaks havoc with your sleep cycles and makes you jumpy and crave sugar—they affect your sex hormones, too. Sex hormones are inextricably synchronized with your insulin and melatonin for accuracy in timing mating.

In summer, the weightless, invisible energy of the sun saturates plants and fruit, they ripen, and we eat them. Any sugar is a carbohydrate and any carbohydrate is just sugar. When the plants and fruits as "solid sunlight" enter the body, over time the sun's energy becomes very visible as *insulating* weight around our middles and backsides. In the natural world, which still has seasons, we would reburn this weight, this solar "charcoal," in winter, when summer's carbohydrates were gone. But when winter never comes because we have indoor heating and electric lighting, we continue to crave the carbohydrates of summer and become exhausted, and sexually a little crazy.

We go to the grocery store and buy fruits we would never have seen in winter before, plus thousands of recently invented forms of sugar that would never have been available to us seventy-five years ago.

Unfortunately for us, all that nature allows is *one* period of high insulin a year—the three months or so of summer. Since we evolved and adapted to this rhythm, when we are exposed to heat, sugar, and light for all twelve months of the year, we naturally experience accelerated *biological* time. Every year for us in the modern world has *four* summers, because just one of our modern years is twelve months of light and heat and sugar. That's why one year today is like four years to our Stone Age bodies, because our sensors for aging register "four trips around the sun" instead of just one.

We collaterally experience accelerated aging.

The hallmarks of being old, increasing blood sugar, arthritis, macular degeneration, and so forth, are also, not coincidentally, the hallmarks of Type II diabetes. This adult onset form of diabetes is on the increase in adolescents as of this writing. Human timing mechanisms read the endless summer cues literally and respond *automatically*.

If this behavior goes on year after year, well, you do the math.[109-110]

The fact that we enjoy all this light and heat doesn't mean our biology won't respond to it in the only ancient way it can. The false cues of endless summer affect not only our appetite for food but also our appetite for sex. In our brave new world, it's always mating season. We are experiencing a forty-year mating frenzy. It's not only apparent in our cultural obsessions, but in our ovaries, "party" has become a verb, and there are only so many eggs to go around.

Tune In, Turn On, Drop Out

This sleep/sugar/survival equation is *the* control mechanism on how fast we age, and how fast we age determines how fast we deplete the eggs in our ovaries. As children we matured faster and began ovulating sooner than our grandmothers did. The average age of menarche at the turn of the century was seventeen, for us it was twelve, for our daughters, it's down to ten years old.[111-116]

Higher insulin levels not only mean faster maturation sexually, they mean that the reproductive machinery is on overdrive. We weren't meant to ovulate twelve months a year, every year, year in and year out, from a very young age. If we should have our first period at about seventeen years old and then, in the natural world, we would be pregnant soon afterward, and then breast-feeding, we'd save a lot of eggs and be exposed to high levels of estrogen and progesterone as a bonus. Birth control pills didn't save our eggs by stopping ovulation; instead, the androgens (testosteronelike hormone drugs) actually caused egg cell death, as the eggs aged at an increased rate.[117-128] Picture a carton of chicken eggs left out in the heat for a couple of months. That's where we are.

Menopause, or "egglessness," causes the breakdown of the estrogen and progesterone feedback system that controls all the cell cycles in your body. Remember the narrowing Slinky? That's the real problem. As we said earlier, estrogen leads to progesterone by way of released eggs, and progesterone regulates the genes that cause cells to grow, differentiate, or die. Cancer is not really about *too much growth* of one kind of cell or another.

It's about *not enough death* of one kind of cell or another.

Life and death is a three-act play consisting of genesis, florescence, and decay—the endless cycle of birth, life, and death. Cells are born, they live, but they must die so new cells can come again. When cells don't die cyclically, *we start to.*

While we are young, the ups and downs of estrogen and progesterone month after month strike the beat that keeps us rocking and rolling with the stresses of life that could negatively affect our health. When the cycling rhythm of "on and off" ceases, we can no longer handle germs, fatigue, and hot or cold weather; maintain our body temperature; or control our appetites under stress. We are beginning to die. Sometimes death can happen in as little as three years, or it can take as long as an agonizing twenty or thirty. When our hormones stop humming the tune of the Sun and the moon and start keeping the beat of an artificial environment, our internal systems—which have evolved over millennia to adapt for survival—are being driven by *artificial signals.*

When this happens, what was the dance of life becomes a malignant pas de deux. Those of us more genetically predisposed to be light- and food-responsive suffer first and most from the altered rhythms. But in the end, losing the beat gets us all.

Hormonal timing mechanisms, including the ones that control the genes that regulate cell growth and cell death, were laid down millions of years ago when the earliest mammals split off from reptiles. Darwin's theory of evolution shows us that a tiny invisible thread binds us to monkeys and amphibians and fish, to insects, and to the bacteria from which it all began. Darwinism is sort of a theory of universal brotherhood in which mankind is a product of contingency.

We see this premise in evidence in pictures taken of the human fetus in utero. In *Being Born,* a beautiful book of photography of the developmental stages of the human fetus, Lennart Nielsson shows us vivid glimpses of the phases of fetal development of ourselves as fish, birds, and eventually primates.[129] The miracle of transmogrification—all evolution, in fact—is attributable to the interplay of estrogen, progesterone, and testosterone on the genes that sculpt eyes, arms, legs, fingers, and toes.

It's these hormones that tell genes like homeobox and Hox genes,[130-132] which are in control of the grand body plan, whether they are to create arms, wings, or flippers, depending on what species mom is and what modifications the environment demands for the survival of the offspring.[133-136]

In the case of a human fetus, it is progesterone's message to certain genetically preselected cells to die that ultimately sculpts a baby into the likeness of its parents instead of another species. The reason your fingers on your hand holding this book right now aren't webbed, as they were when you were a four-week-old fetus, is that the amount of progesterone your mother produced during her pregnancy said to the fast-dividing bundle of cells that became you, "*Human*, not chicken, not fish, not insect."

The unnecessary cells, for a human baby, between your fingers were "removed" by the interplay of estrogen and progesterone on regulatory genes as those hormones rose and surged throughout your mother's pregnancy. The ever-rising estrogen that your mother made created more and more progesterone receptors; in turn, progesterone reached through its receptor the controls on the Hox and homeobox genes that caused preselected cells to take a suicidal path, each one sacrificed for the good of the many.

Estrogen grows life, and progesterone refines and stabilizes it.

These two hormones always act in tandem to control cell growth for normal function. Cancer researchers call progesterone's end of the job *apoptosis*.

Apoptosis is derived from Greek and roughly translates to "falling away from life."[137] In science it's known to mean "cell suicide." Progesterone, through the process of apoptosis, is in charge of just the right amount of death to keep things living. Anything alive must grow and die and grow and die within the sphere of its own lifetime. Bone cells, blood cells, even brain cells begin in an embryonic form, mature, and die, all in a matter of days, and then the process of life starts all over again—in your leg or spleen or brain, if you have hormones to regulate the pace. Science has shown time and again that no higher organisms can grow in a healthy way unless they are time-controlled and differentiate to a purpose.[138-139]

It is the *unregulated* growth of cells that characterizes what we identify as cancer. Cancer cells not only proliferate and multiply without ever going beyond the embryonic state, they can even go backward. Cancer cells actually dedifferentiate, or lose their individuality.[140-141] The reversal to the oneness of universal life, along with unstoppable growth, is the defining property of cancer. Since all of the cells in our bodies have had a distinct job since Day One, the rapid takeover of purposeless cells destroys the integrity of the coordinated efforts of all the other systems and organs and siphons off precious metabolic resources.

Not Fade Away

If the rhythmic ups and downs of estrogen and progesterone over the twenty-eight days of a normal lunar cycle create genesis, florescence, and decay—the three-act play of life in all the tissues of your body—why do medical experts call that estrogen produced in our own bodies a carcinogen? In *low* concentrations, 17-beta estradiol, the strongest-acting estrogen found in our bodies, is proliforative. The low levels in the early part of the menstrual cycle grow the lining of your uterus and change breast tissue. The low levels of early pregnancy control genes and growth in an explosive way. And the trailing-off of normal estrogen rhythms in perimenopausal women with no progesterone could be the trigger of the unchecked growth of cancer.

It's this evidence that has made "estrogen blockers" the new standard of care for breast and ovarian cancer patients.[142-143] These relatively new drugs are called selective estrogen receptor modifiers (SERMs) and are now being prescribed *prophylactically*, as the television commercial for raloxifene[144] states, "to eliminate cancer worries." That means medicine is willing to block the receptors for what little estrogen we are still producing on the off-chance that it could cause cancer someday in the future.

The justification for this premise is based in the petri dish studies of estrogen's growth-enhancing potential and the unscientific assumption that any extra estrogen in your body, for your age, or any estrogen that stays in your body too long, will encourage, not cause, the growth of any cancer that might already exist. However, there is no evidence to that effect in large studies of women who take estrogen after cancer diagnosis. In fact, studies show the opposite effect.[145-149]

Women on natural hormone replacement after breast cancer diagnosis in a large study published in the *Journal of the National Cancer Institute*[150] in 2001 were reported to have 50 percent lower recurrence rates and 30 percent less mortality. The erroneous assumptions medical science has about estrogen are drawn from the evidence that it acts as a growth factor in petri dish experiments. But in our bodies that fact is only half of the equation.

Many growth factors exist that alone are not sufficient to cause cancer. Insulin, for example, is one of the strongest growth factors on earth. Insulin by injection or pump is hormone replacement in Type I diabetics, who, because their pancreases have failed, regulate their blood sugar with a synthetic version of the same insulin that occurs in all of us. Now it is well known that in *Type II* diabetics, who have so much insulin around that their insulin receptors become nonfunctional because their pancreases overproduce, their excess insulin production is a factor in their increased incidence of breast[151] and prostate cancers. There is no movement afoot to refuse Type I diabetics insulin because the same hormone is likely to be associated with cancer in Type IIs.[152-153] In the case of estrogen, a dose-dependent response and the absence of its partner hormone, progesterone, could be the actual cause of cancer, not estrogen alone.[154-157]

Coupled with estrogen's propensity to grow tissues, the undeniable evidence that breast cancer occurs less frequently among women who have experienced pregnancy and lactation[158-159] has led researchers to conclude that it was the egregious estrogen produced by unending menstrual cycles in women who didn't have children that is to blame in cancer-stricken women. It has not occurred to them that pregnancy and lactation might have been beneficial, which would also account for those statistics.

But the simplest answer continues to elude them, and unfortunately for us, the jury is in. The advice from medicine and science to date is that the less you are exposed to your own estrogen, the better. That was the moment in time when hormone *ablation*, otherwise known as chemical castration—and once reserved only for extreme cancer treatment—entered the medical or prophylactic spectrum somewhere between vitamins and sunscreen.

It will be available over the counter any day now.

Sometimes I Feel Like a Motherless Child

Once again, the salient point that escaped their logic in this new wave of the war on cancer is that the very protective states that statisticians identified—pregnancy and nursing—are states in which a woman is exposed to more than ten times the amount of estrogen and progesterone than a normal menstrual cycle ever generates, and that it steadily climbs for nine months.

Early menstruation, one of the other risk factors, isn't even about estrogen. Early menstruation, "precocious puberty,"[160-161] in its scientific guise, is a function of a high-carbohydrate diet (causing high insulin, an enormous growth factor in cancer) fostering accelerated aging, hence the term *precocious*. In this case, they've vilified the wrong hormone *again*.

The issue of the risk factor of late menopause gives the truth to the "scientific" lie. Although on the surface it would appear that the later you reach menopause the more hormones you must be exposed to, the fact of the matter is that those extra cycles are not real cycles. Although a woman may still be having a period, shortened or exaggerated bleeding is not evidence of ovulation, and ovulation is the real indicator of whether you are in menopause or not. Any period of bleeding less than four days long is anovulatory,[162] meaning eggless. So bleeding for just two days on a regular or irregular basis, even just two or three times a year, is enough, by medical standards, to say you're not in menopause, but *you are*.

And that is a perfect scenario for cancer.

Women who arrive at menopause late have had just enough estrogen to cause cell proliferation, but not enough to peak and cause an egg to pop. If there's no ovulation, there's no progesterone to cause apoptosis, or cell death. And, of course, *late* menopause means even more years of low estrogen without progesterone than is the norm.

That would cause cancer.

The biggest clue is found in the statistics showing that in our grandmothers' generation, breast cancer struck one woman in twenty-eight and in our mothers' generation, one in sixteen. In ours, it's one in eight or nine. In our daughters it's expected to be one in five.[163-164] The escalating numbers reflect the pandemic proportions of this killer of women.

While various special-interest groups look for lack of exercise,[165] fat in your diet,[166-167] or estrogenic pesticides and plastics[168-169] as the cause, the real reason is never examined because it's too politically incorrect. It's as politically incorrect as citing the leading cause of infertility to be aging.[170] Breast cancer is evidently caused by a woman's lack of childbearing.

Look at the numbers again.

Our grandmothers had the children who became our parents and our mothers had us. What exactly do we have? Will we have grandchildren?

Will we live to see them if we do?

It looks like the Summer of Love has become the winter of our discontent.

two

CHILD OF THE MOON

Many women in their forties and fifties today didn't reproduce at all or reproduced once or twice late in life. Medicine defines "late in life" as over twenty-six years old; in fact, any pregnancy after the age of twenty-eight is called a geriatric pregnancy in the reproductive endocrinology textbook.[1] This is being brought to your attention because the age at which you reproduced—or didn't—has an impact on your overall health for the rest of your life.[2-5]

A woman's reproductive résumé is a profile of her hormonal history. The picture it paints can predict how she'll age. It can also predict how healthy she'll be for the rest of her life. The hormonal symphonies involved in reproduction and lactation bring about changes in a woman's breasts, ovaries, brain, bones, and heart forever, right down to the genetic level. This is a significant issue, especially when it comes to cancer.

But no matter how alarming some of the information in this chapter may be to women with one or no children, there is a *logical* answer. We promise. While it may be as serious as it sounds, you need to know what the cause of cancer, heart disease, and Alzheimer's is in order to fully take advantage of the remedy. We haven't sounded the alarm after the doors have been locked. The evidence we've found all points to the possibility that hormone replacement can still save you from all we fear medically.

Although it's not well publicized, there are over 300 bodily processes and more than 9,000 gene products requiring estrogen in order to happen that are not directly involved in reproduction but are most certainly involved in good health.[6-11]

Reproductive or not, women still must have estrogen.

The ups and downs of a normal young hormonal scenario turn groups of regulatory genes on and off all over a woman's mind and body to time the next phase of her life—or as a precursor to her death. In the natural order of things, women have very brief windows in time to start the machinery. If the time between twelve and twenty-eight is our fifteen-year window to reproduce, then, logically, we wouldn't be fertile at twelve if nature wanted us to reproduce after thirty.

Women need to be aware of this. It's a given, biologically.

Our health depends on it.

Infertility treatments are statistically effective only 35 percent of the time after thirty years of age. The numbers plummet in short order to 15 percent effectiveness by thirty-five, and drop all the way down to 2 percent by forty.[12-13] A woman almost has a better chance of being hit by a snowmobile after forty than she does of getting pregnant naturally or unnaturally.[14] From nature's point of view, it makes sense. In brutal nature before now, and in developing nations today, human beings rarely live to be fifty years old. To be forty years old, in the scheme of things, was ancient. Without modern conveniences like clean running water, grocery stores, heat and electricity, strollers, cars, and disposable diapers, the rigors of taking care of a baby in the real world back then would be too much for most of us.

Then we neither had nor needed the capacity to have a baby after thirty, let alone forty. Unfortunately, for us "then" is still "now" in our bodies. The average age of death for women at the turn of the twentieth century—before anesthesia, blood transfusion, antibiotics, and surgery—was about forty-eight years old.[15] Once we fully realize these numbers, it gives some perspective to infertility statistics, today.

And She Was

In a world without technology, not here today, a girl is born and then she's fattened for growth and immunized by antibodies in mom's breast milk for three to seven years. In developing nations, even today, most babies are breast-fed for a minimum of two to two and a half years.[16] Nursing in the past would have lasted as long as possible because food was scarce. Back then, at somewhere around age eight to ten, she enters adrenarche. This milestone, which marks the end of childhood and the onset of a series of events that culminate in puberty, is so named because it is when a girl's adrenal glands, if she's healthy, kick in.[17-21]

A woman actually has a triad of glands—hypothalamus, pituitary, and adrenal glands (called the HPA axis)—that act in concert to read the cues in her environment. The HPA axis has marked off the years she's lived by adding up all of the summer days of her life, when she had high levels of cortisol and insulin, and coming to the conclusion that she is old enough to begin the next phase of her life.[22-25]

When a girl has passed enough summers, her adrenal glands, which sit on top of the kidneys, take the cue from her brain's calculations of her age in relationship to time passed and pump more testosterone faster. In our world, adrenarchy often begins as early as age seven or eight, instead of ten to twelve,[26] because artificial light and food have sped up our internal clocking mechanisms, hence the surge of precocious puberty in our time. The problem is that in today's world your chronological age may not necessarily be your biological age. The first sign of adrenarche is what medical textbooks call *secondary sexual characteristics*—armpit and pubic hair, for example. Eventually, leg hairs get coarser, and even head hair changes.

When testosterone reaches a certain threshold, or crescendo, it converts, or becomes something else. An enzyme made in your fat base, called *aromatase*, controls the conversion of testosterone into estrogen. That's why "baby fat" is important to normal development and why young women athletes often don't menstruate when they're too thin. With no fat, they have less estrogen to build a uterine lining to start that first period.

The conversion of testosterone to estrogen is the beginning of puberty.[27]

At first, the system begins to turn over slowly, like an obstinate starter in a car. It takes a while for it to rev up to speed. These low-level fluctuating sex hormones make it hard for you to sleep, and you begin to stay up later and later. This behavior is your brain and body's attempt to gain weight. Just like in summer, the longer you are exposed to light in a day, the more cortisol you make. Circulating cortisol levels mobilize blood sugar stored in your liver and muscles.

All of the extra blood sugar raises insulin production enough, over the course of just a few days, to make you insulin-resistant *enough* to gain weight for winter and to make the enzyme aromatase appear to increase estrogen.[28-29] As we said above, aromatase from your fat base is needed to convert more testosterone to estrogen. Your body, by gaining weight, is trying to optimize that mechanism.[30-32] Staying up late enhances weight gain, and by being awake later and later, you shorten your time to produce melatonin.[33] Melatonin is made while you sleep and blocks estrogen receptors. There would be more melatonin, naturally, in the winter, since the days are shorter. Short, colder days mean almost no carbohydrates, so fertility would be down, too, thanks to less estrogen reception and less insulin.

Not sleeping enough means less melatonin and puts you into summer or mating mode, with estrogen receptors listening and insulin high.[34] On the way to menopause we run through this very same scenario of increased appetite for carbohydrates and decreased ability to sleep because this is the only template nature knows for raising estrogen levels. But without eggs in place, it doesn't work.

When enough testosterone finally converts to estrogen,[35] the pituitary gland responds with follicle (egg) stimulating hormone (FSH). The point of increasing FSH is to ripen eggs (actually, the follicles holding the egg). The ripening eggs throw off even more estrogen. At this point in puberty, a girl will go through a few anovulatory periods, but each time estrogen will peak higher and higher, until it actually peaks high enough to make the pituitary send luteinizing hormone (LH) down to her ovary to release her first viable egg.[36]

Love, Love, Love

The key to understanding life and death rests in being mindful of nature, and we're not mindful anymore. In the world we live in, we've blurred the distinction between summer and winter and day and night. We can barely tell what season it is, let alone when the full moon is coming or going.

But your body still reads nature very clearly.

Otherwise, the artificial triggers wouldn't play such havoc with our systems.

The light of the moon in its various phases has always controlled and "phased" the hormonal interplay of our menstrual cycles.[37] That's why most women cycle between twenty-eight and thirty days. In our brave new world, where we are no longer governed by natural light, including the natural timing of moonlight, our fertility is not as reliable. One hundred years is not quite enough to effect extinction through infertility.

But two hundred is. We're getting close to the point of no return.

We've only really been exposed in any great way to artificial light after dark since the turn of the twentieth century. Although we've had candles and then gaslights longer, the expense and mess of those forms of light made them less ubiquitous to the masses than cheap, easy electricity.

Moonlight is really the reflected light of our sun—still shining, out of our view—on the other side of the planet at night. The moonlight at night inhibits melatonin release just like sunlight in the daytime, the lightbulb in your refrigerator, or the light from your computer screen does.[38] Any light at night changes natural rhythms. It is melatonin, in turn, that controls the amount of estrogen you receive by destabilizing the estrogen receptor.[39-44] When the moon is bright and melatonin is low, you can feel your estrogen, and, conversely, when the moonlight is dim and melatonin is high, you can't. The reason, psychologically, that moonlight is so universally romantic is because we have evolved to feel sexy in the extra light of the moon and act on those feelings.

Romance is *hardwired.*

The program for reproduction is run by the light and food supply. Just as the summer sun makes food and hormones more available for mating, your menstrual cycle of twenty-eight days has a "fruiting" period, too, guided by the amount of moonlight your skin and closed eyelids absorb.

In the darkness of the new moon, melatonin is high because it's not being inhibited by moonlight. This means that no matter how much estrogen you have, you can't feel it because your cells can't receive it, because high melatonin has destabilized your estrogen receptors. Before electricity overpowered the light of the moon, women living by natural light bled four to six days *after* the new moon. Until fire lit our caves after dark and we could individually control the amount of light we were exposed to, we all cycled together just like other animals exposed to natural light rhythms.

From the new moon to the quarter moon, FSH is busy ripening at least 150 eggs. All of those eggs ooze estrogen.[45-46] A program of actual bio-identical hormone replacement with natural plant-derived hormones would also start increasing your dose of estrogen now, aiming for a "peak" dose by next week.

As the moon's light brightens, melatonin wanes, so estrogen can talk to its receptors. The estrogen rising in your bloodstream makes the lining in your uterus thicken with new layers of cells, your breasts swell, and your attitude becomes downright charming. Your lips and the pseudolips around the vulva redden, as do your nipples. Your hair looks thicker and shinier and your skin is perfect, like a baby's.

In the current vernacular, you look *hot*.

You're also putting off heavy pheromones,[47-53] those invisible airborne molecules of attraction that bounce among all things living, plant and animal, speaking volumes. Pheromones are how we read each other's immune system's potential for mating.[54-57] The genetic rules that lead to your choice of mate reside in your immune system and your nose. Immune sensors called *major histocompatibiliy complexes* (MHC) and *human leukocyte antigens* (HLA) encode cells with *immunological* "individuality markers." MHC and HLA can determine the behavior of an individual from specific odor cues. MHC controls mating preferences and nesting behaviors in humans. In studies, it has been shown that we prefer to mate with MHC-*dissimilar* individuals because olfactory signals can mediate kin recognition. You really don't want to accidentally mate with a relative because your genes are too similar and would double your risk of genetic disaster.

So it's really his immune system that mates with yours.

Flowers speak to each other of love in the same way, with airborne hormones. Powerful volatile regulators of gene expression, pheromones contain the same *esters* used in perfumes. Certain orchids, for example, produce pheromones that mimic sex hormones, and through hormone receptors in the olfactory bulb in the brain,[58-60] they elicit copulatory behavior in bees and wasps. That's why we're much more likely to respond when he brings flowers, and it is quite probably the ancient reasoning for why we bury our dead with flowers, hoping to revive them.[61] The attempt to use the power of hormones in the brain to "get a rise" out of someone is instinctual.

Recently researchers gave two groups of modern women the sweaty (fermented in Ziploc bags) T-shirts of men unknown to them and asked them to choose which ones smelled best. One group of women was on birth control pills and the other group wasn't. The object of the study was the communication potential of pheromones in regard to immune system control on miscarriage rates.[62-63] Couples with "like" immune systems have a higher rate of miscarriage. In order to reproduce *successfully,* you need to score an opposite immune system. That way a greater possibility of survival is brought to the genetic table.

Since women's hormonal status controlled the women's preferences, the group of women not using contraceptives, across the board, chose men with complementary immune systems by aroma alone. The other group didn't. The synthetic hormones in the contraceptive pill not only prevent pregnancy, but they also preclude the possibility of women choosing the genetically optimum mate,[64-66] because mate selection is a function of immune response to pheromones, controlled by your hormones. Could this physiological premise be the reason for the dramatic increase in the divorce rate of the late 1970's and early 1980's? Did we all take birth control pills and pick the wrong guy?

Let It Be

As the light from the moon goes from a quarter full to half to full, melatonin is more and more suppressed and estrogen rises higher and higher, until, in the full light of the moon, estrogen peaks. Several things occur now. First, the high level of estrogen tells your brain that the nest is ready and it can stop growing the lining of your uterus. Growth abruptly stops, literally, everywhere inside you, all the way down to your DNA. Actual rhythmic hormone replacement with natural plant-derived hormones would have to have this peak of estrogen, which makes progesterone receptors for the next two weeks of the progesterone phase of the cycle.

Just like in the fits and starts of puberty, when estrogen peaks, your pituitary floods your system with *luteinizing hormone*, causing the very best egg out of the 150 or so available to burst out of a blister that has formed on the ovary.[67] The blister in which the egg has been waiting is called a *corpus luteum*, which means "yellow body." This transient, relatively ephemeral endocrine gland leaks progesterone for about two weeks.

A little testosterone is in play in a woman's body now, too. Just as testosterone is what compels men to mate with anything and everyone all of the time, the woman's testosterone compels her to use that egg. Now that hormones have peaked your interest, so to speak, the timing of mating is in sync for both of you.

Last, under the full moon, estrogen's peak doesn't just stop growth and tip off your pituitary to release that egg. When it's at its highest, estrogen also makes progesterone receptors for the next phase of the cycle. By the waning of the quarter moon, progesterone is as high as it ever gets except in pregnancy. Therefore, when actual natural hormone replacement is attempted for you, a progesterone "peak" dosage is as necessary as making a peak of estrogen in the first half of your cycle.

If no pregnancy has occurred by the last quarter of the moon this month, the peak levels of progesterone will undo all that's been done. All the preparation for creation will come crashing down. When no pregnancy occurs in a normal cycle, progesterone must destroy, from the inside out, every cell in every part of your body that's not supposed to be in an adult woman to clean the slate for another try next month. As long as you *seem* to have a future, reproductively, you will stay in the pink of health. That's why natural estrogen and progesterone hormone replacement must be prescribed to exactly mimic a youthful cycle no matter how old you are.

Estrogen grows cells everywhere (remember the 9,000 gene products and 300 body processes) for two weeks, and on Day 14, progesterone steps in to sculpt and define the nest, while simultaneously *undoing*—through apoptosis and estrogen receptor blocking—all that estrogen has done to you everywhere else in your brain and body, too. If a full-term pregnancy occurs, the soaring levels of both hormones will permanently change the way your body handles food, light, toxins, and stress on the cellular level forever.

Pregnancy, like puberty, is *physiologically* a developmental milestone that must be reached to be completely healthy for your *whole* life. If a young girl never spontaneously menstruates, it is accepted that she's ill or has an extra male chromosome.[68] Puberty and menstruation are obvious developmental milestones, physiologically. So is pregnancy and breast-feeding. It is a continuum of development in adult women that if omitted has serious complications that jeopardize our health. Having never completed a pregnancy or never breast-feeding may mean that you need continual natural hormone replacement more than someone who did.

The scenario of this series of interlocking and mutually reinforcing tensions between the forces of growth and death, governed by estrogen and progesterone, is at the heart of our modern predicament with cancer. Conventional HRT, PremPro, caused unpredictable new disease states and solved none of our problems with aging because in order to restore and mimic the health of youth, we must replace genuine hormones in these time-tested rhythms. Conventional HRT, even prescribed to mimic body

How Moonlight Controls Hormone Reception and the 28-Day Menstrual Cycle

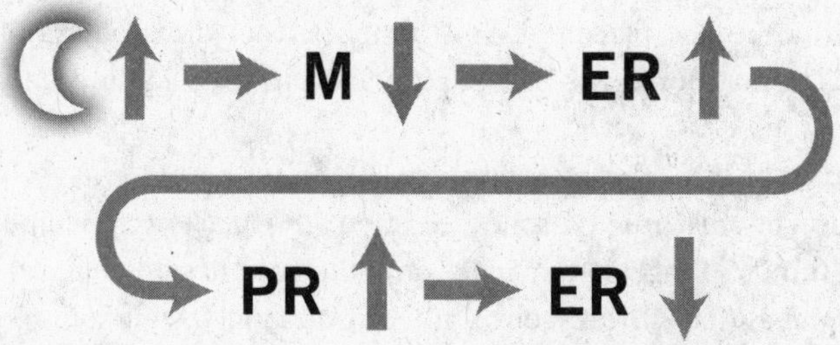

M ER

PR ER

Light enhances estrogen receptors, estrogen action causes progesterone receptors to be created for the next phase of the cycle. After ovulation, progesterone in its receptor turns off estrogen receptors to complete the negative feedback loop of estrogen's and the moon's control over hormone reception.

ER Estrogen Receptor
M Melatonin
PR Progesterone Receptor

rhythms, is still a synthetic drug made from a combination of lab-altered progesterone and the synthesized by-product of a hormone from another species, not a whole, natural substance.

Live and Let Die

In the hormonal interplay of progesterone and estrogen during the menstrual cycle, nature gives us the prescription for health. But most important, in respect to cancer *treatment,* it may be possible to re-create that hormonal interplay that first grows, then destroys unnecessary cells, something that conventional HRT—the synthetic hormonelike drugs—can't ever do.

A good way to examine the hormonal mechanisms at work in a cancerous tumor is to examine the placenta in pregnancy. The placenta, in every pregnancy, is really a well-regulated, controlled "tumor."[69] All of the fetal oncogenes turned on in any kind of cancer are switched on in the growth of the placenta. In fact, placental growth mimics the wild proliferation of any cancerous tumor. But in this case, nature has provided a premise to regulate growth.

This "tumor," the placenta, produces progesterone.

Because of this progesterone secretion, the placenta becomes a self-limiting "tumor." Progesterone locks onto the switches on genes called *promoter regions* that throw cells into self-destruct mode or apoptosis—*mandated* cell suicide.[70-74] That's why, although the placenta of pregnancy has all the criteria of a cancerous tumor, it almost never becomes metastatic or kills the mother. Men are not destined to go through the acute growth phases that women must to produce new life. They never have need of a progesterone-producing machine like the placenta. In men, testosterone converts to dihydrotestosterone (DHT), which is capable of the same apoptotic genetic action. We know that cancer increases as men age and, simultaneously, testosterone falls off.

As we discussed in Chapter One, we humans actually work our way up the evolutionary ladder in utero through this same mechanism; the apoptosis or cell death that sculpts the fetus into a "human, not a chicken" is controlled by progesterone's action on genetic controls.

As the placenta grows, the increasing output of progesterone from the placenta limits the organ's growth so it won't take over the uterus. Simultaneously, progesterone sculpts those fishy webbed fingers into perfect tiny hands. Thanks in large part to progesterone from the placenta, we metamorphose from a tadpole with gill arches until we reach our final human form.[75-78]

The mechanism of control on the genes of morphology—that is, do we have wings or do we have a tail—is directed by our genetics' dose-dependant response to progesterone. An organism adapts to be the fittest in his niche—that is, to fit in the place that has the best food and shelter for him. If he lives by the sea, he's better off with fins and gills than arms and lungs.

Therefore, Hox genes and homeobox genes, by way of progesterone's ability to kill off the cells he doesn't need, be they bones or tissue, give him perfect form. We're all made of the same materials.

Hormones like insulin, melatonin, and cortisol control estrogen, testosterone, and progesterone and communicate the environment's terms to the genes that shape us. In the case of pregnancy, the only difference between the "normal tumor" that is the placenta and the cancer that can kill us is a finely tuned cascading symphony of regulatory genes[79] switching on and off in a rhythm.[80-81] In the creation of a baby, genes offer directional differentiation via progesterone to wildly growing, fast-dividing cells, telling them "you be a liver," "you be a brain," "you be a leg," or "you be an arm." Your baby, in the parlance of molecular cell biology, is a well-differentiated tumor.[82-84]

Let It Bleed

If the nest turns up empty in the last quarter of the moon, progesterone, the destroyer, shuts down the machinery to make life in the now-unnecessary cells lining your uterus for this moon cycle. Just like the cells in breasts, in lymph nodes, and even in the lining of your colon, the nest built in your uterus will now undergo cell suicide and fall away about four to six days after the new moon.

At the end of your cycle, menstrual bleeding is physical proof that apoptosis is in play as you shed the lining that estrogen has created. The overgrowth of cells in your body is discarded, and you're healthy. Now the music can start again.

It's a *moon* dance, a marvelous moon dance.

When you no longer bleed in the cycle of the moon, you have started a process of disruption somewhere in your body or brain. Science's assumption that it is the repeated toxic exposure of your own hormones, cycle after cycle, that must be the cause of breast cancer is drawn from the statistics showing an increased risk associated with early menstruation or late menopause.

The actual cause is delaying pregnancy.

Before modern times, the grow/die, grow/die scenario would have occurred only a few times after the first time a woman bled. Then she'd begin a different rhythm that would overlay the first, a nine-month rhythm of escalating estrogen and progesterone, followed by high prolactin.

She'd be pregnant.

In older times, before artificial light and excess sugar out of season, when menarche, the onset of ovulation, came around at sixteen or seventeen years old, a girl would be pregnant by eighteen. Since delaying pregnancy does expose you to more cycles, and we do delay pregnancy, it may seem to prove the hypothesis, but it doesn't.

Nature meant the amount of time between actual ovulation and pregnancy to be maybe two to three years, at most thirty-six cycles. With "early menarche" occurring at around age ten today, it is possible for a girl to experience ninety-six cycles by age eighteen, with no full-term pregnancy in sight.

That's the math that led researchers to conclude that a woman's estrogen could hurt her. But the truth is vastly different from the conclusion they reached. *A pregnancy before the age of twenty turns on or upregulates the gene for apoptosis (p53) permanently in the nucleus of all your cells, reducing the risk for breast cancer and cancer anywhere else in your body—forever.*[85-87] Like everything else that really matters in life, it's all about timing. Statistics also show that a pregnancy before twenty years of age assures your risk of breast cancer to be practically nil.[88-90]

That's right, a full-term pregnancy before twenty permanently increases the amount and activity of the anti-cancer gene p53, among other things. But if too many cycles pass before conception occurs, all bets are off, in terms of your potential for breast cancer. Another pertinent topic for Women's Studies classes everywhere.

Delaying your first pregnancy—whether it's for twelve years from the date of your first period or until never—does, of course, mean that you are exposed to more menstrual cycles, but it *does not mean* that the exposure to the estrogen and progesterone levels experienced in a normal cycle are the *cause* of the statistical evidence. To make such a ridiculous assumption in the face of the evidence that women who still have normal periods rarely have cancer is just shoddy science.

Nature expects you to start early because 50 percent of pregnancies end in miscarriage. The fetal mortality rate for live births is about the same—meaning that a woman with five children has more likely than not been pregnant ten or more times. In the old days, childbearing *was* a woman's life work. Yes, you went from child to mother in short order, but the payback was that you didn't die on your offspring from cancer, heart disease, or Alzheimer's.

When this rhythm of procreation stops or, worse, never starts, and then its underlying generator, the sine wave of menstrual cycling, stops, it's game over. *Hormone production and reception in a lunar or light-driven rhythm orchestrate your menstrual period.* The same hormone production and reception that control menstruation also control every aspect of good physical and mental health that we enjoy as the "bloom of youth."

Your normal menstrual period was a symptom of being *healthy* because it signified a new chance every month that you weren't already pregnant that you would be given another chance. That's why rhythmic, cyclical natural hormone replacement, now and all the rest of your life, will fool nature into believing that the "prime directive" to be reproductive to be healthy is still in place

An abnormal—or worse, absent—menstrual period, unless you are pregnant and nursing, is hard evidence, biologically speaking, of impending pathology. In the past, women always knew that. The entire practice of gynecology arose from just this premise. There wasn't ever a time before the present when fertility was not prized. Contraception, the obsession of our modern lives, was used very sparingly in the past. Maybe that's how we became so confused about what being a healthy woman is.

Lady Madonna

Nature sees it this way: hormonally, pregnancy is a whole new rhythm. From the moment you become pregnant, estrogen and progesterone start to rise to a preordained crescendo. The exposure to your own hormones will never be higher in your lifetime. At the end of the pregnancy, estrogen and progesterone all but stop.

This sharp fall off of estrogen and progesterone at birth triggers the hormone prolactin for nursing. For most women, the milk comes in within three days to feed the star of the show—the baby. The prolactin triggered by birth stays high for about half a year; after that, it will only stay high as long as you continue to breast-feed.

In *true* on-demand breast-feeding,[91-92] not the six weeks to three months we think of as breast-feeding today, the sleeplessness of the first nine months—which prevents most modern women from working and nursing—enhances prolactin production to make more milk.[93] Prolactin blocks the pituitary's normal rhythmic production of follicle stimulating hormone (FSH) and luteinizing hormone (LH), so no eggs can ripen or be released. The average healthy baby, with no other food supply but mom, nurses approximately every two hours around the clock for at least four months. Breast milk digests in two hours, whereas cow's milk takes about four and a half. From the four to eight months of the baby's life, nursing sessions space out to a little more like every three to four hours apart around the clock. Any supplemental food is not introduced until the baby has teeth, which can be as late as ten months to a year.

In previous generations, women used herbs for birth control and, of course, condoms made from animal entrails. But the safest, healthiest form of contraception, both free and convenient, was breast-feeding—real breast-feeding, the kind where you just sit and nurse to the exclusion of everything except eating and going to the bathroom.

Until the 1970s, scientists puzzled over the birth spacing in traditional societies of hunter-gatherers, until anthropologists visiting the !Kung in Africa recorded just how *often* !Kung babies suckled at their mother's nipples. Anthropologists Mel Konner and Carol Worthman reported that the !Kung babies were carried everywhere and nursed *several times an hour* during the day and off and on while co-sleeping with mom and dad all night.[94] On average, eighty minutes of suckling, spread out into six bouts of nursing over a normal day, should reliably suppress ovulation for an average of eighteen months.

Where there is no suitable substitute for breast milk, no safe water, and no safe place for the baby to be apart from mom, weaning as a necessity must occur late. The actual world, outside in nature, where our bodies, brains, and breasts evolved, fit those criteria to a T. Only the nipple stimulation of "natural" incessant nursing over at least fifteen months per child provides contraceptive protection and protection from breast cancer. Babies take nine months to ripen on the inside and perhaps another three years on the breast outside to be healthy. Since mother and baby are an ecosystem unto themselves, nature has made your good health contingent on what's best for the baby.

That's what the small print in the prime directive of life says.

Breast cancer statistics support the small print.[95] Every baby you have lowers your risk of breast cancer by 7 percent. Every year earlier than age 28 that you have that baby lowers it by another 3 percent. Every twelve months of your life that you breast-feed lowers your risk by 4.3 percent.

The longer you breast-feed without supplementation, the lower your risk of cancer.

This is how evolution ensures the survival of the species, and this is how it works: The high prolactin of breast-feeding, coupled with daytime melatonin from the occasional naps, suppresses ovulation very reliably. If food were scarce, you'd continue to share your body with your baby for the benefit of both of you. The baby eats well and you avoid another pregnancy. Women today breast-feed, if they do at all, for an average of three months instead of the average of 15 months in developing nations. Women also have no children or at most 2.7 on average.[96]

Before modern times, giving birth was just the beginning of "the hard part." You had to keep the baby alive outside of your womb with your own body for nourishment. Lactation, the most exorbitant phase of reproduction, lasts longer in all primates, the class of mammal that human beings are assigned to, than in any other mammal of comparable body size.[97] In primates, without access to baby formula, if mom succumbs during the process, her infant most likely dies with her. No one, then, could feed your baby but you.

"Wet nurses" are women who rent out their breasts to feed other women's babies. These surrogates were the only alternative. Unless you died in childbirth or were extremely wealthy, a wet nurse wasn't *really* an option for the average mom. Bottle-feeding did not exist for most of history. No one even tried, with any actual success, to feed the milk of one species to another until about a hundred years ago. In 1864, Louis Pasteur discovered the process for sterilizing animal milk, and by the 1880s wet nurses were all but forgotten in Europe. Breast-feeding continued to be the norm in America until the 1930s. A short fifteen years later, only 25 percent of mothers in this country were still breast-feeding, and then for only a few weeks or months. The marketing and promotion of formula or milk substitutes by both industry and the medical profession lined a lot of pockets in this country between 1940 and 1975.[98] Those years show the greatest increases in breast cancer, too.[99]

A 1975 study showed that American culture has become intrinsically hostile to breast-feeding.[100-101] American women face two sets of conflicting demands: Do they stay at home and nurse their babies, or compete with men for jobs without regard for sexual difference? The tension between nursing and earning a living shows in the statistics.[102] With reasonably long paid maternity leaves and on-site nurseries being very rare in America, the American Pediatric Association's recommendation that mothers nurse for at least a year is a hopeless goal.

Two-thirds of mothers with infants are employed full-time, and barely 20 percent of all mothers in this country breast-feed for even six months. In 1987, statistics showed that 60 percent of white mothers tried to nurse while still in the hospital versus 25 percent of black mothers.[103-104] We think that when breast cancer statistics show a higher death rate for black women, the assumption is always that the differences in health care options for black women mean less early detection and therefore less intervention being the cause of the difference in survival rates. The difference could be attributable to the diminished economic potential to breast-feed.

As far as we can ascertain, the health of the baby has always been the motivation for doctors and governmental public health agencies to get involved in any widespread promotion of breast-feeding to mothers. The distinct evidence that not nursing long enough and well enough is likely to be the cause of breast cancer in mom has heretofore been ignored. The anecdotal wisdom of previous times and cultures seemed very clearly to understand that the symbiosis between mom and baby, as far as good health was concerned, went both ways.

Ancient Egyptians prized breast milk for its healing powers for people of all ages.[105-106] They may have been accurate in ways unimaginable to them. In 1999 the Institute for Laboratory Medicine at Lund University in Lund, Sweden, published an astonishing piece of work reporting that the human version of alpha-lacalbumin, a protein found in all mammal milk, induces apoptosis in cancer cells but spares healthy cells.[107-108] In cancer research, that's referred to as a "magic bullet." This news should have made the front pages of newspapers globally, but it didn't.

First, the Lund University people tried a breast milk bath on the bacteria pneumoccoccus, which kills infants in respiratory distress, and of course it worked. Then they found that the protein in breast milk in vitro also killed every kind of cancer they tried it on—lung, throat, kidney, colon, bladder, lymphoma, and leukemia. The evidence that breast-feeding protects children from lymphoma has been around for some time, along with reported protection from diarrhea, ear infection, bacteremia, meningitis, botulism, urinary tract infections, necrotizing enterocolitis, SIDs, Type I diabetes, Crohn's disease, and all sorts of allergies.[109-110]

The Greeks believed, as medicine did for thousands of years, that menstrual blood changed course, went up through the breast, and magically became breast milk.[111-112] The modern-day assumption that HIV can be transmitted through blood products like semen and breast milk makes the ancient Greek conclusion seem not so far-fetched. Because of this medical mandate, women in the West with HIV have been advised not to breast-feed. But medicine may have gotten it wrong again.

S. Sabbaj et al. reported in the *Journal of Virology* that it has been found in sub-Saharan Africa, *unexpectedly*, that about 85 percent of the babies with infected mothers *who nurse* escape the disease. Apparently there are immune cells in mother's milk (cytotoxic CD8 + T cells) that recognize and bind to the HIV protein to kill infected cells.[113] In reality, studies show that the infectious HIV viral particles are most often spread through abrasions to the baby traveling down the birth canal during vaginal birth.[114-116]

For us as newborns, mother's milk creates our "first one's free" addiction to the taste of *sweet*. The milk of all mammals is pretty much like melted ice cream laced with antibiotics. The antibiotics come in the form of anti*bodies*. When you're nursing, your immune system is on overdrive. It's downloading antibodies into your baby via the breast milk, actually transfering the collective memory of your immune system about your environment to your baby—and if *you* were breast-fed, your mother's environment and her mother's environment and so and so on since before time had a name.[117–118] This ancient function of antibody inheritance means that your breast is as much of an immune gland as your spleen, thymus, or bone marrow.

The next baby wouldn't come until you'd nursed three or four trips around the Sun, maybe as many as seven if the food supply was scarce. Then, after a few more new moons, you'd be blessed again and again and *again*. Riding on the luck brought to you by the Sun and the moon and the stars, your daughters and their daughters and their daughters would have a life as rich as yours. We may not be able to imagine the sheer power of matriarchy then, but *we had it*. Everything in life is a trade-off. Maybe, at least physiologically, we really can't "have it all." Then, we controlled life and death.

Now, it controls us.

Heartbreak Hotel

In the last century and a half, the abundance of farmed food, anesthesia, surgery, and antibiotics has extended our lives far past nature's norm, just as animals in zoos outlive animals in the wild. We've lost our innate sense of what should come next. In the world of zoology, it's called *instinct*. When animals lose their instincts for survival—mating, eating, and sleeping—they become extinct.[119-120] That's why the birth rate is down in general. It's strange that only 150 years, really no more than a spit in the eye of time, could wipe out 150 million years worth of collective memory.

But apparently it has.

At the beginning of this chapter we discussed the fact that any pregnancy after the age of twenty-eight is determined to be a geriatric pregnancy. *Geriatric* is defined as "the medical study of the structural changes and diseases of old age." Medicine labels us geriatric reproductively after twenty-eight because thirty to forty years is old in nature. Female apes live about forty-five years if they can dodge germs and sharp objects. We, too, lived until about forty-five until about seventy-five years ago, before surgery and antibiotics.[121]

Biologically speaking, what we refer to as "midlife" is, reproductively, the end of life and definitely *not* the time to settle down and hope to reproduce. The machinery, by then, is outdated and broken. "Broken" can mean any condition from fibrocystic breasts, hypothyroidism, diabetes, a bad gallbladder, fibroid tumors, or cysts to depression and cancer. These conditions are the hard evidence that we have not evolved around our biology.

Although we have the same rights and potential as any man, if a woman is born with two X chromosomes, she is a female and as such was designed by evolution to reproduce, which includes breast-feeding, in order to be truly healthy in the long term. Reproduction is an elemental force that you can use or that can destroy you.

Before our time, it was a given that women would reproduce. Of course, there were always some who did not. Nuns, for example, are known to have more breast cancer than any other group of women.[122] But in our generation, for the first time in *all* time, we refused to reproduce—wholesale.

What could have changed in women to goad them into forsaking the prime directive at the cost of their physical well-being? What changed in women to lead us make choices that leave us so powerless in the face of nature? We were lied to.

Therefore, our refusal was indirect, in most cases, and misguided in all.

We were led to believe that we could have sex without pregnancy, and the drugs, birth control pills, were provided to allow just that. We were encouraged culturally to "shop around" for just the right mate no matter how long it took, but *nobody consulted our bodies* about these premises.

We were pressured to pursue higher and higher education, leading to careers that put us in competition with biologically different creatures—men. More recently, we have been assured that fertility, like some sort of science project, could be reproduced in a lab.

Now that many women have become ill, the only thing they tell us about breast cancer is that we need to be patient and keep raising money for a cure. What no one ever thought to ask were the real questions: Is it more dangerous to have a first pregnancy after thirty than it is to have no children at all,[123-124] or could delaying childbearing until we "couldn't" have children make us sick in ways we could never have imagined?

three

TWO THOUSAND LIGHT-YEARS FROM HOME

Our relationship as animals with the Sun, moon, and tides is slipping away. The hormonal symphonies that have been worked out over millennia to control our hearts, minds, and fate are growing faint. We don't live in sync with nature anymore, and we haven't for several generations. Women have never reproduced so little in all of history.[1]

A great many women in our generation have availed ourselves of the opportunity to live our lives like men do. Even if we married, we've worked outside the home, and have had the opportunity to have our laundry, housecleaning, and, if we gave birth, child rearing done by other women. A lot of us, even with families, eat a large percentage of our meals out or in the form of prepackaged food. By earning our own incomes, we've been able to pick and choose the details of our lives.

That wasn't how our great-grandmother lived. In the 1860s, she woke with the sun and worked all day with children and animals, cooking, cleaning, and managing the resources for her family—a family created in tandem with her husband and fed with her own body. At the end of her day, which came when the sun set, she had worked hard, eaten little (compared to us), and slept long and soundly at night.

Her risk of breast cancer was 1 in 91, not the 1 in 8 that we face.[2] It is over ten times more likely that one of us will be diagnosed with breast cancer as it was for her only 130 years ago.[3]

How could this be?

After the Industrial Revolution, around the middle of the nineteenth century, the world kicked into fast forward and has never slowed down. At about the same time, electricity brought extended periods of bright light and reliable refrigeration, two things that dramatically changed both our sleep patterns and the food supply. The rising tide of technology, bringing even more light and more food, ultimately changed not only the behavior of women, but the definition of what it meant to be a woman as well.

Behaviorally, our great-grandmothers, grandmothers, and mothers were moving up and out into an undiscovered country where few women had gone before—more importantly for our investigation, where few women had *wanted* to go before. We assume that our frustrations—our desires for equal pay and for an equal opportunity to leave our families and go to work, and even, in some of us, to fight like men—has been shared by all women in all times.

But that's not true.

Of course, there have been some women across time who have achieved world-class milestones outside the home, but now most women wake up positive that they *have* to. We are *different* from the women in the paintings, who waited to be courted and hoped to exchange eggs for resources to gain a lifestyle that would allow them to have children—just like the birds and the bees on the Nature Channel.

But please remember, this book is about biology, not politics.

Born to Be Wild

There's more of a difference between our lives and our mothers' than there was between our grandmothers' and our great-grandmothers'. Examining the female-led changes in mating and reproduction of the last half-century give us staggering statistics: Only forty-five years ago, or about as long ago as we are old, 97 percent of twenty-one-year-old women were married.[4] That figure rests at less than 50 percent today. In our mothers' day, there was virtually no divorce, comparable to today.[5] It was a couples' society. Home for most of us was the suburbs. Life was about conformity and stability, about "farming" children, and about pair-bonding for safety. Two parents guarded the territory (tract home) better than one, just like our gibbons in Chapter One.

Not anymore.

Did we really decide not to get married and have children *one day*? Was the change one of attitude and attendant behavior? Or was our environment changing our physiology—which then altered our attitude and changed our behavior and goals? There must be a compelling reason why women suddenly—in evolutionary terms, a nanosecond—began living against the grain of our very own bodies. What was it?

It is an evolutionary truth that when food and sleep patterns change, our offspring reflect those changes. If you change the environment, the environment changes you (and your descendants). That concept is the essence of adaptation for survival.[6]

When the environment—food supply and seasonal light exposure—changes around a pregnant woman (like grandma and mom), the baby she delivers is *different* from her. Survival is based on the premise of adapting quickly to your environment, preferably before everyone else, so you can live and outpopulate the competition. This phenomenon is known as "survival of the fittest." So adaptation is a big evolutionary asset. *Unless*, of course, the environmental cues you are adapting are a cosmic impossibility. In that case, you just die.

Viewing the mortality rates for cancer in our generation in light of this etched-in-stone law of evolution certainly puts a different spin on the moniker "*new* woman." How can we live long enough as new women to get to become old women?

Material Girl

We started this chapter by comparing and contrasting our reproductive life span with great-grandma's because the best way to extricate ourselves from this evolutionary squeeze is to figure out how to re-create what was meant to be in our bodies. The biological truth is that we, who are now stricken with cancer, have spent our reproductive life span on other things.

We were not continuously pregnant, and we weren't nursing or ovulating regularly, either. We've gone through decades of unnatural drug-induced contraception—that is, contraception that was not a side effect of breastfeeding or cultural abstinence. These twenty years—from eighteen to thirty-eight—must be accounted for in the musical score that is our female lives.

The small, steady beat of estrogen and progesterone, overlaid by the sweeping arcs of new rhythms that chime in during the years of pregnancy and nursing, are the song the female body is designed to sing to stay healthy and age slowly. The real guts of the song, a series of interlocking and mutually reinforcing tensions, the part that really evokes the emotional health in you, is held in the pull between the two hormones, estrogen and progesterone. That's the beat. That's the rhythm. What our generation has experienced is more like a skipping record. It's affecting our health in a myriad of different ways.

Unfortunately for us, the truth about breast cancer is that biology *is* destiny. Nature is all about life, making it, expanding it, and taking it from you if you fail to produce. "Producing" children and making new life in the past was a lot harder to avoid. Equal sexual rights for women were still always controlled by the prerequisites of pregnancy and lactation. Even though you *could have* any and all the partners you wanted (as long as you could "date" while you were pregnant and nursing for about five years at a time), nature made sure that you were too busy to be available for mating any more than once every five years. We were meant, biologically, to drive in the slow lane. Cross-cultural taboos on promiscuity for women were derived from biological logic that is now coming back to haunt us. As surely as men aren't going to give birth anytime soon, we aren't going to turn into nonreproductive women. But a lot of us are going to die trying, unless we figure out how to make it seem like we could still reproduce, if given a chance.

In choosing to opt for reproductive freedom, with no evolutionary architecture in place for such a choice, we became "velocitized." The driver's ed teacher uses this term in class when referring to accidental speeding in your car. Velocitized is a state of being where you become inured to how fast things are rushing by.[7] Velocitized is what happens on a long highway car ride at night. After a while, aiming toward your goal, you lose track of just how fast you're going and how far you've gone. Then all at once you look up and you've missed your exit. A lot of us have done just that. The options available to us—delaying mating and childbearing, maybe not nursing at all—have skewed time perception in all of us. We thought we had more time than we did to live our reproductive lives. A lot of us have missed more than a few "exits."

In the premise of using bio-identical, natural hormone replacement with estrogen and progesterone in a cyclical rhythm, we get a chance to turn around and go back. We can't take quite the same road that we missed, but maybe, just maybe, we can keep driving to see what's out there.

It's Too Late, Baby

We need to examine what destiny awaits us now if we don't replace our hormones. From the biological perspective, it's called *debilitation*. The falling hormones you experience in perimenopause drop you back into the same range that you rose through in the period between adrenarchy and puberty.[8] It's sort of déjà vu all over again. On the way down, you will experience the same symptoms that you lived with as you were building up a head of reproductive steam the first time.

As your estrogen decreases into that same range again, you may still have "regular" periods or periods that come at fairly regular intervals, but you're not actually ovulating anymore. These perimenopausal periods are like the ones you experienced as your reproductive engine was revving up the first time. Then, your adrenal glands were trying to jump-start your brain to turn the burners on in your ovaries. Once your ovaries kicked in, you had enough estrogen generated by a full egg basket to run for at least twenty years.

In perimenopause, you're nearly running on empty.

You still have just enough estrogen to make a thin lining in your uterus and cause unopposed hormonal growth elsewhere in your breasts and body, but not enough to peak. That's why your periods are getting shorter and shorter, your breasts lumpier and lumpier, and your mind far less agile. The fact that you don't peak estrogen with any regularity anymore, and you haven't since your late twenties, is the hallmark of perimenopause.[9-10]

As we stated earlier, you need a peak of estrogen to stop growth of cells and make progesterone receptors. With no peak of estrogen, your brain can't send the signal to release any of the eggs you have left. With no peak of estrogen, there's no feedback information to shut off FSH, so follicle stimulating hormone pours constantly, overstimulating your ovaries[11] and ripening all at once most of the eggs you have left. The loss of this rhythm in perimenopause actually triggers the destruction of the rest of your eggs through the action of excessive FSH, using up the remainder of your eggs. At about this time, you begin to feel the heat of hot flashes. That's how the system effectively shuts itself down for good. This proc a decade.

The clinical diagnosis of menopause is a finding in your bloodwork of an FSH score higher than 5. Ask your doctor what yours is. You can stop the destruction and essentially achieve feedback and shut off FSH with estrogen replacement.

Having no more eggs means having no more estrogen, which of course leads to no more progesterone anymore, either. Since you've stopped regularly producing the small amount of progesterone that you would from a normal menstrual cycle, and there's no steady increase of it, either (that is, you're not pregnant), nature "thinks" that you're back in adrenarche. Because your estrogen is so low, and you're producing even more testosterone than before, thanks to your sleeplessness, the pubertal picture is complete.

After we reach thirty, nature identifies falling (low) estrogen and higher than normal (rising) testosterone as the beginning . . . *again*.[12-17] This is a perfectly reasonable conclusion on the part of nature. *You must be in adrenarchy, because nature knows no other template for not ovulating except pregnancy and lactation*—unless, of course, you're a man. Now nature tries to send you on your way to puberty. Only it can't.

The whole point of puberty is to get you to the next level of existence—ovulation. There's the hitch. That developmental milestone takes eggs, and we don't have any. It's too late to start puberty again, but the outcome of puberty, a normal rhythm of estrogen and progesterone in youthful quantities, is something you can achieve, with natural hormone replacement. You can try to fool nature by covering the fact that you're missing eggs if you replace the hormones that they would generate in exactly the amounts and rhythm in which they would occur.[18-21]

Helter Skelter

Perimenopause is problematic because women are *hormonally* in first-trimester pregnancy range. That is, the specific hormone ratios of insulin (high), estrogen (low), and thyroid (fluctuating) of early pregnancy are mimicked by perimenopause. This triggers "fetal" oncogenes to start flipping *on*,[22] but perimenopausal women are stranded with no source of progesterone to give the growth or death command[23] to turn those same genes *off*, because they don't have enough estrogen to make a peak to ovulate anymore with any regularity, and there's no placenta on board. Without the progesterone from the remains of an empty egg sac, their low chronic estrogen is never turned off, either.

The state that they are in now is life-threatening.

It is *the* backdrop for cancer.[24] The regulatory hormones for growth and death in your body are waning.[25-28] Without your sex hormones in place to *read* the environment, the environmental cues have become static noise. Without ovulation and its attendant progesterone to keep the balance between life and death in your cells, your life itself is in jeopardy.

If we follow the clues backward, we can see that the symptom of sleeplessness (of pseudopuberty) was the beginning of the end of ovulation. Although the growth potential—from either *low* levels of estrogen or *high* levels of insulin without progesterone on board to keep it in check—might have been enough to cause any number of kinds of cancer from lymphoma to ovarian to liver, the real danger is in the overproduction of prolactin[29-33] out of rhythm outside of nursing. Prolactin is a relative in the family of growth hormones known as *somatostatins*.

Stairway to Heaven

Without hormones, it is really impossible to sleep. Without sleep, prolactin keeps escalating. You'd never be awake off and on all night otherwise unless you were nursing. At the end of perimenopause, cortisol soars and estrogen and progesterone hit bottom . . . *just as they do during labor and delivery*.[34] At this point in the template, your immune system revs up so high that it may attack your cartilage and mucus membranes, and that scenario creates joint pain (arthritis) and allergies, and an autoimmune disease called *Hashimoto's Thyroiditis* can happen now, too. Once your immune system has attacked and halted thyroid function, with the insulin resistance from sleeplessness, you just keep getting fatter.

The lack of progesterone coupled with dribbling estrogen and sky-high prolactin is the trigger to make milk, just as it is at postpartum. All of the ducts in your breasts are "festering" from the mammary gland stimulation of this hormonal scenario. Noninvasive or precancers, called *ductal carcinomas in situ* (DCIS), are diagnosed on mammograms for a lot of us at this point in the play. DCIS are sparkles of calcification and inflammation in your "rusty pipes." Nature assumes that when your estrogen plummets and progesterone is nonexistent, pregnancy is over and it is time to turn *on* your breasts.

When, in reality, this time it's just the finality of menopause.

But Mother Nature rules, and her rule says: With your hormonal profile, you'd better be nursing. If you still had a thyroid and enough growth hormone, you might actually make milk. But at your age you won't. However, under these circumstances, already high levels of prolactin continue to increase *past* the trigger point of real lactation. Your breasts are now all turned on with nowhere to go.

Instead, your milk ducts just get stimulated and overgrow epithelial cells—*lactotropes*—that never get to produce milk to feed a baby because there is no baby, and there is no baby coming. The tragedy occurring here, breast *cancer*, happens because prolactin is in charge of *all* the growth factors now identified by modern science as active in breast cancer.[35-38] On the molecular level, the growth activity in breasts to produce milk is *embryonic* in fervor, just like cancer; the same genes and growth factors that make milk foster the unstoppable growth of cancerous cells. These growth factors fuel milk making because, on the cellular level, *lactation is a cancerous state* that gets to resolve itself over time.[39-46]

If you were really going to breast-feed for the time necessary to get a child off to a good start in a world where there was no other option for food but you, you would pass through *developmental stages* in the process of lactation, too. You would continue to breast-feed until your estrogen came back almost a year later. Then it would take another year of "revving" the hormonal engine to get estrogen levels high enough to tell your brain to tell your ovaries to ovulate again. The normal rhythm of ovulation would bring the return of estrogen and progesterone to turn *off* growth factors.[47-52] We postulate that that's how bio-identical, natural hormone replacement could resolve this life-threatening situation.

In breast-feeding, postpartum estrogen rises to almost prepregnancy levels after about nine or ten months. At that point, prolactin is produced right in the breast by the baby's sucking alone. When estrogen rises, it, alone without progesterone, turns off a powerful cellular growth controller called *epidermal growth factor* (EGF 1 and 2). This particular growth factor, when it's left turned on, is the major player in Her2-neu breast cancer.[53] You need the estrogen rising to high enough levels to turn off EGF 1 and 2[54-55] or you may end up with cancer.

Your estrogen has to keep rising over the following year to ovulate again. The point here is that a young woman will ovulate again. And if, in the scheme of things, she gets pregnant and breast-feeds at least eighteen months at minimum, all's right with her biological world.

If, however, she gets pregnant and does not breast-feed, two things will happen—first and foremost, her breasts will assume her baby has died. Then she will become pregnant again as soon as possible (unless she uses contraception). The large families of ten to twenty children that occurred in the early part of this century are a phenomenon that does not occur in nature. Women during the Industrial Revolution here and abroad couldn't breast-feed for child spacing while holding down jobs in factories and were often literally used up physically by unrelenting childbirth. Until the Pill, women always ovulated again after birth unless they breast-fed, if they were young.

A menopausal woman won't. She is out of eggs and their attendant hormones.

By the time a woman is in her late forties, she's spent anywhere from ten to twenty years in this hormonal confusion, depending on whether or not she's reproduced. And reproduction assumes lactation. In nature, the option of not feeding your baby from your body does not exist. By the time you are in your forties, your hormones are all over the place; none of them are in the right place, unless you've lived a very different life with many more births and decades of nursing than most of us have. But even then, you can't just stop being a woman, biologically, or there's hell to pay.

In this macabre reenactment of life so benignly called *the change*, a woman doesn't quite make it through puberty, never gets to be pregnant, has provoked the hormonal milieu of labor and delivery (sky-high cortisol ending in the absence of progesterone and estrogen), and is now on her way to "pseudo"-lactation.

That's the last phase of her life.

All Along the Watchtower

Just when you think you know the rules, you realize this is no game. The problem with the lives we've tried to live is that nature still knows the real song of survival *because nature wrote it*. When you try to change the tune of truly ancient songs written specifically *for our survival,* nature will win—no matter what feminism, economics, or pharmaceutical companies tell you.

You can't hormonally be in a place to breast-feed and not do it for decades without experiencing repercussions of great magnitude. If you weren't diagnosed with cancer *before* menopause, in perimenopause, from a lack of progesterone due to hit-or-miss irregular ovulation from the falling levels of estrogen (because you're running out of eggs, which would produce that estrogen), you get a second chance when you finally run out of everything but insulin and prolactin.

Postmenopausal breast cancer can be diagnosed in women into their nineties.

There seems to be no defense in mammography[56-57] or exercise,[58] low-fat diets,[59, 60] thousands of dollars' worth of supplements, prophylactic tamoxifen,[61-62] or genetic screening.[63-64] Cancer is a natural phase of life that just happens to end in death. The terrorism of the constant threat that you might be next never stops. Fortunately, there is hope, and it is in the very thing women are being warned against—hormones, not the synthetic drugs being marketed as hormones, but real, bio-identical, natural hormone replacement that may take you out of this cancerous state.[65-69]

Tombstone Blues

After watching the progress made by science and medicine in the war on cancer over the last five or six decades, it's pretty clear that research isn't going to save us anytime soon, or cancer would be cured or at least decreasing in incidence by now. The statistics for breast cancer mortality have stayed steady for over sixty years.[70] Modern medicine's newest treatments for cancer, from monoclonal antibodies to vascular inhibitors to gene therapy to stem cells, don't just border on science fiction, *they are science fiction*.[71-72] None of them can ever effect a "cure" because in your body, new genes or somebody else's stem cells must still be regulated by hormones you don't have anymore.[73] The old science fiction treatments still being used on us, like radiation, chemotherapy, and surgery, evidently don't work, either. In a massive study of vast cancer data by R. Fossati et al. published in *The Journal of Clinical Oncology* in October 1998, under the auspices of the Laboratory of Clinical Research in Oncology, Italian Cochrane Centre in Milan, untreated women lived only three months less than treated women with metastatic breast cancer.[74] The suffering for those extra three months from the treatment is unacceptable in a field whose motto is "do no harm."

As we were altering the environmental cues that changed us hormonally, modern medicine discovered germ theory, antibiotics, and anesthesia, making successful surgery possible. It all comes together, in respect to medicine's approach to cancer, when we consider that the original cure was surgery.[75] This fact speaks to medicine's perception of what they're trying to fight. The original premise was a local disease that could be eradicated before it spread. Chemotherapy was utilized when it became apparent that there were "nested metastases," or distant sites of cancer far from the original tumor. It's never discussed in modern medicine that if the cancer is already so disseminated in you that your mastectomy or lumpectomy will routinely be followed with chemo, you don't need to lose your breast.[76] The chemo should take care of the cancer's site of origin, too, or it isn't going to work anyway. Radiation never made any sense, because the one definitive *cause* of cancer on this earth is ionizing radiation. According to all the laws of physics and biology, the treatment in the case of radiation can only cause more cancer.[77]

When we consider that those very *recent* advancements are the sum total of the arsenal of modern medicine besides antibiotics and blood transfusion,[78] it's not surprising that the standard of care treatment for cancer is still just surgery to remove the tumor and a chemotherapy regimen based on the model of infection—that is, cancer "spreads" and can be killed, like a virus or germ.

Cancer doesn't "spread." It's not an infection, it's a bodywide phenomenon of change that happens in a pattern of occurrence in the absence of genetically regulatory sex hormones after midlife.[79]

The element of contagion even comes into play with the notion of "catching" cancer from pollutants or, oddly enough, from your own estrogen. They even call it the "war on cancer" and shoot radar *guns* at it. Medicine wages the same *kind* of war on cancer that was once waged successfully on tuberculosis and pneumonia. But it can't work this time because cancer comes from within, not from the outside like a germ or virus.

What medicine has never considered is the possibility that cancer is an evolutionary state on the same metabolic disease plane as, say, diabetes. The enemy is within us, not just outside us. That's why no matter how hard medicine tries, there seems to be no definitive defense against it.

Science has begun to identify which regulatory genes are active in the formation of tumors. They've even gone so far as to name them *fetal* oncogenes.[80-84] This is, of course, because these genes are switched on in the first trimester of pregnancy. (As we've seen, in pregnancy there is a mechanism for switching them off.)

This should have been a clue.

But although they've named them fetal oncogenes, they have yet to apply the hormonal models of puberty, pregnancy, and lactation to the actions of those cancer genes. When the compare-and-contrast exercise plays out, it becomes startlingly clear what's gone wrong, and what women can do about it.

In the last three generations, we have become something we are not biologically evolved to be—essentially *childless* during the apex of our reproductive years. That fact, all by itself, accounts for the increase in reproductive cancer in our generation, and in our mothers' and even our grandmothers' generations.[85]

It's time to unravel what's happened to women, from the pseudohormones that constitute birth control pills to the fertility treatments we've undergone, the time we've spent not nursing, and, now, the false hormone-like drugs that we're told is HRT. We're going to have to take a long hard look at the health implications and try to save ourselves, because we're really in this all alone.

We can't go back and do it differently.

We are who we are.

But we don't have to die for it.

part **two**

LIES

four

YOU CAN'T ALWAYS GET WHAT YOU WANT

What exactly was the trade-off for free love, in terms of your health? Politically incorrect as the realities may be, in order to save your life we've got to tell you that if there's no free lunch, then there's no such thing as free love, either, in terms of biology.

No one in 1968, the summer of love, had any idea that birth control pills would lead to the need for fertility drugs, or that fertility drugs would lead to ovarian cancer.[1-8] By 1968, we conclude, 1.5 million human guinea pigs had been on the pill for over five years, as participants in the biggest live drug experiment ever run. This was self-inflicted mass infertility. Such a thing had never occurred before in history.

We had always controlled fertility with herbs on a monthly basis, or for religious purposes, but never on a scale like this. That old standby abstinence worked day to day, and breast-feeding worked month to month. Interestingly enough, mistletoe berries, containing natural progesterone,[9] were used as contraceptives thousands of years ago in the same way we now use the synthetic progestin RU-486 and the "morning-after" pill. In our generation, after a decade of easy contraception, by the mid-1970s a lot of us would choose not to become mothers or wives for at least a decade more, if at all.

The message of equality sent to women by the feminist movement was interpreted to mean that marriage and children could wait on a back burner behind accomplishments outside of marriage. Needless to say, the feminist icons who sent women the message either to forgo men as life partners or to eschew childbearing, and to continue to have sex for no purpose (in the evolutionary sense), were not evolutionary biologists, infertility specialists, or cancer researchers.

There was no way they could have predicted the psychological distress brought by multiple partners, the infertility from delayed childbearing, or the dramatic increase in our generation of breast and ovarian cancer[10-19] resulting from the lack of extended periods of placental progesterone—that is, from pregnancy. After all, having the ability to avoid bearing children before you wanted them and getting to have sex without consequences, just like men, seemed like a good idea at the time.

Given that this is our reality, our evidence points to the reasonable assumption that cyclical, rhythmic natural hormone replacement may be even more important for those of us who did not have more than three children young in life and those of us who weren't breast-fed by our moms and those of us who didn't get to breast-feed our own children for three years each.

Why Don't We Do It in the Road

The sexual revolution of the 1960s was a paradigm shift that had an intimate cause-and-effect relationship with the invention of oral contraceptives. We know that the contraceptive pill is the single most important evolutionary endocrine disrupter of all time. The introduction of an oral contraceptive facilitated the loosening of sexual mores, which had been largely enforced by the fear of unwanted pregnancy. Thanks to the Pill, magazines like *Playboy* stepped up and began to sell the idea, for the first time in human history, that "nice girls" liked sex, too. *Playboy* magazine, founded by Hugh Hefner in 1953, was pushing sex before the Pill arrived on the scene, but naked women were so hard to come by in the mid-1950s that Hefner's first centerfold, Marilyn Monroe, was a secondhand photograph purchased from a local printer of naughty calendars.[20] The world was still pretty tame compared to our lives today.

It's interesting, and more than a little coincidental, that oral contraceptives just popped into existence when they did. Why, in all time, then? After all, synthesizing sex hormones from animal and plant sources is almost as old as civilization itself.

The Chinese collected and dried in the sun the urine of pregnant women over two thousand years ago.[21] The steroid salts dehydrated out of the urine were pressed into ancient pill presses and used as treatment for a number of diseases in the elderly. These metabolites and used-up hormones were really a precursor to Premarin, which consists of the same kinds of metabolites and used-up hormones from pregnant mares' urine. If the possibility of easy, reliable birth control in the form of natural plant and animal hormones had always been at hand, why hadn't humanity taken advantage of it earlier in our history, instead if saving it for special occasions, like orgies and treatment of diseases?

Was there really a lack of interest in recreational sex until now?

Probably not.

The birth control movement and Planned Parenthood would argue that it was the frightening rate of population growth, that the Earth was heaving under the weight of so many of us and it had to be stopped. But that's just not true. Ever since the 1970s, demographic forecasters have been scaring us with population figures that appear to wildly outstrip even the most optimistic projections for resources (food, water, and land). It *is* true that during the twentieth century the world's population ballooned fourfold from 1.6 billion to 6 billion. But what if that increase in human heft was a result of death-defying health care measures, not the birth rate?

The truth is that in the background of the baby boomer population explosion, fertility has been falling steadily since the turn of the century. In 1950, worldwide (despite pockets of crowding in China and India), the average woman had five children. Today, she has just 2.7. In fact, the numbers show fertility rates looming in our future that are far below replacement levels.[22-23] Replacement fertility requires 2.1 children per woman (the excess 0.1 compensates for the girls who do not live long enough to have families). The United Nations population forecasts, to be finalized by the end of 2002, are expected to conclude that within two generations four out of five of the world's women will be having two or fewer children. Even in countries like China and India, the birth rate is declining.[24]

If it wasn't the need for recreational sex, which has always existed, or global overpopulation, which seems to have never existed, what is the reason for the sudden appearance for the first time in history of reliable, day-in-and-day-out-for-decades global contraception?

Something besides the need for unencumbered sex was happening to us.

Women have been changing on some fundamental evolutionary mental and physical plane. And, so have men.

Don't You Want Somebody to Love?

Behavioral changes related to population control triggered by environmental cues are always related to mating because saving the group inevitably requires a reallocation of resources. The best way to do that is to put the brakes on reproduction by altering mating rituals, which will ultimately mean fewer mouths to feed, and thus enhance survival. A smaller population is often more viable. What's happening to us now—the changes in attitude and behavior that have resulted in a reluctance to mate and have children until it's too late—is simply a way of culling the herd for the sake of all of us, that is, to ensure the survival of the species as a whole.

While the planet is not really heaving under the weight of us all and although no asteroid has hit, by creating artificial light rhythms and an unending food supply we've triggered a stress-induced "save the population" scenario that seems to be playing out in mating strategies.

In the interplay between the environment and your hormones, nature can cue certain hormones through environmental stimulus to make you behave in a way to survive or die.[25] The part of this time-tested solution that's problematic for us as human beings, with our intense sense of individuality, is nature's use of pronouns. When nature says "you," she doesn't mean *you*, she means your group. Nature always "selects" (natural selection) for the group, *not the individual*.

When a group is under stress,[26] that is, in trouble—signified by a sudden temperature change (an out-of-season fire or drastic weather); an extended growing period (endless summer) for carbohydrates; or "crowding," triggering a rise in cortisol (the stress hormone), which alone can imply a potential food shortage—then a cascade of hormonal events that are hardwired responses in each individual for the survival of the group will cause changes in the uterine environment of the reproducing females.[27-30] These "stress" hormones cause changes in the offspring's behavior that will continue in each new generation until the stress is gone.[31-37] The only environmental stress big enough to set off population controls would be drastic changes in weather (like the Ice Age) or in the food supply, or attack by another group.

We have triggered the stress scenario over the last 150 years by eating too much carbohydrate and creating long hours of artificial light.[38-39] In our bodies, all of the insulin we're producing creates insulin *resistance*.[40] While our bodies just get fatter and fatter, our brains can't access any of the sugar we eat because *in the brain* insulin resistance reads to the controls on behavioral cues as "famine," because of the lack of access to the body's own blood sugar[41-43] (this mechanism is why overweight people are generally hungry people), and because all of the cortisol we're producing from the incessant light just reads as "fear."

Because of these artificial triggers, our environmental sensors honed by evolution lead us to keep eating sugar and trying to mate twenty-four hours a day because it seems like summer in our heads. Since year-in and year-out eating and mating is not a template on this planet, nature perceives a "bug" or glitch in the program and so shuts down for repairs. The way it shuts down is to slow reproduction by changing the individuals *sexually* in the group under stress.

The major "hormonal players" activated in the individuals of the group during any of these possible stresses are always *cortisol* (which reacts to light, temperature, and fear) and *insulin* (which reacts to light and the food supply).[44-45] Our insulin and cortisol mechanisms always act in tandem in stressful situations such as mating, famine, or fear. Mating season, because of sexual competition and aggression, is a biologically stressful event.

Remember that mating season is, in nature, *always* summer, because the light creates food and food makes reproduction possible. In summer, your insulin is up from the abundance of carbohydrates and your cortisol is up from the extended daylight. When the long light of summer relays to your brain the signal "Eat sugar *now* and get fat enough to make it through winter," a simultaneous hormonal pathway says "Mate *now,* so your baby will come in the spring when there is more light and food." Anyone who watches *Animal Planet* on TV knows this about bears, fish, and penguins. It's true about humans, too.[46-47]

Thrifty nature uses the same "summer scenario" of hormones—insulin, cortisol, and testosterone—used in mating to control population density, too. When nature has to decrease the population by culling the herd with rising infertility and metabolic disease, we have the rise in diabetes and infertility we see now. By 1960 this event had been one hundred years in the making.

The status of the food supply, in the form of carbohydrate energy, is always represented in the body by the "when" and "how much" of insulin. The food supply literally writes the story of human potential, since human life and its accomplishments, like being able to work and to be able to have

Environmental Control on Mating and Sexual Behavior

NORMAL PATHWAY:

STRESS PATHWAY:

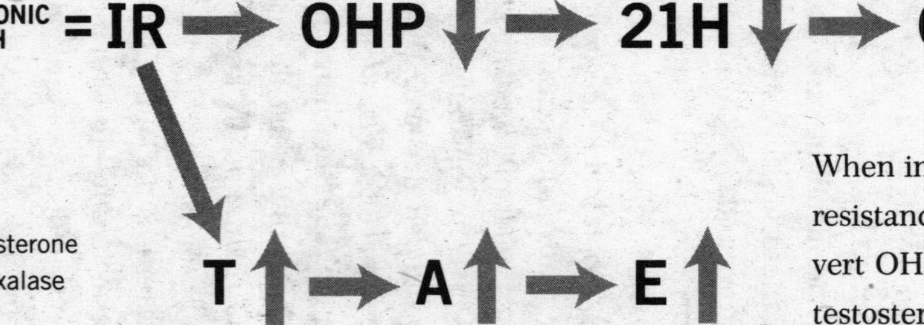

I Insulin
OHP OH progesterone
21H 21-Hydroxalase
C Cortisol
T Testosterone
A Aromatase
E Estradiol

When insulin can't be read (insulin resistance), there is no 21H to convert OHP to C. Instead, it becomes testosterone androgenizing mother and offspring children, are based on the availability of food to give you the energy and latitude to do both. The way the food supply can change the outcome of the story is by controlling the "punctuation," in the form of *enzymes*.[48]

Enzymes can cut pieces off of molecules like progesterone and turn them into testosterone, or turn testosterone into estrogen or DHT (dihydrotestoterone).[49] That means that enzymes can change the meaning of a molecular, physiological, informational sentence—that is, a directive to brain and body—just like a well-placed comma.

The enzymes are controlled by insulin,[50] the amount of which is a result of the quantity and abundance of carbohydrate energy, provide the fine-tuning on your sex hormones. Whether or not we mate is a result of whether or not there's enough food for that kind of energy expenditure. This is how it's done: in summer, the carbohydrates available boost insulin. Insulin not only stores the sugar as fat for winter, it also enhances the production of an enzyme called *21-hydroxylase*[51-52]—this enzyme converts a form of progesterone into cortisol under normal stress like fear or weather changes, episodic conditions of short duration. Extra cortisol helps us deal with the stress.

However, in the presence of prolonged insulin secretion, nature assumes that it's mating season.[53] In other words, nature, or your body, reads prolonged high insulin (insulin resistance) as summer because in nature that's the only time it's that high for that long. By the end of summer, we should be fatter for winter and have a bun in the oven—be pregnant.

In response, at the requisite threshold, "stress," which is read as light and food insulin resistance (no insulin action), stops the production of 21-hydroxylase,[54] and instead of adrenal progesterone converting to cortisol, it becomes testosterone,[55] which you need to reproduce. Because the food supply (insulin) is the control on reproduction (testosterone), it is insulin that controls the choice between the production of cortisol or testosterone. This mechanism of testosterone can either enhance masculinity in females in utero or, if it's too intense, cause male hormone *resistance* and actually feminize men.[56]

Something's Happening Here

If you think back to our collective childhoods, was it really good old American middle-class, Midwestern Protestant repression that kept us from recognizing gays and lesbians in our parents' peer group or among our grandparents' friends? Or is it possible that they really weren't there, in the way they are now? We *assume* that the sexual freedoms we "enjoy" as the norm have contributed to shining a light into everyone's closet, but maybe not. We all assume that all of the gender-bending we encounter in a day had just been waiting all this time for the freedom to express itself openly, but what if, back then, it really was just a different world, populated with different people, than the one we live in today?

While there are always pregnant women under stress and there have always been shades of gray in their offspring and always will be, we have come to live in a brave new world where heterosexuals need a parade to be noticed. It's a world where the women are strong, the men are good-looking, and the children are all above average. This is not the norm. Garrison Keillor was right. In the world before now, all the men were strong and, for the most part, heterosexual, and the women were good-looking and, for the most part, heterosexual, and the children were all just about average.

It's the only world *we* know, but that doesn't mean this is how it's always been.

What we're living through now, in our lifetimes, is the way nature saves us from ourselves: because cortisol and testosterone are at the heart of the process of sexual orientation, male hormones called *androgens* in varying degrees make us what we are.[57-58] The study of population control via breeding patterns is called *population dynamics*. Sex hormones, insulin, and cortisol are all involved in the breeding impetus as it applies to population dynamics.

All fetuses start out as female.[59-61] Then, at about nine weeks gestation, the Y chromosome turns what seem to be all girls into some boys. Boys have an X and Y, and girls have two Xs. However, the amount of testosterone (androgen) seasoning mom's womb can actually turn an XY boy into a girl by affecting hormone reception and brain and body architecture in the baby.[62] Even though the baby girl has not XX, but XY lineage.

In extreme examples, the resulting male XY "female" child will look, act, and think like a girl. There's absolutely nothing to betray her Y chromosome, until her teens pass and her period never comes—because she has no uterus or ovaries, and has a "blind" vagina with small testicles high up in her abdomen. The testosterone from her tiny testes that, at week nine in utero, should have worked its male magic went unread by androgen receptors.

In cases like this, stress on mom,[63] any kind of stress—physical, mental, or light and food—promotes testosterone and soaks her in high cortisol (which made her insulin-resistant by way of cortisol mobilizing blood sugar, and took away her 21-hydroxylase,[64] which made her testosterone pour). Then, the ultrahigh androgens (testosterone) in mom make the baby boy's androgen receptors retreat.[65] This leaves only receptors that can read estrogen, making the little boy forever feminine. In the same way that insulin receptors can retreat and cause insulin *resistance*—the insulin receptor becomes resistant to the attempt by insulin to get blood sugar into the cell—*testosterone resistance* can happen[66] the same way.[67]

This is an evolutionary mechanism of great power.

This protocol can act in three tiers to control reproduction for limiting population. The first tier of minimal stress on a population can turn baby boys into very unlikely reproducers and extremely creative individuals. We know this phenomenon as male homosexuality. These men could reproduce, but they probably won't. This is often an aftermath of war, when women are left during pregnancy to guard themselves in a vulnerable time. That may be why we have had a population bulge of homosexuality after World War II.[68-71]

The second tier of increased stress on mom increases androgen resistance in baby boys to make some of them the gorgeous, tall, voluptuous women with little or no body hair—the XY females of the previous page. Since they can receive little or no androgens, they are highly estrogenized and seem extremely female.[72]

Nature seems to have two jobs for these infertile "women": first, as nonfunctional decoys, they distract still-fertile males from fertile females, and second, since they are soaked in estrogen, they are incredibly maternal, love children, and become devoted nursemaids to children who may become orphaned in whatever crisis the group is up against.

The third-tier option—the most drastic in nature—turns girl babies into boy babies via brain architecture only. We know this phenomenon as female same-sex preference. Lesbians are women who, as they are not attracted to men, would not (until the advent of artificial insemination) have reproduced. These templates exist to create planetary homeostasis with regard to space and food supply.

A Hard Rain's Gonna Fall

We are different from the women who came before us because the increasing light and sugar of the last hundred years or so has been read, hormonally, as *stress*. Our brains have been reprogrammed with behavioral mandates to slow down population growth in our group because strange unending light and food nonrhythms are "stress." Our grandmothers and mothers gave birth to children who in every generation are reproducing less and less. That's how nature estimates the environmental stress we're under and then changes the product produced by women to reduce the population. To an evolutionary endocrinologist, if one existed, it would be very clear that we are undergoing an episode of evolutionary bottlenecking wherein for the good of the many, there have to be fewer of us. This will not only affect our ability to pair-bond and our rate of giving birth, but in the end our rate of death as well.

Things that seem to be one thing often turn out to be another. What seems like choice, what would appear to be rights (our ambitions, our desires, all of the equality and political clout that rests under the umbrella of feminism), is really just part and parcel of an evolutionary template to slow population growth. It's happened before, in Egypt, in Greece, in Rome, and during the Renaissance.

The dirty little secret of evolution is that individuals who are not part of the project—life—die first, to leave the most resources for the reproducing women and the offspring, because that gives the group a better chance of survival as a species.[73]

So although we've been programmed by the environment to choose work over child rearing, to benefit all of us as a group, we are destined to die early for it, too—unless we replace our hormones in a way that makes us look as if we could still reproduce.

Then we may not have to die.

This world, this cosmos, and our individual bodies are all run on programs, routines, and subroutines triggered by melodies that are played by the instruments of light and food. When we changed the environment with artificial light and extended growing seasons, we disturbed the music. Now, according to the programming, we will die.

A Hard Day's Night

Most of us believed we would have children *someday*.

Most of us just wanted enough time to be able to make "choices." But the Pill, diaphragms, sponges, and abortions all gave us the manifest impression that we could wait and wait and wait. Because we *could* wait, the implication was that it was okay to wait.

It wasn't.

If we're going to unravel the implications (for our health) of the methods that we've employed to stay infertile, we're going to have to examine exactly what we've ingested, internalized, or excised.

Maybe we should first ask what (or who) were the driving forces behind the concept of *terminal* (forever) contraception. The cast of characters is a motley crew, all but one of them homegrown. They include Margaret Sanger, Gregory Pincus, Carl Djerassi, Ph.D., Father John Rock, M.D., Beverly Strassman, and a misguided doctor-scientist named M. C. Pike, whom we'll get to later. Without the individual contributions of these six individuals, our lives would have been vastly different.

There would have been no sexual revolution.

Times would have been bawdy for a while, as they have been many times before in history, but they would have swung back the other way to a more conservative lifestyle, as they always have. But the wholesale dismissal of the "original bargain" between the sexes—the trade-off of children for resources—would never have happened. While there have always been some women to whom childbearing did not appeal, their options were limited if they wanted the sexual company of men, because they might get pregnant, and limited professionally, because until recently the only profession open to them was wife and mother or a caretaker in some form.

You Say You Want a Revolution

Margaret Sanger[74] set out to change all that and she did. Her name is familiar to most of us as a feminist icon who brought the message of "choice" to women all over the world. She fits nicely into our timeline because she was born in 1879 into an Irish Catholic family in Corning, New York. She was seventy-one in 1950, just exactly the right age to be our great-grandmother.

She was at the cusp of change. She was a new kind of woman.

She was the sixth of eleven children, and she was born *different.* If she had followed in her mother's footsteps, motherhood would have been a given, but instead, her older sisters' spouses helped Margaret attend Claverack College, the Hudson River Institute, and the White Plains Hospital's Nursing Program.

In 1901, at the ripe old age of twenty-two (remember, women at the turn of the century married between the ages of fifteen and nineteen), she married an architect and immediately had three children. Her architect husband soon thereafter quit his relatively lucrative profession to try his hand at oil painting. In a role reversal, Margaret returned to nursing as a visiting nurse on New York's Lower East Side, to support the family. She is the model of the gender-bending new woman.

Both of the Sangers were immersed in the Bohemian, intellectual, activist culture thriving in Greenwich Village at the time. Influenced by the ideas of anarchist Emma Goldman, by 1912, Sanger began to argue for family limitation as a tool for the poor women of the Lower East Side to liberate themselves from the economic and physical burden of unwanted pregnancy. Two years later, in 1914, she published the first issue of her radical, militantly feminist magazine, *The Woman Rebel.* She was promptly arrested for violating the 1873 Comstock laws prohibiting the dissemination of obscenity through the mail. She jumped bail and left her husband, all in the same year, then traveled to England, where, in keeping with her views, she had simultaneous affairs with psychologist Havelock Ellis and writer H. G. Wells.

This was not normal post-Victorian behavior.

When Margaret got home, she was convicted. But the New York State appellate court exempted physicians from the Comstock laws if "the patient needed contraceptive information for her health." And this loophole allowed Sanger to open the first legal birth control clinic in 1923, a year after she married much older oil magnate James Noah H. Slee.

Slee, who died in 1943, the year after Margaret founded the original International Planned Parenthood Federation, was the main source of funding of the birth control movement. It seems that Margaret, the original feminist, got her fortune the old-fashioned way—by marrying it. It's at this point in the story that Margaret's motives get a little murky, too. To this day, prolifers contend (with no small amount of documented evidence) that Margaret's real intent was to limit reproduction in the poor, uneducated immigrants of New York City's Lower East Side—that, in fact, Margaret Sanger was a eugenicist.

In her tour de force of scientific investigative journalism, *Women and the Crisis in Sex Hormones*[75] (which was published in 1977), Barbara Seaman reprints a fund-raising letter written in 1951 by Margaret Sanger to her friend heiress Katharine McCormick.

Margaret stated her thinking very clearly:

> *I consider that the world and almost our civilization for the next twenty-five years is going to depend upon a simple, cheap, safe contraceptive to be used in poverty-stricken slums and jungles, and among the most ignorant people . . . I believe that now, immediately, there should be national sterilization for certain dysgenic types of our population who are being encouraged to breed and would die out were the government not feeding them.*[76]

Margaret lent her name, her money, and eventually her political clout to the liberal wing of the eugenics movement. Eugenics is the science of breeding—people—to a purpose. To this group, birth control was a means of reducing the genetically transmitted mental and physical defects passed on from parent to child.

These were also the people who supported the forced sterilization of the mentally incompetent, which was, at that point in time, a very broad category of disease that included illnesses as treatable today as epilepsy.[77] Margaret Sanger had the Pill in mind for very specific groups of people. The founder of Planned Parenthood intended it for the people we call "Third Worlders."

Sanger used $150,000 donated by Katharine McCormick (McCormick ultimately spent $2 million) to challenge Dr. Gregory Pincus of the Worchester Foundation for Experimental Biology to find an effective oral contraceptive. Pincus located a scientist named Russell Marker who, in 1939, had changed a plant cholesterol from sarsaparilla roots into human bioidentical progesterone.

It took all of the 1950s and a priest for Margaret and Pincus to turn natural progesterone into the drugs in the Pill called progestins. Margaret's plan to slow population growth among the poor had one big hurdle to overcome—Catholicism—because almost all the groups that she intended to market the Pill to were, at the time, Roman Catholic, and Catholics, in 1950, hated contraception.

The quest moved to Mexico, when Marker found that Mexican yams were an even better, cheaper source of natural progesterone. Marker eventually left the project for other financial opportunities, so Pincus pursued Carl Djerassi, Ph.D., a Viennese chemist working in Mexico, and research chemist Frank Colton, Ph.D., in Chicago. In 1954, Pincus and Sanger enlisted John Rock in their mission, a Harvard gynecologist who, serendipitously for Margaret, happened to be a priest, just the right person to convince Catholics to try contraception.

He had taught obstetrics for three decades at Harvard Medical School. His association with the Pill gave it respectability. The Pill chosen for submission to the FDA was called Enovid. Father Rock appeared before the FDA in 1959 to testify to its safety. It was approved in 1960.

In the years immediately after the FDA approved the Pill, Father Rock was everywhere—*Time, Newsweek, The Saturday Evening Post*. He published a much-publicized, highly controversial book in 1963 called *The Time Has Come: A Catholic Doctor's Proposals to End the Battle Over Birth Control*.[78] At the time, as now, abortion was a hot topic with Catholics, who interpret the willful end of a potential Catholic's life as murder. Father Rock felt that the Pill would be welcomed by the Church because it intervened *before* life occurred.

Father Rock's church disappointed him. The papal commission, established by Pope John XXIII and continued by Pope Paul VI, said no.

But the rest of America didn't.

Within two years, 1.2 million women were using it, within five years, 5 million, and by 1970, about 10 million. In 1960, when the Pill was approved, we, as potential customers, had been led to believe that it had been tested for years on thousands of women in Puerto Rico, when in fact nothing could have been farther from the truth. A Senate investigation in 1963 revealed that the Pill was tested only on about 132 women who had taken it continuously for a year or longer. Three of the 132 young women died during the testing but were never autopsied.[79]

The FDA later exonerated themselves with the premise that the Pill was a special case, since powerful drugs are prescribed for powerful diseases and pregnancy is not an illness.[80] On this momentous occasion in pharmaceutical history, the birth control pill would be the first powerful drug ever prescribed to normal *healthy* women for long-term use. In essence, the FDA sanctioned a drug to medicate half of the population for something that wasn't a disease. By the way, for those women born in 1970, thirty-three years ago, now ready to have a baby, infertility stands conservatively at 6.1 million.[81]

There's a direct connection.

Father Rock's church wasn't the only thing he was mistaken about. In his collaboration with Pincus, Rock was working on the premise that ovulation was suppressed by the artificial progesterone (progestin): convincing the brain that the body was already pregnant. In reality, the low level of estrogen plus the progestins put the body into a sort of controlled menopause.[82-85] Since menopause is the beginning of the end, healthwise, this was a tragedy to perpetrate on eighteen-year-olds.

Putting eighteen-year-olds into a controlled menopause with the same hormones used in conventional HRT accounts for the increase in breast cancer and vascular events in women on the Pill.[86-88] By 1962, there were 132 reports of blood clots and 11 deaths.[89] Pill users were beginning to show abnormal glucose tolerance and some diabetes from altered metabolism.[90-91] Today we know, from a study in 2002 involving 103,027 women in Norway and Sweden, that even users of the "mini-pill" have a 22 percent increase in breast cancer versus childless women who haven't used oral contraceptives.[92]

There are fifty-nine different versions of the Pill on the market today, as well as a contraceptive patch called *Ortho Evra* that you can "preview" by tearing a sample out of a variety of women's magazines. Drug companies found another market, a few years ago, as a cure for acne. The latest audacious marketing move is a version called *Yasmin* that is being touted as a weight-loss aid. Some infinitesimal group of women lost an average of two, count 'em, two pounds over the vast stretch of time of six months.[93]

Now that's a weight-loss aid.

Right now, sixteen million women in America are on the Pill,[94] approximately one third of those sixteen million for perimenopausal symptoms. The Pill can in no way ameliorate the real and present dangers to health before, during, and after menopause. Our evidence shows that, at best, it masks the real symptoms of impending disease and enhances low-level estrogen-driven cell proliferation in breasts, liver, and cervix.

Birth control pills contain higher doses of estrogen than regular hormone replacement therapy. The very same progestins' thrombotic action (forming of blood clots) in birth control pills has been seen to be caused by the "Pro" in PremPro in the recently canceled HRT heart trials.[95]

No one in forty years ever tried to recall the Pill.

Since its introduction in 1960, over 468 million women in America have used oral contraceptives. The number in the rest of the world is only 100 million. We in America have taken almost five times the amount of birth control pills as all the other countries in the world combined.[96] Add to that hormonal picture that when we do have children, we breast-feed the least of any other nation in the world. For our health's sake, this is all very bad. We don't breast-feed the ones we have long enough. And we can't breast-feed the ones the Pill prevented us from ever considering having. Contraceptives have been the key player in our lack of childbearing and, by degree, our subsequent lack of breast-feeding, but there are a couple more pieces to the puzzle of breast cancer.

The Times They Are A-Changin'

In 1935, the same year that Russell Marker isolated the progesterone from plants that through Djerassi and Rock ultimately led to the Pill, Sir Charles Dodds in England synthesized a steroid called *diethylstilberol*[97] that they believed had effects similar to, but not exactly like, the estrogen made in your body. The effects of this synthetic estrogen go right down to genetic inheritance. In the same year, the artificial baby food we came to call formula was introduced into the U.S. market.[98] The Pill, DES, and infant formula—together these three events have contributed almost exclusively to the epidemic of breast cancer seen in the last fifty years.

It's not pesticides or your diet or your lack of exercise.

We know Dodds's estrogenlike steroid as DES, the devastatingly multigenerational carcinogen given during the 1940s and 1950s to pregnant women who were in danger of miscarriage. But its first use, in the early 1930s, was *lactation suppression*, so that modern women could bottle-feed.[99] Why, suddenly, would women not want to nurse their children? Part of it was the zeitgeist of the times. Germ theory and the model of infection was the big scientific news after World War I; the major killer of Western man, pneumonia, had just been cured by antibiotics. Science began to equate health with the model of germ theory: Germs make people sick; if we can kill germs, people will get well. After the discovery of antibiotics, all diseases were wedged into this model whether they fit or not.

Unfortunately, medicine just took a new idea too far. Health authorities at the time told women breast-feeding was unsanitary because breasts are dirty.[100]

Breast milk was unsterile.

Henri Nestle had invented an artificial baby food in Europe in 1867, and by the turn of the century bottle-feeding had spread all over continental Europe and the British Isles. The medical profession was in large part responsible for the dramatic decline in breast-feeding in America between 1940 and 1970; they handed out free formula to new mothers as they left the hospital, and they still do. New Zealand is the only country in the world today where a mother in hospital must sign a release form before anyone can feed her baby formula.

The drug vernacular "first one's free"—giving nonaddicted people drugs to hook them—applies completely in the instance of breast-feeding because of the window of time for breast milk to "come in." The term *come in* refers to a delicately synergistic symbiotic dance done between the mother and the newborn to establish a milk supply. Enough formula in the first days or weeks makes successfully nursing a baby permanently impossible. Mom's milk dries up and the baby will die without the substitute. That's the textbook definition of "hooked."

Pushers always keep their eye on the money, and in the case of breast milk substitutes, the acceptance and growth of bottle-feeding can be attributed to the profits made by the industry that created them and by the medical profession's endorsement.[101-103] Breast-feeding is one of the hardest things in the world to learn to do. It's messy, you're disrobed most of the time, and working at anything else is neigh to impossible. Doctors at the time, and in their characteristic enthusiasm to "help" women, no doubt pushed formula-feeding as a better option from day one.[104] Because canned milk had been sterilized, with mother's milk, they felt deadly germs could infect the baby. In 1998, the annual sales of formula, or synthetic milk, for babies raked in $8 *billion* in America alone.[105]

In 1935, 17 percent of babies were bottle-fed exclusively when they left the hospital. By 1946, it was close to 35 percent, and by 1966 the numbers had more than doubled to 73 percent. *At the end of the 1970s, 95 percent of babies were bottle-fed exclusively from day one of their lives.*[106-110]

Those babies were us.

Oh, Mama, Could This Really Be the End?

A study conducted at the National Institutes of Health (NIH) in Bethesda, Maryland, and published in 1997 in the journal *Epidemiology* reported a "7% reduction of risk for breast cancer in women who were breastfed as babies."[111]

Remember the fine print in the nature's prime directive?[112] We said that breast-feeding immunizes the baby against death from the outside—germs and the like. This study supports the statement that breast-fed girl babies seem to be immunized *against breast cancer,* or death from the inside. Breast-feeding immunizes *you,* as a mother, too, against breast cancer. The benefit of singing the song of your own biology is not only for your baby. It makes you a *fit* mother, and survival belongs to the fittest.

In July 2002, the British medical journal *The Lancet* published an article entitled "Breast cancer and breastfeeding: a collaborative reanalysis of individual data from 47 epidemiological studies in 30 countries, including 50,302 women with breast cancer and 96,973 women without the disease."[113] This is a ponderous analysis by any measure. It took sifting the data from forty-seven studies gleaned from thirty different countries to find out whether breast-feeding has any demonstrable effect on your risk of breast cancer. The authors say their study contains 80 percent of all of the worldwide epidemiological data on breast cancer. "Epidemiological" means the scientific data represented by actual disease and events in real *people*—not mice, not monkeys, not even esoteric molecules.

The conclusions state very clearly that a woman's risk of breast cancer decreases by 7 percent for every birth she experiences and 3 percent more for each year under twenty-eight years old she is when that child is born, and most importantly, another 4.3 percent for every twelve months of her life that she breast-feeds. Add to that another 23 percent for whether or not she was personally breast-fed by her mother.[114]

That's science, not politics.

The numbers culled by this study will enable women to calculate their percentage of risk in a new and more accurate way—versus "how many miles do you run a week," "how many fruits and vegetable servings do you eat a week," "are you living under power lines," or the ever-popular "do you take the right vitamins and supplements in the right amounts?" All these questions have answers that you can implement with money—new running shoes, expensive imported out-of-season fruit, a new neighborhood, and only God knows how much at the health food store.

The reality is that if you think money is the answer, you didn't understand the question. We can't buy or run or eat or move our way out of this one.

You can't breast-feed babies you never had.

But you can put natural hormones back in a cyclical rhythm, so it seems like you might still have them. That may be all it takes to fool all of your systems into staying healthy for that potential.

Margaret Sanger wasn't really a proponent of choice for women. Her approach to restricting family size has been twisted into restrictive social and economic dogma for women that can endanger your health. We believe that choice for women should constitute the ability and freedom to exercise all of the options you are biologically capable of before it's too late. It's hard to exercise your options when you're on chemotherapy or have Alzheimer's. Biological choice must come first, before lifestyle choices. Margaret Sanger's idea of choice was to have the capability to avoid having children, and she wrote articles supporting safe abortion to that end. From our point of view, as researchers into women's health, someone needs to tell our daughters what no one told us, that first-trimester abortion increases breast cancer risk by an overall odds ratio of 1.3.[115-119]

No one in medicine took into consideration that when it comes to the life forces in nature that keep the planet spinning and all of its creatures fruitful and multiplying, nature isn't really big on choice. But giving the women's movement the benefit of the doubt, we will presuppose that the point of forty years of feminism is, in fact, real choice, and will continue to be, although evidence from the past and the present doesn't support it.

Here's a quote taken from an interview in *Newsweek*[120] magazine with Kim Gandy, the president of the National Organization for Women (NOW). She was responding to a question about the American Society for Reproductive Medicine's (ASRM) new campaign to warn women of the possibility of impending infertility from delayed childbearing. On the sides of big-city buses all over the country, they ran and paid for an advertising campaign utilizing the clever image of an inverted baby bottle dripping milk like sand through an hourglass.

The text reads, "*Time is running out.*"

When queried as to what she thought of the campaign to urge women not to put off childbearing until it's too late, Ms. Gandy said, "The idea that you can choose at what age you'll be able to have your children is a ludicrous proposition for most women."[121]

We found that an interesting response because that was exactly what Margaret Sanger moved heaven and earth to do—give women a choice about *when* to have children. That was the original premise for taking the Pill. But Ms. Gandy, in her response, has spilled the beans, as it were. She's made it crystal clear that to make one choice pretty much negates another. That, in fact, choosing a path at all means you didn't take the others open to you—that just maybe, biologically, we can't *have it all.*

She goes on, "We don't want to give the message to young women that if twenty-eight is good, then twenty-three must be better, and eighteen must be better still."[122-124]

This book was written to address just that issue, in terms of your health. The research in epidemiology and evolutionary and molecular biology agrees that while we can attempt to stop the epidemic of breast cancer with rhythmic, cyclical natural hormone replacement in us and the generations before us, repeating the same mistakes in future generations, now that we have the knowledge of *why* breast cancer takes the lives of those we love, would seem self-serving. To risk our daughters' lives by suppressing the truth to justify our choices is not what being a mother is about.

Ms. Gandy will be receiving a copy of the *Lancet* and the journal *Epidemiology*, which reported twelve years ago, in 1990: "Participants were between the ages of 20 and 54 at the time of the study. Based on the results for 2,492 childbearing women newly diagnosed with breast cancer and 2,687 childbearing controls from the general population, a 15-year increase in maternal age was found to be associated with a 29 percent increase in breast cancer in daughters."[125-127]

In the *Los Angeles Times*, Ms. Gandy went so far as to say, "I don't think the younger-is-better message is the right message to be sending."[128]

Really? Whose body is it, anyway?

This study and literally thousands of others like it[129-131] prove conclusively that the Pill, breast-feeding, and menopausal cancers are inextricably linked and *no one ever told you*. Did somebody else decide it's not the right message to be sending?

If there had been a way to profit from lactation, even NOW couldn't have stopped you from knowing. It didn't make it to you because there's no money in it, and even the people who take the position of guarding our right to choose may not make the knowledge public if your biology intrudes on their politics.

Women must appeal to the leaders of the women's movement to make it clear, no matter how difficult it might make our choices, that reproduction is an elemental force that you can use or that can *destroy you*. With the political clout they wield in 2002, we'd like them to concern themselves with what happens to women when they don't reproduce, or when they reproduce late, or when they don't breast-feed long enough to protect themselves and their children.

As women, we must put the women's movement on notice: We are dying of breast cancer and heart disease and dementia, and it seems as if we're all in this alone. With the political clout we've garnered over the last four decades, women can truly save their own lives. NOW can lobby for easy access to natural hormone replacement, for more scientific studies using natural hormones in a cyclical rhythm, for educating doctors on how to prescribe them, and, most importantly, for long enough paid maternity leaves—eighteen months, just like in Scandinavia—so women can "have it all" and not die for it.

It is a genuine miracle that there may be a solution. There is another study as authentic and impressive as the depressing ones. It's from the journal *Proceedings of the National Academy of Sciences* from October 2001.[132] It reports what we already know from vast sources of epidemiology and molecular biology:

> Full-term pregnancy early in reproductive life is protective against breast cancer in women. Pregnancy also provides protection in animal studies against carcinogen-induced breast cancer (i.e., toxins in the environment), and these effects *can be mimicked by using natural hormones estrogen and progesterone.*

There are many more studies concluding the same thing.

It's going to be all right.

Just make an appointment and tell your doctor what you want.

Show him or her all the research and assure him or her that these treatments are what you wish.

Tell him that you are a reasonable, voting-age adult of sound mind and you've considered your options and done your homework and you would *still* like to try hormone replacement, maybe a *lot* of hormone replacement, natural transdermal hormone replacement, creams, prescribed in a natural rhythm, probably for the rest of your life.

Then watch him tell you, "*No* way."

five

SYMPATHY FOR THE DEVIL

Medicine is one of the last hierarchical systems in the modern world in which an elite at the top still set the standards for the rest of the group. In this guild system, when a researcher/doctor or academician makes a pronouncement, it is rarely challenged by the specialists and family physicians who will, in turn, direct the course of treatment in their patients. As a patient seeking a chosen treatment, you will rarely challenge the wisdom of your doctor because, as a patient, you assume that visiting your doctor means an expert opinion garnered from a wealth of sources.

When you go seeking natural estrogen and progesterone to be prescribed for you in a cyclical rhythm, it won't be a slam dunk, because your doctor's mentors have indicted synthetic hormones. To physicians who have been educated by the researcher/doctor/academician—who is most often funded by a drug company—the hormones most readily available are synthetic. Not only has your physician not been made aware of any other kind of hormone, she has no instructions on how to prescribe them.

Why? Because very few *human* studies have been done using natural hormones for treatment. Since the late 1960s, there have been more than twelve million articles published in medical research journals around the world.[1] Searching on the Internet through the National Library of Medicine site and PubMed,[2] which provides on-line access to all research published globally, we could find only one very small Italian study using natural estradiol and natural progesterone in women, not rats, mice, or monkeys.[3] Why? Because drug companies, and people who work for the drug companies at the National Institutes of Health (NIH) in Bethesda, Maryland, couldn't patent anything they would discover using natural hormones, because you can't patent a natural substance in this country, so there's no money in using natural hormones on human subjects. A patent is where the money is because as long as your patent is in force, no one else can use the knowledge that led you to it without your permission. The only way to patent natural hormones is in a "use patent." A use patent is a way to patent the natural substance *for use* as, say, hormone replacement. Vivelle and Climera patches have minuscule doses of natural estradiol in them. The drug company, in this case, has patented the delivery system—the patch—to make money. As it became obvious that synthetic hormones exacerbated premenstrual syndrome symptoms in young and perimenopausal women, the drug companies had no other solution than to file a use patent for natural progesterone for premenstrual tension, in pill form. Solvay Pharmaceuticals, Inc. called it Prometrium. There's also a vaginal suppository used called Crinone. Oral natural progesterone, Prometrium, has a much different effect physiologically than the transdermal potency of Crinone's suppository.[4-5]

Natural substances are herbs, vitamins, minerals, water, and hormones that are derived from plants. Almost every drug that has ever been proven useful—like aspirin from tree bark, penicillin from mold, or digitalis from deadly nightshade—came from a natural substance that would have done the job as well or better than the synthetic, altered form.[6-7] Although you could chew bark, leave your bread to mold, or make a tea from any plant, people in this country would rather just take a pill. As far as the drug companies are concerned, without a patent, there's no point in marketing a substance that you don't hold the exclusive rights to.

Your doctor will be very unlikely to question what he or she has been told or read. He's even more unlikely to rock the boat because only very rarely, in his line of work, does anyone ever do so. In fact, the medical guild system is so entrenched in this country that it has a name: "the standard of care." If a physician is confronted with a patient demand that he or she is uncomfortable with for any reason, such as she's unfamiliar with the research, or is familiar with it but has no instructions on how to prescribe it, or disagrees with it, or feels it's too radical to be accepted by her peers, she will defer to "the standard of care."

Your doctor will tell you, or anyone trying to help you get these hormones, which *you* have chosen to be treated with, that they are *not* the standard of care, because they're not. Of course, these hormones never could have been the standard of care because they are not part of the medical/industrial/research moneymaking machine, even though they are quite possibly the solution to breast cancer and more.

Although you can't acquire the hormones you need without a prescription (because the FDA has deemed them so potent that they are not sold over the counter), you won't easily get a prescription because your doctor is only going to prescribe what the drug companies offer him. This is the rule because he believes they've been tested or the FDA wouldn't approve them (remember birth control pills?), and they come with *instructions*. Natural hormones aren't used in randomized clinical trials (RCT) either, because they are the "raw" materials, not the drugs donated by the drug companies for research.

In this country, medicine is practiced very differently than it is, for example, in Europe.[8] In most European countries there is a form of nationalized medicine that can be as tedious, slow, and restrictive as our own experiences with HMOs, but that's where the similarity ends. Once you are assigned a physician in Europe, your doctor decides *with you* on a course of treatment, which in many cases can veer into some realms considered laughable in this country—like "energy work," acupuncture, or even magnet therapy—and then she sticks with you and your mutual decision.[9-10]

That's not how it happens here.

A Change Is Gonna Come

Because of the guild system in medicine as well as the remarkable costs borne by doctors in our litigious society, your specialist—an endocrinologist, urologist, or oncologist—feels most comfortable and secure following the standard of care. Doctors are understandably panicked because straying from the standard of care means that patients' families can sue them if the treatment fails. Defense attorneys actually invented the standard of care premise to reduce damage awards to plaintiffs in malpractice lawsuits.[11] Instead of going to trial and relying on expert witnesses from the accused doctor's peer group, the standard of care premise required very little name-calling by doctors who had to work together. And as time passed, more and more procedures and drugs began to fall under the mantle of the standard of care.

The standard of care model[12-13] in this country has given rise to a "hive mind" that all doctors are intrinsically tuned in to. By all thinking the same thought, there's no individuality of care, either. What the standard of care prescribes in your case is most likely going to be the most ubiquitous and profitable (for the drug companies) treatment available, not necessarily the most effective or newest or easiest treatment. By following the standard of care, your doctor has a safety net that means he or she can never get it too wrong, at least according to the system.

Surprisingly, since your doctor will refer to this standard of care as though it's the law, it isn't actually written down in any one book. So, although the phrase insinuates that it is "the," or only, standard of care, that is, in fact, not true. There are many debatable and negotiable standards of care depending on where you live and what you've been diagnosed with.

The closest medicine comes to the premise of the various standards of care is the degree of consensus contained in what's known as "practice guidelines." Practice guidelines are particular to each specialty—that is, the guidelines for oncology are slightly different from those for, say, gastroenterology. In the case of oncology, the National Cancer Institute has some say in what practice guidelines will be. So, in fact, what the standard of care will be for you is really just the agreement of some, not even necessarily most, of the doctors in the particular specialty assigned to your disease.

Thanks to the lawyers, in America the only treatment decision that can safely be made by your doctor—in every case, no matter what the details or what the patient may want—is the decision that most other doctors would agree with. It demands ironclad compliance; the penalties for your doctor for straying are far too high. There is no creative or inventive medicine if your doctor intends to be taken seriously and protected by his peers if, God forbid, something should go wrong. In other words. Clearly for your physician, in this country, *it's acceptable to prescribe a treatment that may have no proven value or little positive effects on a disease as long as all of medicine prescribes it together.*[14] For example: chemotherapy for metastastic breast cancer has no proven increase in survival.

It's safer that way.

At least for your doctor. That, however, may not be the safest thing for you.

Many doctors are coming around to the notion that their jobs might be a lot easier and less emotionally draining if, in fact, they weren't all "alone in this." To try to sort out the ponderous amount of cutting-edge research and then to try to be a clairvoyant in terms of colleague covenant is an untenable job. That's why the guild system and the standard of care continue. Dr. Kevin Patterson, in his article in the *New York Times Magazine* of May 5, 2002, entitled "What Doctors Don't Know (Almost Everything),"[15] declared that "This pecking order is now in the throes of a revolution known as evidence-based medicine, which asserts the supremacy of data over authority and tradition." The problem here is that most doctors have been convinced that "evidence-based medicine" is only a result of the randomized controlled human trials engineered and paid for by the drug companies using only their own products.

Real evidence-based medicine can only be had in a discussion to the facts at hand as they pertain to natural hormone replacement versus drugs called HRT that would cover everything available—basic research (animal and human) that consists primarily of epidemiology, mulit–center case-controlled, and randomized controlled trials, as we have done in this investigation. What we're saying is that many doctors practice medicine in this country, literally on handed down and agreed-upon hearsay knowledge, not on any particular examination of the scientific research pertaining to the specific case at hand. To be an oncologist and treat breast cancer, for example, your doctor would need to be a reproductive endocrinologist, geneticist, and pharmacologist in order for him to make any educated decision except to order chemo, radiation, and surgery.

All the restrictions found in the standard of care model regarding hormones and their link to cancer are based on studies done with low-dose *synthetic* drug-devised "hormone" derivatives.[16-18] The trouble with that is that studies in molecular biology and the genetics of cancer using synthetic products do show synthetic estrogen as carcinogenic,[19-23] but natural hormones *in the same kind of studies* show just the opposite result.[24-26] Natural estrogen and progesterone in physiological amounts, especially in a rhythm, are known to cause apoptosis—to cause cancer cells to die naturally. Even estrogen in "peak" amounts causes a complete break of cell-cycle proliferation, called *G1 arrest*.[27] At the moment, the standard of care treatment for breast cancer just doesn't hold up to a rigorous scientific examination of evidence-based medicine.

Patterson, an advocate of evidence-based medicine, continues, "You can count on the fact that people, doctors included, have a tendency to see what they expect to see. It's the premise of every sleight-of-hand game." It's certainly the premise of *this* sleight-of-hand game—testing with synthetic hormones instead of the bio-identical molecules in plant-derived natural hormones that your body would read as your own.

In this demonstration of "the hand is quicker than the eye," *there are two different beans under two different walnut shells.*

These synthetic hormones are usually offered to doctors by the drug companies as the only option for treatment. They are offered as the only option because they've been tested. But the only reason that the synthetics have been tested is because the drug companies have offered them to researchers to use in experiments in order to prove their worth. This is a win/win situation financially for the drug companies.

Synthetics are *intentionally* switched for the real thing in the study in question[28] because the drug companies are the source of the materials being studied. They could just as well donate the natural hormone materials that they worked with to make the drugs, but they don't. That's why we say that the natural hormones are *intentionally* switched for synthetic products. The drug companies have used the natural hormones to invent the drugs, but instead offer the synthetic hormone drugs to researchers to test and often pay them to do it with "grant" money.

If the synthetic hormones come up a winner—that is, look to promote health or solve the problem being tested for—so much the better. But if they produce pathology[29-30]—that is, cancer or heart disease or Alzheimer's—then researchers can legitimately declare, in their studies, that hormones in general have been proven to be deadly because the only "hormones" that they've ever tested were. This situation gives the drug companies the opportunity to invent five new ways to block the natural hormones that you have in your body, *which were never actually tested in the first place,* because "hormones show in studies that . . ."

That's the old shell game in a nutshell. It's pretty slick.

Patterson concludes, "In the world of medicine, if it makes sense that a treatment will work—or if one stands to make money if the treatment works—then the doctor will, with alarming and disheartening reliability, perceive that it *does* work. What is surprising is that a profession that dresses itself up in the garb of science has taken so long to acknowledge a principle that every small-town Carney understands."

Remember, a *doctor* said that.

His point is that the conclusions doctors reach from clinical experience and "day-to-day observations" are often not completely reliable. People, who just happen to be doctors, usually see what they *expect* to see. He also agrees that "The vast majority of medical therapies, it is now clear, have never been evaluated by systemic study and are used simply because doctors have always believed that they work."

We'd like to add, *even if they don't work now and never really worked in the past.*

Treatments like surgery, radiation, chemotherapy, and hormone ablation have no leg to stand on in evidence-based medicine.[31-38] Evidence-based medicine should be the practice of integrating the best basic research with clinical expertise. A thorough review of the statistics in any and all of these "standard of care" treatments reveals a sorry margin of success.[39-40] If cancer is caused by hormonal falloff, radiation, and sometimes chemically induced DNA breaks, all of the treatments above can only cause cancer, not help you. Surgery is the only one left, and there's evidence for injury-induced breast cancer,[41-43] too.

Surgery is quite an injurious assault to the breast and body.

Do You Want to Know a Secret?

If we and other researchers have actually provided *scientific* evidence[44-46] to this effect for some years now, why isn't *real* hormone replacement therapy for cancer, let alone menopause, readily available to women?

There are many reasons. The drug companies own the patents on all of the chemotherapy drugs and anti-nausea drugs and, now, anti-anemia drugs; the current standard of care is remarkably profitable for them. Your doctor's acquisition of information after medical school comes in bits and pieces from medical conferences and drug company reps and literature pertaining to his specialty and something called *throw away* journals by doctors that are sent and supported by drug companies that may not be read in detail at all. It is unlikely that your doctor personally does any research. Running a medical practice is too time-consuming. It's like being a mother and a CEO of a corporation and managing employees at the same time. Most pertinent of all, the American medical establishment assumes that it knows what the causes of cancer are, even though they can't quite isolate the cure.

And because they say so, we believe them. We are indoctrinated to believe that the causes of cancer are mutations caused by toxins in our air, water, and food. We also believe that high-fat diets, insufficient exercise, and the one thing everyone seems to agree on, estrogen *naturally occurring*[47] in your own body, must act to mutate DNA in your cells and cause unregulated cell growth. The one thing everyone agrees on is that cancer cells have mutated DNA.

That's the first big lie your doctor has swallowed.

Doctors are taught this theory in medical school. In reality, less than 10 percent of very early cancers of any kind are found to have mutated genes, which science knows develop later in the disease process.[48] In their view, a normal mutation rate does explain the mutations that actually occur in a cancer. Accumulation of mutations can be seen as a natural process within the human body and cancer as a normal part of the human life cycle.[49-50] The process of tumorogenesis therefore is a form of evolution: mutation and selection are the essential components of this process.[51]

The biggest deal in cancer research right now is the gene p53, the granddaddy of a family of genes that regulate cells. Regulatory genes are not only in charge of the cell cycle and tell the cell to grow, stay, or die, but are also in charge of other groups of genes in an upstream fashion where point X will control Y + Z.[52-53] Science and medicine are convinced, at this point, that it is the *mutated* version of a regulatory gene, such as p53 that must be dealt with in most cancers because mutated p53 is often found in tumors.[54-56]

That's why has the search for the cure focused on finding the one gene controlling that mythical "renegade cell" responsible for mutation and metastasis when it's well known that no *one* gene is ever responsible for any singular function in the body.[57-58] Certainly not p53 or any other gene for the 90 percent of early cancers without gene mutation.[59]

The reason for this dogma is the theory of multiple mutation, which researchers cling to against all logic. This theory posits that consistently dividing cells consistently make mistakes over time, leading to the accumulation of multiple deletions and mutations over the course of your life. The idea of time-driven cellular derangement explains, for those who believe in this premise, why the predominant occurrence of cancer is in people over forty—the notion is that the longer you live, the more chance there is that you'll develop a cancerous mutation from being exposed long-term to your own hormones.

There are more than a few problems with the theory of multiple mutation as the cause of cancer, not least of which is the fact that, as we said, 90 percent of all cancers *do not* start with mutated genes—either regulatory genes like p53[60-63] or any other mutated genes.[64]

But the biggest problem is that the math just doesn't hold up.

It's a matter of probability. Probability is the branch of mathematics used to explain things like how the occurrence of seemingly random events is distributed. For example, every time you flip a coin, you have a new and equal 50/50 chance to get heads or tails, *unaffected by the previous flip*. If a cell divides once, it always has a small chance of mutation. If that same cell divides yet again, it still has the same small chance of mutation. And even if it divides a third time, it *still* has only a 50 percent chance of mutation . . . and so on, and so on. The point is, the chance of mutation never goes up, no matter how many times a cell divides,[65-66] because the probability just isn't there. However, over time the accumulation of events means that the probability of a single mutation having happened is the sum, not the product, of all those little probabilities. But even that doesn't matter.

Although it seems somehow logical to assume that the more and faster a cell divides, the more chance it has for mistakes, it is a faulty premise for more than one reason. In fact, your cells divide fastest and most frequently from conception to age five, *not in old age*.[67] If the theory of multiple mutation were correct, it would mean that babies and children would be at the greatest risk for cancer.

This is clearly not the case.

If you do their math, the peak age for all tumors would be about sixteen years old. This is also not the case.

In point of fact, at the time cancer is most likely to strike you, when you're in your forties and fifties, your cells are dividing more *slowly* than at any previous time in your life. Since young people *rarely* get cancer and old people *often* do, *it must be something that happens in the in-between time*.

It is not coincidental that cancer happens at the time in our lives when our sex hormones are going, going . . . gone. Menopause is the hallmark of aging, and all the graphs in all the research on cancer show a steep incline in all cancers beginning at age forty for men and women.[68]

The first victim of this new view would be the widely cherished idea that estrogen causes cancer. How can old people get cancer from their own hormones—hormones supposedly so high that we have to block them with estrogen receptor blockers like tamoxifen as a prophylactic—when in fact *they don't have any hormones anymore*? This view—that it's the absence of estrogen—certainly explains the age of onset for cancer in a much more rational way than the theory of multiple mutation.

Instead of causing cancer, accurate hormone replacement in physiological doses should put you back where you were when you were young—in effect, in a place with *no cancer*.[69] The proof is in the cohort study of all young women because cancer, of all sorts, is very rare in young women. Sex hormones are the regulators of gene activity; you can afford a mutated gene, because as long as it's turned off, you're okay. It shouldn't matter how many mutations you have in a day as long as you have the hormones of a young person to keep growth in check.

The point of spending billions of dollars on research for the last two decades to find the gene for breast cancer is moot. When and if we find those genes, and it won't be just one, if we can't turn them off, we still haven't accomplished *anything*. Studying "a gene" will never tell us anything because any disease state is the result of *many* losing a regulatory brake, not just one. And since sex hormones are the regulatory brakes on genes that produce everything from growth factors to death commands,[70-75] we will always find that the errant genes are just "out of control" without hormones.

Bringin' It All Back Home

There was one very important man who thought to test natural hormones. His name was Dr. Charles Huggins. He built the Ben May Cancer Institute at the University of Chicago back in 1946. Dr. Huggins was a surgeon and urologist who looked at the effects of testosterone administration on bone metastasis in prostate cancer patients. Based on the findings from his eight-man study in 1941,[76] Dr. Huggins was awarded the Nobel Prize in 1963 for his work proving that cancer—all endocrine cancer—is hormonally controlled.[77-79]

He *did* prove that cancer is hormonally *controlled*. What he *did not prove* is that hormones *cause* cancer. We may seem to be playing linguistic games here, but we're not. There is a difference between "control" and "cause." To "control" is to hold authority or dominion over the object being controlled, whereas to "cause" is to induce or instigate or bring about. These are two very different actions, especially in cell biology.

This confusion is the second reason your doctor will say, "No way."

Dr. Huggins reported that the addition of testosterone, a sex hormone, made the bone metastases of prostate cancer grow in three of the men in the study.[80] The problem he created in our lives stems from human nature's proclivity to see what we *expect* to see. This was 1941. We hadn't even dropped the bomb yet. There was no MRI or body scan technology, just indefinite X-ray. So how could he report any change in these men so soon after administration of testosterone? He reported his findings in terms of alkaline phosphatase elevations in plasma.[81]

In those days, the only blood test for a solid tumor/epithelial cell cancer like prostate cancer was a cellular assay of an enzyme called *alkaline phosphatase*. Today, if you were to have bloodwork to diagnose a cancer, it might be a test called CA-125 for ovarian cancer or a blood panel looking at hematological (red cells/white cells/immune cells) factors for various leukemias.[82-83]

The biggest scientific problem for us, in the case of whether Dr. Huggins's work proves that hormones cause cancer, is that alkaline phosphatase is produced all over the body, *not just in rapidly dividing bone cells*.[84-85] So what if it went up in response to hormone administration? It proves nothing definitive.

There were other problems, too. The study was run on eight very sick, very old men. Huggins did not give all of his test subjects testosterone. Five of the men received DES—*synthetic* estrogen.[86] Only three men actually received intramuscular injections of testosterone, and the testosterone Dr. Huggins gave these men was "dirty"—in other words, it was synthetically altered bovine-derived from bull testicles, hardly bio-identical to human testosterone.[87]

Do not misunderstand. Dr. Huggins was awarded the Nobel Prize for proving cancer was hormonally *controlled*, not *caused*, which, we certainly agree, is a cosmic truth. However, the outcome of his study in 1941 on testosterone enhancing cancer was not the truth of his *body* of work. It took us a while to find the truth because it was hidden in his studies on women, not men.

Déjà Vu

With all of the molecular, epidemiological, and historical evidence we have uncovered, we wondered who in the world could ever have thought it would be a good idea to remove a woman's ovaries (oophorectomy) to ablate her hormones and put her into *surgical* menopause to treat breast cancer. We found the first reference to this procedure in a 1901 issue of *The British Medical Journal*,[88] reporting on procedures carried out in 1889, a few decades after anesthesia was invented. The issue of anesthesia matters because oophorectomy is a major, open-up-the-body's-entrails kind of procedure that was impossible before anesthesia and antibiotics. In 1889, there were still no antibiotics to protect the wound from systemic infection, so when Beatson conducted the procedure on three women in their forties, it was bizarre, risky science.

Although he reported an impressive regression in the tumors, not only was it a transient effect much like chemotherapy, he reports a relatively rapid recurrence within two to three years in all three women. He thought that perhaps the thyroid supplementation he administered—he gave them 300 mg or 15 grains of Armour thyroid—had been the magic bullet that caused regression. We think he might have been on to something with thyroid, too. Beatson said, "I do not think that oophorectomy and thyroid will effect a secondary deposit [of cancer], sooner or later its harmful effect will be felt and eventually to such an extent as to completely overshadow any beneficial effects on the local disease in young women." In other words, surgery was no cure.[89]

So why is this surgery and its follower, mastectomy, still the standard of care?

Dr. Huggins is why. In 1952, sixty-two years *after* Beatson's experiment, Dr. Huggins published a paper on his newest area of interest—adrenalectomy, which is, simply put, removal of the adrenal glands of living people.[90] If you recall from previous chapters the importance of adrenal informational feedback to the brain, ovaries, heart, lungs, and kidneys concerning the homeostatic state of your environment externally and internally, then you'll agree that adrenalectomy can't ever be a good idea.

But because of his work in 1941 with testosterone,[91] Dr. Huggins contended in 1951 that oophorectomy failed to stop breast cancer in Beatson's women because their adrenal glands were still producing estrogen from the conversion from testosterone. Now, the only place Huggins could have gotten the idea that estrogen *fueled* breast cancer was from the transient effect Beatson reported after the removal of the ovaries and his own work with testosterone in men. Although Beatson himself had concluded that the Armour thyroid supplementation might have been the cause of regression, Huggins concluded that the cessation of estrogen following the removal of the ovaries was the reason for improvement.

Huggins should have been aware of research that took place in the fall of 1947, four years earlier, known as the Therapeutic Trials Committee of the American Medical Association.[92] This was a cooperative investigation undertaken by sixty different investigators on "the effects of steroid hormones in the treatment of advanced or disseminated carcinoma of the breast." This investigation was coordinated by a subcommittee on Steroids in Cancer. This was a retrospective study of 1,944 patients over twelve years that reported in 1951,[93] 1953,[94] and 1960.[95] They concluded that hormone replacement showed great promise in the treatment of breast cancer. This was a reasonably long trial.

The Therapeutic Trials Committee of the American Medical Association met every two years from 1949 to 1960 to review and publish incoming results on the "objective responses of the neoplasm [cancer] to estrogenic and androgenic hormones when administered to women with disseminated mammary carcinoma."[96] The complete and total evaluation of effectiveness rested in the "distinct and measurable decrease in one or more dominant metastatic areas by clinical or radiographic examination, without progression of any other metastatic lesions and no new foci of disease having appeared." *They used real estrogen, estradiol.* In conclusion, the committee stated uncategorically that "There can be no reasonable doubt concerning the advantage of estrogens in the initiation of regression [of cancer] in post-menopausal woman." It also stated that "The younger the patient is at the time of recognition and treatment of her primary disease the longer the evidence of metastasis is likely to be postponed."

While the American Medical Association was studying replacement of a sort (not cyclic, not rhythmic), Dr. Huggins was still removing organs—ovaries, prostates, pituitaries, and adrenals. Although Dr. Huggins's patients more than occasionally died from the surgery, he still reported that when they didn't die, they often improved, briefly.[97]

"Improve" is an interesting word. In Dr. Huggins's 1952 adrenalectomy study, in seven cases of advanced breast cancer, two women died from the surgery, three had no improvement (got worse), and two "improved." This does not mean they "recovered." One of these women experienced "relief of symptoms," and the big "improvement" in the other one was a weight gain of a few kilograms.

This study by Dr. Huggins testing hormone ablation (ablation means to wipe out your hormones entirely) is the kind of study that led to today's standard of care. It's that kind of thinking that created the hormone-ablating drugs known as Lupron, Casodex, and Arimidex, and selective estrogen receptor modifiers (SERMs) like tamoxifen, Femara, Evista, and Faslodex. Lupron destroys feedback in your pituitary permanently, and Casodex destroys the production of testosterone from your adrenal glands. The more recent drugs, Arimidex, an aromatase enzyme inhibitor to stop testosterone from converting to estrogen, and tamoxifen and Faslodex,

SERMs, are just as brutal to your brain's feedback systems as castration, but they take surgery out of the equation.[98-106]

Of course, the question remains: Can removing the glands whose intermittent failure may have given you cancer in the first place cause any sort of improvement? No, but surgery and drugs make more money in medicine than natural hormone replacement.

But no one then (or now) seemed aware of the implications of previous AMA research that took a pro-replacement stance. They just knew the Nobel Prize winner was still removing glands. That's why they kept doing it, too.

Mr. Jones

Dr. Huggins, it turns out, went on to do further work that showed the same results that the AMA saw in 1949. After reviewing the work Dr. Huggins did in 1941 and again in 1951, as researchers and journalists trying to investigate his past choices, we were willing to give him the benefit of the doubt. We were willing to assume, like others, that Dr. Huggins was just misguided . . . until we found his 1962 paper in the premier journal of the *Proceedings of the National Academy of Sciences*, published four years before he accepted the Nobel Prize for proving the hormonal controls on cancer. Dr. Huggins's paper was entitled "Extinction of Experimental Mammary Cancer: 1. Estradiol-17b and Progesterone."[107] Its conclusion is implicit in the title.

He gave two natural hormones to rats, 17-beta estradiol (the kind of estrogen that we are going to recommend, the very same one that the establishment says causes cancer) and progesterone. He used natural bioidentical plant-derived hormones dissolved in alcohol and suspended in sesame oil. The concentrations were 10 percent. The doses were physiological, or the normal amounts found in the young body of the female rat.

He used six hundred rats bred from genetic lines known for a *high incidence* of "spontaneous" mammary tumors. That means that their moms had bestowed on them a genetic predisposition to breast cancer. First he gave all the rats a known carcinogen, a substance called *DMBA*. Rats fed DMBA always develop tumors within a few weeks. Then he gave them estrogen alone, progesterone alone, estrogen and progesterone together, and gonadotrophin (the pregnancy hormone) alone. The experimental animals were healthy young virgin (meaning no previous pregnancies) females kept in air-conditioned rooms and fed commercial ration, sort of like all of us, and then they were mated.

His results staggered us.

First, progesterone *alone* and what Dr. Huggins termed *late-age* pregnancy "vastly *accelerated* the growth of mammary cancer."

Second, young pregnancy "*reduced* the appearance of cancer of the breast."

Third, using estrogen alone at physiologic—that means normal—levels, however, "*delayed* the appearance of mammary cancer in all of the rats and the time of onset was prolonged and the growth depressed in comparison to females not injected, but the tumors were not extinguished."

Most startling, estrogen *with* progesterone resulted in "a *decreased* incidence of mammary cancer and 52 percent of the rats treated this way were completely cancer-free even six months later, whereas all of the untreated rats had already succumbed." In the ones that did develop cancer, the number "of active centers was small." We have calculated the appropriate dose for human women based on the same dose in women by mg per kg of body weight. The equivalent dose of estrogen in a 150-pound woman is 3 mg, ascending in graduating doses to 7 to 10 mg twice a day, and the progesterone dosage is huge. The progesterone levels were equivalent to 600 to 1,000 mg in a 150-pound woman—or pregnancy levels.[108]

Huggins was eager to find out why there was a "threshold effect," in other words, why if he gave too little estrogen, the progesterone didn't work. Science now knows about 17-beta estradiol's ability at its peak to make progesterone receptors turn on, but Huggins had no idea of receptor reciprocity in his time. Yet his study proves you can't take one without the other and get the same effect.

More importantly, *Huggins knew.* He even published it in the rat study, and then he attempted rhythmic replacement later the same year in women. His paper, published in the *Journal of the American Medical Association* in 1962, is entitled "Estradiol Benzoate and Progesterone in Advanced Human Breast-Cancer."[109] His findings were the same in humans as they were in rats: The replacement of estrogen and progesterone, cyclically, in a rhythm in the high doses that would normally occur in youth, prevented and treated cancer better than anything else ever tried. Imagine our surprise, we thought no one had ever known before.

When he accepted the Nobel Prize in 1966, he had the perfect forum to correct the mistakes of all the researchers and doctors who were removing glands and inducing surgical and radiation menopause following his earlier papers. Instead, he just recapped his studies, and chose not to elaborate on the ramifications of his later work. We can't tell you why.

We're knee-deep in irony again. If a single man was truly responsible for the last sixty years of the agony of hormone ablation for cancer, and now for the "witch hunt" surrounding estrogen that prevents all of us from saving ourselves, it was the very same Dr. Huggins who published the first beautifully simple pieces of science that really laid out the template very clearly and confirmed the premise—the way to deal with cancer is to be too young *inside* to have it happen to you.

Dr. Huggins created the standard of care we all must live with today, because he never spoke up. We will find out why. We're continuing our investigation into what really happened with Dr. Huggins all those years ago. This is just a small piece of his story here, and it only addresses how he touched women's lives and, in retrospect, men's, too.

Highway 61 Revisited

Why didn't doctors respond by actually reading the Nobel laureate's papers? It's a mind-set fostered by the amounts of science that doctors are buried in on any given day. Any oncologist, right now, reading the rat study, unaware of the human experiment, would object to Huggins concluding *anything* from a rat study. But the entire field of oncology was actually launched on the results of a study on *one mouse* with lymphoma.[110] If there's any justice, six hundred rats should buy us at least one huge long-running human trial, and we can promise our study subjects would live longer than theirs did.

We're pretty sure your doctor hasn't read any of the studies that we've presented in this book. He might if you show them to him. If he has time, and *if he can understand them*. Although we've carefully selected human studies, like the massive evidence in Chapter Four proving that lack of lactation is the overriding cause of breast cancer, the real wealth of evidence and information that is rarely offered to *clinical* practitioners is in the realm of molecular medicine and evolutionary genetics. New, young doctors are just starting to be taught what it takes be able to read molecular biology and genetics papers.

In 1992, Dr. Gordon H. Guyatt led doctors to debate ethics, responsibility, and power in his watershed piece published in the *Journal of the American Medical Association*.[111] Dr. Guyatt stated that, "If you said to most members of the general public, 'Physicians have been trained in such a manner that they have no idea how to read a paper from the original medical literature or how to interpret it,' that would surprise the public." Dr. Guyatt was referring to what a medical education should be.

Physicians have always tried in some way to quantify their "art." The "art" is the physician's intuitive sense of the patient, the diagnosis, and the possible responses to possible treatments. In reality, the standard of care is a bad attempt to merge art and science by achieving a consensus practice of the art of medicine.

While Dr. Kevin Patterson, in the *New York Times Magazine* article cited earlier, is in favor of the coming overthrow of the standard of care in deference to evidence-based medicine, he also says, "a doctor sometimes needs to generalize and to reduce very complicated problems to first principles. It is simply not possible to be rigorously intellectual and consult the available medical data about every single thing, all the time. It takes too long, and if all the intricacies of the medical data on every clinical problem were fully considered before acting, the operating rooms would grow dusty and people would die while the doctor's chins were rubbed into a bright shine." What Patterson refers to here is a doctor's use of his *intuition*.

But we don't have to rely on that anymore. The evidence is now available.

Dr. Patterson sums up, "The essential tenet in evidence-based medicine (EBM) is that patients, working with their physicians and armed with medical data, are better equipped to make decisions that work for them, than the doctors of the Marcus Welby Model are, because they understand their own expectations better than their physicians can.

"Authority is devolved from expertise to the data and thus, ultimately, to the patient. Patients have always had the final say about whether to accept the recommendations of their physicians, but without the actual data in front of them, the decision has simply been whether or not to trust the wisdom of the physician."

Thanks to the research available to the layman on the website *PubMed*,[112] where all of the medical journals from the National Library of Medicine publish the latest research, any and all of us have access to the truth. If we're lucky and information truly subverts hierarchy, medicine will change fundamentally and create a positive, equalizing shift in the relationship between patients and doctors. Not only will a reassessment of authority shift power to the people; it will take the weight off the shoulders of physicians—who are, after all, just people, too.

She's Leaving Home

We're not the first researchers who feel that the boat should be rocked, the standard of care is eminently questionable, and doctors can be educated. This book is dedicated to two women. One of them was at the vanguard of women's rights in regard to bucking the system of medicine when making choices about their own bodies. This woman was Rose Kushner. She was diagnosed with breast cancer in 1974. The standard of care at the time, no matter how great or small the tumor was found to be, was the Halsted *radical* mastectomy.[113]

The hallmark of Dr. Halsted's surgery was its invasiveness. In the past, before the turn of the twentieth century, breasts were removed. Sometimes lymph nodes under the arm or near the clavicle were looked at for signs of tumor, but Dr. Halsted took the premise of localized disease to new heights. Dr. Halsted was responsible for the notion still in place today among surgeons and doctors of "we've got to get it all." In his attempt to get every last cancer cell, he removed more and more tissue, until by the 1950s surgeons were removing almost one quarter of the entire body of a woman with breast cancer.[114]

Post–World War II improvements in intraoperative and postoperative care enabled surgeons to perform extensive procedures, bordering on vivisection, that had previously been fatal to the patient. Antibiotics, blood transfusion, and improvements in anesthesia and surgical techniques that had been honed in wartime on battlefields came home to treat America's women with breast cancer. One surgeon, Dr. George T. Pack, perfected the scapulothoracic, or "fore-quarter," amputation, which entailed the separation of the clavicle or collarbone, scapula or shoulder blade, and an arm when the lymph nodes contained any cancer.[115] All of these surgeries were lumped under the category named for the man who inspired them—the Halsted radical mastectomy.

Dr. Halsted promoted the theory of localized neoplasm cancer that spread by way of the lymphatic system, radiating up and outward from the breast. The only way to get "every last cancer cell" was to cut away more and more of the patient's chest cavity and arm. Eventually, other surgeons in the 1950s and 1960s removed ribs, leaving only a thin layer of skin between the patient's beating heart and the outside world.[116] Physician Ronald N. Grant, editor of the American Cancer Society's journal, wrote a 1963 editorial in which he compared randomized controlled trials on radical and simple or modified mastectomy to "scientific Russian Roulette." He also wrote in the same editorial, "physicians are likely to be toppled into the morass in which the Nazi physicians found themselves as a result of their ventures with human experimentation during World War II."[117] In other words, gruesome, live vivisection.

These extreme, completely unnecessary surgeries had been sanctioned as the standard of care since 1888. By the time Halsted's approach was seriously questioned, it was practically a requirement of membership in the American College of Surgeons to have mastered the Halsted radical mastectomy.[118] Halsted's only detractors were the radiologists who claimed his patient's survival rates were less impressive than theirs; of course, their patients often had lung fibrosis and broken ribs from the radiation.[119-120]

In 1927, Dr. Ernest P. Daland published a study[121-122] that charted the outcomes of one hundred untreated women with advanced breast cancer, too advanced for surgery. Daland discovered that these women with no treatment at all lived an average of 40.5 months, more than three years, after being diagnosed with cancer. Their overall five-year survival rate was about 22 percent. He compared them to treated patients, whose survival rate, at three years, at 42 percent, was less than double after all of their suffering and physical and psychological pain. The Halsted radical mastectomy was disfiguring. It left women with a hollow, deformed chest wall and armpit, which was often the site of persistent pain and a condition known as lyphedema swelling. Between 1935 and 1942, another group of doctors reviewed 495 radical mastectomies, finding that more than half of the women had either died or were in the throes of a recurrence.[123]

Rose Kushner lived in Washington, D.C., when she was diagnosed with breast cancer. A part-time journalist (after raising three children) who once entertained the idea of medical school, she went straight from her doctor's office to the Library of Congress to assess her options. One of the most damning pieces of research uncovered by Rose was a review of 950 breast cancer patients treated at Johns Hopkins between 1889 and 1931 by Dean Lewis and William F. Rienhoff Jr., two of Halsted's surgical heirs at Johns Hopkins. Seven hundred and ninety-eight of the patients were treated with radical mastectomy. The authors began their paper with the rather remarkable admission that Halsted's original fifty patients back before the turn of the century had a local recurrence rate not of 6 percent, as reported by Halsted in 1898, but of over 30 percent.[124] Moreover, of the 420 Hopkins patients known to be dead, less than one-third had survived as long as three years. Lewis and Rienhoff, after pointing out that Halsted's meticulous dissection did not reliably prevent local return of breast cancer, still, unbelievably, ended the paper with a favorable nod to the continued use of the Halsted radical mastectomy rather than "a less radical operation supplemented by the very questionable effect of radiation."[125]

From the time Halsted falsified[126-129] his data on localized recurrence, in 1898, until after his death, no one realized that he was a cocaine, and later morphine, addict.[130] In all those years, too—although some of his peers slowly unraveled the fraud of his work—his patients and the patients of the surgeons devoted to his method *never knew the surgery doesn't work*,[131] until Rose Kushner told them.

Rose found the research proving there never was any benefit to the Halsted radical mastectomy and publicized it until the system changed.[132] Rose Kushner stopped the Halsted radical mastectomy. We intend a similar outcome for our current standard of care—hormone ablation.

It Takes a Lot to Laugh, It Takes a Train to Cry

Rose's cancer is what medicine today would call a neoplasm, or "carcinoma in situ." The full name is *ductal carcinoma in situ* (DCIS). Only about one-third of these tumors progress to invasive cancer within twenty-five years. There was hot debate among physicians twenty-five years before Rose was diagnosed about whether these small lesions were even cancer, or if, in fact, they should be classified as "benign pathological-clinical entities."[133]

Rose went through eighteen doctors before one agreed to a *modified* radical mastectomy. A modified radical mastectomy removes only the breast and lymph nodes involved. When her ordeal was finally over, her pathology report stated that her cancer was only 1 mm in diameter and there was no lymph node involvement. Not only did Rose take dominion over her own body, but she wrote a book exposing the truth and then lectured for the rest of her life on what she'd found.[134]

A decades-long veteran expert in the trenches of the war on cancer, Dr. Cushman D. Haagensen at Columbia-Presbyterian Medical Center in

New York, argued in the 1960s that "the proper 'treatment' of these neoplasia was to examine the patient's breasts every four months."[135] The condition was often eventually found in both breasts, signifying what we, as researchers, know to be normal hormone deprivation of glandular tissue as we age.

Rose had already been treated for uterine cancer; she is the perfect example of multiple cancers arising as we age from the falloff of hormones. That's the connection between breast, uterus, and ovaries when it comes to cancer—the hormones and regulation. She may have needed complete bio-identical hormone replacement. She was, quite naturally, falling apart, or deevolving, in the absence of hormonal controls on regulatory oncogenes.

But that's not how science and medicine think. Instead, Rose became a candidate for a new (really old)[136] procedure—mammography to keep her remaining breast "safe." Using X-rays to "see" abnormalities in breast tissue had been around since 1913, but had never really become a diagnostic tool until the mid-1970s.

For the Halstedians, who were aging and ascending to leadership positions in the 1950s and 1960s, and who embraced the notion of cancer as a local lesion to be stopped at the earliest possible point—like a germ that could infect the whole body—mammography's ability to find cancers earlier and earlier made it the next big thing in prevention.[137]

Enter the radiologists.

As researchers and journalists, we looked back 150 years at the numbers. The statistics Rose Kushner unearthed also proved that early detection is worthless because breast cancer, statistically, kills half of all women diagnosed with it within five to ten years after diagnosis *no matter how early it's detected.*[138-139] The statistics have never changed. If women never experienced the hormonal fall-off known as menopause, these cancers might never develop.

When a pinpoint-size lesion appears in your breast, there may already be cancer cells multiplying in the shin of your leg,[140] in your bone marrow. The pinpoint-size lesion that a mammogram picks up is only a symptom of what's happening everywhere else in your body.

The other problem with mammography is obvious: Science only knows of one absolute carcinogen to human tissue on this planet, and that carcinogen in ionizing radiation.[141] If the exposed cells don't die, the DNA breaks and they mutate. Cancer, as we've explained and footnoted, rarely starts with a mutated gene; but a gene certainly can be mutated by an outside-the-body influence like the ionizing radiation of power lines or mammography.[142-151]

Mammography *is* ionizing radiation.

When Rose became a patient in 1975, the Breast Cancer Detection Demonstration Project (BCDDP), which was to enroll 270,000 women age thirty-four to seventy-five, had just begun. Their doctors, who were recruited by the BCDDP to be partners in the study, offered free mammograms to women. Twenty years earlier, in 1955, during the first big push for mammography, a Dr. McKinnon had commented that early detection and treatment are meaningless. In the face of the fact that 50 percent of all slow-growing lesions have little if any tendency to give rise to metastases, "curing non-lethal lesions does nothing to reduce mortality."[152-153]

On October 1, 1975, excerpts from an unpublished medical article alleging that the mammograms done by the BCDDP might be causing more breast cancer than they were helping to cure was published by *Washington Post* columnist Jack Anderson.[154] Anderson received the tip about the article from the National Cancer Institute's Deputy Associate Director for Cancer Control, John C. Bailar. With respect to the hazards of mammography, Bailar himself published an article in the *Annals of Internal Medicine* pointing out that there was "experimental and clinical evidence that ionizing radiation can cause breast cancer."[155-158]

This natural effect of radiation is dose-dependent. The more radiation a woman receives in her lifetime, whether it's during a dental exam, at the airport, or during her yearly mammography, the more likely it is that she will have breast cancer ten to fifteen years later.[159-161] In 1976, Benjamin F. Byrd Jr., president of the American Cancer Society, admitted that the 245,000 women enrolled in the BCDDP had not been told of any potential risks.[162-164] To this day American women undergo mammography not knowing that fifteen years down the line they could get breast cancer from an attempt to prevent it. Rose Kushner died in 1990 of metastatic breast cancer, a coincidental fifteen years after her diagnosis. She refused chemotherapy in 1975, because her instincts were good.

Even at the end, in 1988, when her cancer recurred, Rose said no, to chemo.

Considering the company she kept during the rollout of the new theory of chemo-*prevention*, Rose might have spent the 1980s taking tamoxifen.[165] Tamoxifen is now known to precipitate contralateral breast cancer in the breast you have left after mastectomy and radiation.[166]

Rose only had one breast left.

SIX

PLAY WITH FIRE

Given the evidence, in addition to not having children and not breastfeeding, there are three other definite ways to risk your life healthwise a decade or two into the future. These three other ways to increase your chances of being diagnosed with breast cancer are: have a mammogram every year, have a mammogram every year if you have hereditary BRAC I or II defect, or take tamoxifen.[1-10]

Mammograms are delivering ionizing radiation to your breast, which causes breaks in the double-stranded DNA *and injures breast tissue*.[11-13] The historical literature reviewed by Patricia Jasen in *Breast Cancer and the Language of Risk, 1750–1950*[14] was replete with physician-reported, injury-induced breast cancers. This means that if your breast is injured or bruised, an immune reaction of cellular proliferation happens.[15] As we'll demonstrate, whether a random accident befell the victim or spousal abuse was the basis of a woman's injury, it was well known that many turn-of-the-century cancers were injury-induced. And those incidences were not additionally exposed to the ambient electromagnetic waves that we now encounter in a day, like electric blankets or cell phone megahertz.[16-18]

If it was true then, it's most certainly still true now. In mammography, the radiation dose to the breast varies considerably depending on the technique and the film used and the number or frequency of repeat examinations.

In 2001, the *British Medical Journal* published findings from the National Health Service's Breast Screening Programme, begun in 1989, in which 44,430 British women[19] born between January 1, 1926, and December 31, 1940, were invited to participate. The final study population included 40,939 women. Of this number, 33,706 had at least one mammogram and 7,233 never attended and so never had a mammogram. In the group of 7,233 "never irradiated women," the incidence of breast cancer, after 69,098 person-years of follow-up, was found to be 121 women.

This number is significantly *less* than the 147.2 cancers *expected* to naturally occur in 7,233 women, and the expected number was almost certainly an underestimation because the incidence of breast cancer had been inexplicably steadily increasing before the screening program began. The women *who never had a mammogram* had less cancer than the women who had had mammograms.[20]

From the evidence that we've gathered and reviewed, it appears the risk of breast cancer in the nonattenders was lower than that of the population targeted for screening because mammography, which combines the effects of both radiation and injury, can cause breast cancer.[21-28] The group that did the study seemed to be aiming more toward the conclusion that women with breast cancer in their immediate families were more likely to get mammograms and that that assumption, alone, explains why the women who attended had higher rates of breast cancer. However, since only 5 percent of all women with breast cancer have a first-degree relative with breast cancer, that's probably not it.[29-30] However, the findings of this and many other studies lead us to conclude that mammograms, in principle and in effect, do much more harm than benefit.[31-37]

Surgeons two hundred years ago speculated that "whenever cancer was blamed on a blow, there was almost certainly some internal predisposing latent Cause in the Blood and Juices. A blow received early in life might produce a lump, or scirrhus, which posed little risk until the woman reached a more vulnerable stage in her life, namely menopause. At that time melancholy of the blood might cause the scirrhus to degenerate into a Cancer."[38-39] We'd like to suggest that "melancholy of the blood" is a poetic way to say *no progesterone*.

Jumpin' Jack Flash

To this day oncologists are very reticent to concede that there is a body of literature confirming the fact that a simple bump or knock can cause cancer.[40-43] As we said, there would be a panic if doctors admitted that an accidental blow to the breast could cause breast cancer.

Many women, after more than one mammogram, underwent genetic testing for what science determined to be a "marker" for breast cancer—a mutated or altered form of the regulatory genes BRCA I and BRCA II.[44–45] Mutation is always assumed by science to be a bad thing, which is not the case, because it makes no sense that an organism would ever mutate to die. Mutation is always for good, to enhance survival.[46–48] In fact, research shows that breast cancers in women with the altered form of the BRCA gene are far less invasive and aggressive than breast cancers in women who possessed the functional forms.

An examination of BRCA I and II also shows clear evidence that, far from *causing* breast cancer in its "mutated" forms, *un*mutated BRCA is in charge of the repair mechanisms for radiation damage done to double-stranded DNA.[49–50] That means that if you have a mutated copy of BRCA I and II, getting a mammogram is particularly dangerous because you have no repair mechanism for the radiation damage that enhances cancerous growth from the injury done by the machine to your DNA.[51–56] Any constant source of ionizing radiation would be worse than the episodic nature of exposure in a once-a-year mammogram.

That may mean that living under power lines on Long Island,[57–58] a famous cancer "hot spot," would be particularly dangerous for women genetically predisposed to BRCA I and II mutations. Many of the highly prone cancer families that participated in early breast cancer genetics research were of Ashkenazi Jewish descent. Because the relatively small population of Ashkenazim had inbred for centuries, in both their native eastern Europe and later throughout the world, they turned out to (as any group with highly concentrated genes would) have an extremely high rate of three specific gene mutations—two in BRCA I and one in BRCA II. Estimates are now suggesting that as many as one in forty Ashkenazic women carry one form of the mutation or another. Many of these women were terrorized by these statistics into volunteering for *prophylactic* mastectomies when genetic testing confirmed that they carried the altered form of the gene,[59–65] but they were only given half of the information. Many of the women lived under excessive radiation from the power lines crisscrossing small Long Island communities where they lived.

We believe that the evidence of the BRCA I and II mutations leaving these women particularly vulnerable to radiation points to the possibility that radiation from the power lines exacerbated, as mammography would, a gene deficit that would never have mattered *except* under power lines,[66–69] under light exposure after dark, or on the occasion of being injured by the pressure of the X-ray machine. Since breast cancer can still occur in women after prophylactic bilateral mastectomies, it's safe to say that mastectomy will not necessarily prevent breast cancer. The women who were sold on prophylactic mastectomy really just needed to sell their houses and move, and still do.

Or get bio-identical cyclical hormone replacement—pronto.

Rose Kushner was a Jewish woman who could not have been aware of BRCA I and II. She lobbied for free, accessible mammograms for all women, which means she, too, as a breast cancer "survivor," would have had more than a few over the years. But after Dr. Bailar exposed the BCDDP for not informing women of the risk of mammogram in 1975, Rose, as a friend and colleague of surgeon Dr. Bernard Fisher—the driving force behind tamoxifen's approval—became a candidate for the next big thing: chemo-*protection*,[70–74] now known as adjuvant "hormonal" therapy or tamoxifen. In the early 1970s tamoxifen was promoted on the premise we've now shown was never valid, that healthy levels of estrogen cause cancer and that blocking your estrogen receptors to stop estrogenic action would stop breast cancer.

It just doesn't work that way.

Around and Around

Tamoxifen has not really been proven to prevent breast cancer,[75–77] and while its long-term effects on healthy women are just starting to be documented, its cancer-causing properties are well documented.[78–81] Nevertheless, in a stunning move, on October 30, 1998, the FDA approved the use of tamoxifen (Nolvadex) for chemo-prevention in healthy women, allowing AstraZeneca Pharmaceuticals[82] to tap into a market potentially worth $36 billion annually.[83]

When the advisory committee, consisting of researchers, politicians, doctors, and CEOs of various drug companies, recommending the approval of tamoxifen was asked whether the Tamoxifen Prevention Study had demonstrated that the drug had "a favorable benefit-risk ratio for the prevention of breast cancer in women at increased risk as defined by the study population," the committee unanimously said "no," and went on to new hearings on a drug called Herceptin. The FDA approved tamoxifen anyway.[84–85] We can only speculate why.

Approval was based on a *single* study run under the auspices of the National Cancer Institute. It was an outgrowth of the National Surgical Adjuvant Breast and Bowel Project (NSABP), begun in the 1980s.[86] The study purported to show that tamoxifen was prophylactic, even though two simultaneous European studies in Italy and the United Kingdom "failed to confirm the US findings," as of this writing.

European researchers actually found no preventive effect of tamoxifen in women.[87–89] In fact, *there was no difference in survival for the women taking tamoxifen versus women taking placebo in the NCI study*.[90] The justification for AstraZeneca's claims of a 50 percent reduction in breast cancer lies in the difference between a 1.4 percent incidence of cancer taking tamoxifen versus a 2.7 percent incidence of breast cancer in women taking the placebo. This was also the reason for canceling the study early. They said that in the arm of the study in which women were not on tamoxifen, lives would be unnecessarily lost. What an interesting perspective for the coordinators of a drug company–run trial to take about the efficacy of their product. If the makers of tamoxifen have their way, this substance they've created to wipe out your estrogen reception will soon be prescribed without a diagnosis of cancer ever happening, on the premise that it prevents cancer just as fluoride in the water supply was put there on the premise of saving us from tooth decay.

It turns out that the price for the niggling 1.3 percent was very dear.

Tamoxifen quadruples the risk of endometrial[91–96] and uterine cancer in women over fifty and causes blood clots in the lung,[97–102] liver cancer, colorectal and stomach cancer, twice as many cataracts, sexual dysfunction,[103–105] excess free radical production, weakened heart muscle, hot flashes,[106] sleeplessness, mood swings that double the risk of suicide, osteoporosis (4 percent increase), mental deficits (from garden-variety memory loss to actual Alzheimer's-like brain damage through chloride channels),[107] and, *most importantly*, contralateral[108] and ipsilateral breast cancer[109]—*the exact cancer it was designed to prevent*.

Not only does cancer appear in the other breast and next to the first site, but the cancer tamoxifen can cause is a breast cancer that is often estrogen- and progesterone-receptor *negative*. Receptor-negative cancer always has the worst prognosis of all—earlier death. In the study, "women of color," 9.4 percent at the study sample, got a more definite picture of what tamoxifen could do for them: Their risk of breast cancer was doubled. This result never made it into the official write-up of the study because too few "women of color" were enrolled in the study to make it statistically significant.[110]

It does appear that women who take hormone replacement therapy plus tamoxifen experience *some* benefits. That, of course, would be from the hormones. All the aforementioned side effects are predictably estrogen-deficit states: the hot flashes and the aging eyes and memory are a dead giveaway. These effects are all in response to the *real* action of tamoxifen on estrogen reception. Tamoxifen is not an estrogen receptor blocker—only progesterone can do that—but as the term *SERM* (selective estrogen receptor *modifier*) says, tamoxifen modifies the estrogen receptor. Tamoxifen is really a synthetic super-estrogen that hits the receptor so hard it retreats into the cytoplasm and becomes less effective.[111]

This castration effect on the estrogen receptor makes the side effects of tamoxifen almost the same as those caused by ovarian ablation through chemotherapy, radiation, or surgery.[112-119] In the beginning tamoxifen was used for all kinds of things, just like DES. Like DES, tamoxifen wipes out estradiol's reception, but also like DES, it has estrogenic properties, too, but site-*specifically*.[120] Tamoxifen was actually used as a form of birth control in the beginning. Tumors shrink and then regroup and come back stronger and smarter.[121] This is certainly true of tumors that are Her-2 positive, since they regress under estrogen therapy.[122]

Ballad of a Thin Man

Metastatic breast cancer is breast cancer that has appeared in your lymph nodes, other organs, or bones. Metastatic breast cancer is, for the standard of care at this point in time, *an incurable disease*.[123-124] The news-reported medical "miracles" are limited to what have always been considered to be the rarer malignancies.[125-127] Hodgkin's disease, testicular cancer, childhood leukemia, and lymphoma are the only cancers that have yielded to any innovations in chemotherapy or radiation technology.[128-131]

Those cancers are called the *rare cancers* because they rarely occur.

The three biggest killers in women are still breast, lung, and colon cancer, in that order.[132-135] It's important to point out here that the survival rates among the Big Three haven't changed a whisper.[136]

We suspect that the "five-year *cure* rate" was invented by drug companies to distract cancer patients from the well-known fact[137] in medicine that the preponderance of death from cancer occurs in the five to ten years after diagnosis *with or without treatment at all*. Often patients refuse treatment.[138] These patients, compared to treated cohorts, often fare as well or better statistically, not to mention in terms of quality of life.

But what about the stories of survival and cure that attribute salvation to modern medicine?

Ralph W. Moss, Ph.D., says in his crisp reportage of the entire industry in his book *Questioning Chemotherapy*,[139] "Personal stories are compelling, but inconclusive. Sometimes people get the facts wrong, even about their own cases, or sometimes they speak too soon and will not actually survive any longer than the untreated patient. For example, the majority of people with colon cancer, even those with regionally disseminated disease, survive five years with surgery alone. Cancers can reoccur after many years after the person has been officially entered into the 'cure' statistics."

The language of research, when it comes to cancer, fosters and feeds the conspiracy of optimism that pervades medicine. We think this conspiracy of optimism is an accidental invention of the drug companies' "language of risk." Phrases that permeate the propaganda of published literature on breast cancer are routinely switched and updated. For example, the phrase "five-year cure rate" has become the "five-year survival rate" because the word *cure* wrongly implied that the chosen intervention had effected a cure. The word *survival* is better only by degree. "Survival" erroneously implies that patients receiving the drug in question actually survive.[140-141]

Just because a woman is diagnosed promptly and treated with the standard of care and survives five years does not mean that either the early diagnosis or the treatment was responsible. In the realm of drug promotion and bought-and-paid-for research, it is well known that "early detection" does not necessarily equate with "less invasive." An earlier-detected cancer is not necessarily a less deadly one. The reality is that early detection has been the source of "improvement" in the statistics of survival only through the effect of a statistical ruse called *lead-time bias*.

Lead-time bias means that the earlier you find a cancer, the longer you can live with it until you die. In other words, *no time has been added* to the duration of the patient's life. But on paper it looks great.[142-147] In reality, even if you find it later, you still die at the same time as you would even if you'd found it earlier, you just get to know it longer.

Things We Said Today

It is also important to bear in mind that "disease-free survival time" is not the same thing as overall or absolute survival. "Disease-free survival" refers to the period of time one experiences until the cancer comes back so one can die at exactly the same time, yet have a wonderful increase in "disease-free survival time." The phrase "disease-free survival time" does not pertain to quality of life, either. The potentially tortuous treatment regimens that are required to provide disease-free survival time for only some cancers hardly promote quality-of-life survival on the day-to-day scale. The side effects of the treatments cannot only debilitate the patient, sometimes more so than the disease itself, they impact quality of life severely. It is an intentionally confusing and completely meaningless parameter of improvement. While it might tell you how long you *could* live without signs of the disease thanks to a particular treatment, *"disease-free survival time" does not tell you if you will actually live any longer than you would have without the treatment.*

"Stage migration" is another sleight-of-hand; the promoters (drug companies) of various cancer treatments frequently use the numbers to create hopeful statistics.[148] With better diagnostic techniques, lead-time bias puts diagnosis of the tumor in question into an early "staging pool," so when a group of patients with more advanced metastases are compared to groups in which cancer was found earlier, the data can be "massaged" to produce better response rates to treatment over a longer period of time.[149] This could lead someone reading the study to conclude that the drug in question was actually working, statistically. So the drug companies running the trial report the statistics to doctors as an improvement in treatment options.[150-153]

The term *cure statistics* derives from the invention of *randomized clinical* (or controlled) *trials*. The RCT is the main tool used in this country to decide whether a therapy works. A randomized controlled trial is a human experiment in which the effects of one treatment are directly compared either to no regimen or to a different regimen given to patients with the same diagnosis. *Randomized* means that the patients are assigned to an "arm" or section of the study in a nondeliberate fashion, without choice or bias. Then the treatment the patient is receiving is actually being compared not just to the controls, the people not receiving the treatment, but to the *concurrent* controls[154-157] or, in other words, to people living at the same time, instead of to historical data.

This approach didn't become mandated in America until 1962, when the Kefauver-Harris amendment to the U.S. Food, Drug and Cosmetic Act called for "substantial evidence" of effectiveness of any new drug marketed in this country. The FDA meant it to mean at least two randomized studies. In *Questioning Chemotherapy,* Moss states, "This launched a whole new research establishment that provided RCTs to the burgeoning medical-industrial complex and incidentally gave work to thousands of people.

"Eventually, an entangled financial web of government, academia and industry developed. Soon drug makers firmly incorporated or planted principal investigators (PIs) within most of the leading research/treatment centers around the U.S. and abroad."[158] Without the separation of "church and state," so to speak, the drug companies had free rein to drive their own agenda through our leading centers of research and development. This 1960s push for drugs and money was the second wave in the takeover of our health care by the military/medical industry.

The first wave happened between World War I and World War II.

Lucy in the Sky with Diamonds

In 1943, two years before the Trinity Test at Alamogordo, New Mexico, which was three weeks before the bombs fell on Hiroshima and Nagasaki, Japan, a lone thyroid cancer patient in America was served an "atomic cocktail" of radioactive iodine to kill thyroid cancer cells.[159] From just the outcome of this patient, since he did not die from the treatment and his cancer shrank for the time being, radioactive iodine treatment was thereafter considered a success. Cobalt treatments followed in 1948. It only took five short years for *radio*chemotherapy to blossom. The first annual meeting of the Society of Nuclear Medicine met in 1954.[160] All of the leftover toxic chemicals and radioactive waste material from two world wars now had a use in medicine, but not exactly to our benefit.

On July 16, 1945, when we exploded the first nuclear bomb at the Trinity site, Robert Oppenheimer, the director of the Manhattan Project, gazed at the mushroom cloud and said, "God bless us, we have created something more awful than hell."[161] Any cancer patient would agree.

After the end of World War II, the network of radiation and chemical warfare researchers and government and military officials mobilized for the Manhattan Project did not disband. Rather, they began working on various government programs to promote peacetime uses of the science they had uncovered while working on atomic energy, chemical agents, and nuclear weapons development.[162] From its inception in 1947 until they reorganized in 1974, the Atomic Energy Commission produced radioisotopes that were used in thousands of human experiments conducted at universities, hospitals, and government facilities.[163] These experiments led to the radium seeds used in prostate cancer treatment today and the knowledge applied to radiotherapy in cancer treatment currently.

Burnin' Down the House

Today, full-body radiation treatments for cancer destroy bone marrow in a misguided attempt to, as Marie Curie said, "ease human suffering."[164] It's remarkably ironic that as the twentieth century began, the next attempt after surgery to control cancer was, in fact, with the only natural substance on earth known to cause cancer—*radiation*.

In 1895, Röntgen's new X rays were being tested at the French Science Academy to discover any unknown powers that they might have. Those tests were witnessed by Henri Becquerel, the son and grandson of physicists. Henri went back home to his house in Paris to try to reenact what he'd seen and, in the attempt, accidentally "photographed" his wife's hand, wedding ring and all. As if fate had a plan, Becquerel's lab assistants happened to be a married couple named Marie and Pierre Curie.

By the time the Curies came to work with Becquerel, he had already proven that uranium emissions, or "rays," could turn air into a conductor of electricity.[165] Both Pierre Curie, a professor at the Sorbonne, and his student and wife, Marie, were eager to expand Becquerel's research.[166] The Curies tested pitchblende, an ore of uranium, which produced a current three hundred times stronger than processed uranium; they named the ore *polo-*

nium after Marie's place of birth, Poland. In the paper they published on their discovery, Marie coined the term *radio-active*.

The Curies had stockpiled bucketloads of pitchblende for processing. Marie wrote, "Sometimes I had to spend the whole day stirring a boiling mass with a heavy iron rod nearly as big as myself." She admitted that "one of our pleasures was to enter our workshop at night; then, all around us, we would see the luminous silhouettes of the beakers and capsule that contained our products."[167] Marie, during the research, had been exposed to incredible levels of radiation. She died of leukemia in 1934, almost blinded, and her fingers burnt by her "dear" radium.[168]

The first indication of the effects on the body of the new materials they were working with came in 1901, when Becquerel noticed a red area on his chest after carrying a vial of radium.[169] Soon after the turn of the century Alexander Graham Bell suggested radioactive implants to treat "deep lying" cancers because the radiation caused such mutation that sometimes cells died.[170-171]

For much of the Victorian era, physicians and laypeople alike were consumed with radioactive "cures" for everything. There were watercoolers fitted with a chunk of radium, along with over-the-counter products for health such as Vita Radium Suppositories, Radium Bath Salts, the Lifestone Cigarette Holder, to irradiate your lungs with every puff, and even radium-enhanced flour to bake bread to eat with your irradiated water.[172] Every shoe store in Europe and eventually America had a shoe-fitting fluoroscope that X-rayed the prospective buyer's foot. Since history and science record no rash of foot cancer, apparently not much harm was done. This portable X-ray machine stayed in stores until the 1950s, when the Radiological Society of North America demanded it be put to a stop because it "lowered the dignity of the profession of radiology."[173]

Party poopers.

Purple Haze

The intense growth of radiation research with humans after World War II was just the next step in the enormous expansion of an already intact military biomedical research enterprise that began about the same time a ship, the *John E. Harvey*, blew up in the harbor at Bari, Italy, in 1943. The ship was carrying the same kind of mustard gas (actually a liquid) used by both sides in World War I. Mustard gas attacked moist skin like the eyes, armpits, and groin, burning its way into its victims and leaving searing blisters and unimaginable pain. If it was inhaled, it caused bleeding and blistering within the respiratory system.[174]

When the *John E. Harvey* exploded, the sailors who survived later suffered from a severe depression of their bone marrow. A few subsequently died of a near-complete depletion of white blood cells. Navy doctor Peter Alexander reported this strange effect on the blood of his men to superiors.[175] They were hardly surprised because, unknown to Dr. Alexander, human trials of mustard gas derivatives were already under way at that point "under the cloak of war-time secrecy" at Yale when the *Harvey* blew up.[176-177] The effects of nitrogen mustard gas as a liquid were what Yale researcher were looking at in the early 1940s.

As early as the 1930s, researchers applied a form of mustard gas externally to breast cancer lesions.[178-179] But the use of chemicals in cancer goes back at least to ancient Egypt. Castor oil, pig parts, and herbs were the main treatment cited for malignant tumors in the Ebers Papyrus.[180] Over the centuries caustic chemicals like zinc chloride were prescribed topically on tumors; even poisonous lead was injected into women with advanced breast cancer.[181-182] Before World War II, benzene was used in leukemia, the same benzene we now know *causes* leukemia.[183-184] Any chemical that killed tissue but more often than not left the patient alive was used.[185]

Paul Ehrlich, the man who treated syphilis with Salvarsan 606 and originated the sound bite "magic bullet" to refer to a hypothetical drug that would target only diseased cells just as our own antibodies do, first looked at alkylating agents like mustard gas before World War I as cytotoxic (cell-killing) agents.[186-188] When looking for a magic bullet, they overlooked our own hormones for profit.

In 1942, the U.S. government had signed a contract with Yale University and other research centers to investigate chemical warfare agents for medical use. There was an informal network of labs across the United States. At Yale the sulfur atom had been replaced with a nitrogen one, making mustard gas dissolve more easily in water or alcohol.[189]

Dr. Thomas Dougherty, a Yale anatomist, is credited with the idea of injecting nitrogen mustard into a mouse with a huge lymphoma tumor.[190] After just two administrations of the compound, the tumor began to soften and regress. The average life expectancy of an injected mouse was about three weeks. This mouse had lived a month after the treatment when the tumor recurred. They treated him again, but this time achieved a less complete remission.[191]

Others at Yale tried to duplicate the first experiments, but never could. Nevertheless, on the basis of one mouse, human clinical trials were initiated in December 1942.[192] Alfred Gilman, a founder of the National Cancer Institute, admitted, "The selection of a proper dose of a highly toxic chemical warfare agent for administration to a man for the first time (on purpose) was made with unwarranted confidence."[193] The entry on the patient's chart read, "0.1 mg per kg (of body weight) of compound X intravenously," and the chart was classified "top secret,"[194] Ralph Moss reports. "The response in the first patient was as dramatic as it was in the first mouse."[195] The tumor masses softened within forty-eight hours and obstructive signs and symptoms were relieved within ten days. Huge lymph node tumors disappeared. But within four weeks the patient's blood count plummeted and he developed bleeding problems.[196] Then the tumor "regenerated to the bone marrow—a great disappointment," Alfred Gilman, one of the founders of the NCI wrote.[197]

More rounds of chemo brought only fleeting improvement, and then the man died. Still, today, we believe in chemotherapy from just these studies.

Under My Thumb

"The chemotherapists of the new century brought a special zeal to their cause," wrote Brown University historian James T. Patterson. "They believed their magic bullets would be the salvation of humanity." From the start, however, cancer chemotherapy "proved deeply disappointing."[198] The new drugs had "little effect" and were often highly toxic, killing "mice and rats as fast or faster than the cancers."[199]

Sloan-Kettering researcher Kanematsu Sugiura, D.Sc., a pioneer of experimental chemotherapy, said that in the beginning, in the 1920s, "chemotherapists were looked upon as little better than quacks."[200] Alfred Gilman, Ph.D., said, "In the minds of most physicians the administration of drugs, at that point in time, other than analgesics [pain-killers], in the treatment of a malignant disease was the act of a charlatan."[201]

To illustrate this, in one gargantuan study published in 1978, 31,510 women with breast cancer were followed for twenty-two years undergoing various adjuvant therapies—in total, twelve different combinations of chemotherapies, radiation, and surgery. The conclusion of this huge multivariable study was that "the overall extension of life in 31,510 women" over twenty-two years, undergoing only conventional standard of care treatments, "was found to be less than three months" for all of that suffering.[202]

Chemotherapy was probably part of the broader fascination with chemical marvels. The parallels between the new postwar War on Cancer and the Manhattan Project were clear. Beyond the overriding metaphor of war, the terminology of oncologists says it all—"strategies in treatment," "weapons in our arsenal." Moss says, "Combinations of drugs bear aggressive sounding acronyms like BOLD, CHOP, COP, COP-BLAM, ICE, MOP and ProMACE.[203] This military language has become so ingrained, it's difficult to talk about cancer without resorting to war images."[204]

The rationale for this brute-force approach is that the oncologist must, if he is to succeed for the patient, "kill every last tumor cell," or as Moss puts it, "destroy the village to save it."[205] We've heard that from figures of authority before.

Post–World War II, Sloan-Kettering and the new National Cancer Institute tested over 400,000 chemicals as potential patentable drugs; 10,000 new ones are added every year.[206-207] Only 2,000 out of this enormous number have been "reported to have selective toxicity to at least one kind of tumor cell." Critics of this whatever-sticks-to-the-wall approach call it the nothing-is-too-stupid-to-test method.[208-209] Eventually fifty or so chemotherapy drugs were identified and are in use.[210-211]

Tell Me Why

While these major players in cancer research have been busy for fifty years testing everything from Windex to superglue for cytotoxic properties, they have never tested natural hormones in studies on actual women, because once the drug companies tweak the natural molecule to turn it into a patentable drug, the effect is not always quite so striking or even manageable.[212]

Take the case of progestins. In a landmark study reported in the *New England Journal of Medicine* in 1975,[213] which examined endometrial cancers in users of synthetic estrogen replacement (ERT), it became apparent that endometrial cancer was caused by low-dose unopposed horse estrogens in

Premarin. Incredibly for the drug company selling Premarin, natural progesterone solved the problem nicely in the lab. But since there's no patent in a natural substance, and therefore no money to be made, they had a problem. So Wyeth-Ayerst and its predecessor, Upjohn, invented progestins, which they could patent, from natural progesterone solely to stop the endometrial cancer. But once natural progesterone is turned into a progestin, the side effects start to snowball. Natural hormones work the way they're supposed to in nature,[214-216] *unless they are altered in the lab.*[217-219]

The fake progesterone, or progestin, which they named Depo-Provera, acted in a "site-specific" way—that is, it worked only in one place and made trouble in another. Although in the uterus it had a progestigenic effect, medroxyprogesterone (MPA), which became Depo-Provera, actually had a weakly *estrogenic* effect in the breast, increasing rates of breast cancer in women on the Pill, Provera, and PremPro.[220-224] This switch will break your heart and brain, too, it seems.

We're stuck between a buck and a hard place, and we just might die there.

I Thought I Saw St. Augustine

Hippocrates, the father of medicine, had believed that when menstruation ceased, the body remained uncleansed, and hence the breasts became engorged and developed lumps that could degenerate into cancer.[225] Galen connected "melancholy," or depression, to the development of cancer.[226] By the 1500s and 1600s, the only doctors who published anything in the literature of the time were surgeons, previously known as *barbers,* who hoped to advance their reputations through their published works or case studies.[227] Adrian Helvetius of France has the claim on the first reported "lumpectomy." His 1697 optimistic "Letter on the Nature and Cure of Cancer"[228] describes Marguerite Perpointe, who was diagnosed with breast cancer in 1690 at age forty-six. She had come to him several months before her diagnosis after an injury—she had bumped her breast against a key sticking out of a door. She stalled on surgery for six months, until the tumor was "the size of a fist." He removed the hard lump and reported some years later that Mme. Perpointe was still in excellent health. He wrote extensively on the non-necessity of removal of the whole breast, just as Rose Kushner later did.[229]

But surgery became more and more prophylactic as the decades passed.[230] Case histories provide abundant evidence of breasts removed for multiple cysts. A Dr. Rodman, writing in England in the 1880s, concluded that "every surgeon had seen breast cancer in a maiden, whose sexual life beyond doubt had been absolutely negative."

He claimed that "childlessness was risky for its own reasons."[231-232] Dr. Rodman's peer, Dr. Willard Parker, confirmed in England that when "barren" women contracted cancer in disproportionate numbers, it was only because some of the same disorders that prevented conception also promoted breast cancer.[233-234] They seemed to realize something was happening. We believe that what was happening was that the internal aging process had begun to speed up from gaslights after dark at night[235]—making women older sooner *inside*—and by 1837, Nestle's baby "food"—formula—was on the market in Europe.[236-240] Women were hitting menopause sooner, and in the reproductive interval, breast-feeding less because they could. The writers of the time called it "refusal to suckle."[241]

Research into how often breast cancer occurred versus surgery's ability to cure it is predominantly from William Norford, a male midwife who practiced in East Suffolk, England, in 1753.[242-243] The women Norford reported on gave him a medical history of sorts in response to his questions. In every case, the raw data of Norford's recording and each patient's reporting were guided by the fact that the events being examined correctly corresponded to ancient and still-popular notions of why cancer might develop—with problems of lactation, a stoppage of menses, the experience of unhappy emotions, the onset of menopause, or damage done to the breast by a blow.[244]

There was constant disagreement among surgeons and male midwives as to whether or not cancer was a local or constitutional disease. Medical authority was not as monolithic as it would later become, and many women just said "no" to surgery and sought alternative treatments from local "healers." The growing field of gynecology had supposedly claimed the "whole woman" as its sphere of study and practice, and yet largely ignored breast disease.[245]

As the nineteenth century progressed, women's biological destiny, from childbearing to breast-feeding to menopause, was increasingly linked with a "cancerous tendency" in the scientific literature. There was frequent discussion in Europe of whether or not "unhappy emotions" (depression) were a precursor to cancer. Women themselves, even in that time period, knew that if their mother died of breast cancer they were at greater risk than, say, their neighbor, without the benefit of lectures on genetics or CNN.[246]

When we search for clues to previous conclusions and treatments, we find very little, except the journals of the individual suffering of famous victims. Most eighteenth- and nineteenth-century women's health manuals and texts never mention breast cancer. We would love to believe that's because it was still so rare compared to the incidence in our time, but it may be that their silence related more to the sense of hopelessness in the face of the unexplainable.[247]

Although these women of the past married and had children at young ages, during the later part of the century, as breast-feeding in Europe waned, in the wake of Pasteur's sterilization process and Nestle's formula, and breast cancer increased, the search for specific cancer-causing irritants linked to everyday life intensified. For example, the long-term trauma effects of wearing stays and tightly laced corsets were often cited in surgical texts.[248] In our time, a reasonably loud contingent of activists still look to bras and deodorant in the same way.[249]

The continuing failure to solve the mystery of cancer is one reason for its marked neglect by historians. Cancer doesn't make a great story of narrative history like polio, tuberculosis, or Type 1 diabetes, because there's no march to victory, no big ending. We think, on the contrary, that the cause and effect of risk becomes murkier by the decade.

Then as now, when looking for the one factor that might explain a woman's proclivity to breast cancer in "civilized society," it appears that as time marched on, the lack of lactation and/or pregnancy became farther and farther away from modern perceptions of reality. We fail to look at or consider these things as causes because they have become farther and farther removed from life in our time. Although breast-feeding had a resurgence in popularity in the 1970s, the women being diagnosed now were born to women who didn't breast-feed, and they themselves, if they did, breast-fed for very short duration.

Shortly after the turn of the twentieth century, Dr. Rodman, in England, felt compelled to point out that "mammary carcinoma is much more common in young women than it is supposed to be."[250-251] We can only guess that "young" to Rodman might have been a woman in her thirties. Even then women were already living lives very different from the ones that their mothers had lived at their age. The long hours of artificial light at night and the consumption of sugar, along with less childbearing and lactation, point to lifestyle changes at work on women's health. Breast cancer was still understood by some surgeons as a disease with an environmental context. Dr. Walshe said that "cancer, like insanity follows in the wake of civilization."[252-253] We say amen to that.

Eleanor Rigby

Writer Fanny Burney's chilling first-person account of the pre-anesthesia, pre-antibiotic mastectomy she endured in 1811 remains one of the landmark events in the literature of breast cancer. In a remarkable book called *The History of the Breast*,[254] Marilyn Yalom relates Fanny Burney's personal account in stunning detail. Given the times that she lived in, anesthesia was not an option, nor were painkillers. So she told her doctors not to inform her of the day, but to virtually ambush her, lest she lose her courage. She described her panic on the day they selected, which was unknown to her in advance, when she saw her living room outfitted for the surgery. The surgeons and her maids entered behind her and closed the door. They handed her a glass of wine as seven more men in black entered the room. With some amount of force to her resistance, they stretched her out on the bed, her face covered by a thin see-through cambric-soaked handkerchief, and began the surgery.

Now began *"the most torturing pain."*

> When the dreadful steel was plunged into the breast—cutting through veins—arteries—flesh—nerves. I began a scream that lasted unintermittingly during the whole time of the incision—& I almost marvel that it rings not in my Ears still! So excruciating was the agony. When the wound was made & the instrument was withdrawn, the pain seemed undiminished, for the air that suddenly rushed into those delicate parts felt like a mass of minute but sharp and forked poniards, that were tearing at the edges of the wound.

Burney goes on to recall in excruciating detail "the terrible cutting" and the knife scraping against her breastbone. The operation lasted for twenty minutes—twenty minutes of "utterly speechless torture" performed on a fully conscious woman whose sole anesthesia had been a glass of wine.

The question for us is, was it necessary? Did a mastectomy save Fanny's life?

The violence and unnatural assumption that cancer is a localized disease that can be cut away is as old as surgery itself. But is it true? In Rose Kushner's day it was so believed that the standard of care[255] meant that once you were unconscious, if a preliminary lab report found any abnormal cells, you woke up without a breast. As it has turned out, the one-step procedure was both unnecessary and cruel.

Rose Kushner often drew on an old joke told by Johns Hopkins medical students about penis cancer. In the joke, a med student undergoes amputation of his penis after a preliminary "frozen section" reveals cancer. But the good news, the student is told after the operation is over, is that the tumor was benign.[256-257]

More importantly, Rose Kushner's work and ours strongly suggests that it won't make a bit of difference to your survival whether you allow them to take your breast or not, because surgery can't address what caused your cancer in the first place. The premise for centuries was that breast cancer was "local foci," or that cancer started in your breast and once you removed the offending organ, you beat cancer. If that were true, then chemotherapy, whose premise is that it will knock out all the distant (from the breast) "nested metastases," would surely reach the breast in which the cancer started.

So, why would anyone ever cut off your breast, unless chemo doesn't really work? Or why would lumpectomy ever require chemo and radiation? Chemo, if it works, in principal should always be enough. Radiation is and has always been a bizarre strategy for cancer treatment, since the premise of radiation therapy, damaging cells to kill them, is also a potential cancer hazard if they don't all die.

Burney lived thirty years after her surgery. Was she saved by mastectomy? Or would she have lived anyway? Yalom's book also tells us the sadder (if there could be one), almost simultaneous story of another breast cancer victim in history. Abigail Adams Smith, daughter of John Adams, the second president of the United States, underwent a mastectomy in America within days of Fanny Burney's in France.

Abigail did not live another thirty years. Abigail died two years later.

Why didn't the mastectomy save her?

We think the answer is that cancer is a systemic disease that mastectomy can't really touch. The women who live long lives after mastectomy never really had the kind of cancer that would have killed them anyway, just like Fanny.

In *A Short History on Breast Cancer*,[258] Daniel De Moulin points out that despite the proliferation of literature on cancer during the Enlightenment, little progress had been made in understanding the disease, and surgeons' writings both supported and challenged ancient ideas. For example, was the old distinction between "scirrhus" (nonmalignant growth) and cancer still valid—was an "indolent" tumor to be regarded as harmless, as a sign of possible trouble in the future, or as an early stage of the disease itself requiring immediate action? The decision to operate often rested on whether the surgeon believed the removal of the tumor or the breast would halt the disease.[259] Unfortunately surgeons are not clairvoyant.

It seems that in the cases of Fanny Burney and Abigail Adams Smith, their respective surgeons may have been wrong on both counts. Even today, in the age of molecular oncology and genetics, the same judgment call still has to be made about what exactly is and is not life-threatening cancer. And a great deal of the time, we know, medicine still gets it wrong, because all breast cancer is subject to the same treatment, to the same standard of care, and some women live and some women don't.

It's not the luck of the draw. It's the incompetence of the treatments. Fanny Burney's gruesome torture at the hands of graduate school "barbers" back in 1811 only lasted about twenty minutes, if you omit the agony of anticipation and the misery of recovery. But, all in all, she still suffered less than the average chemotherapy patient. The average chemo patient is subjected to sometimes as many as four to six repeated "rounds" of chemo cocktails, consisting of as many as three dozen different drugs in various combinations.[260]

The standard of care for breast and most other cancers is what we've reviewed in this chapter—drugs for the purpose of hormone ablation such as tamoxifen and now Faslodex, aromatase inhibitors like Arimidex, surgery, and cocktails of chemo and radiation.[261-262]

None of these treatments can ever effect a "cure" or guarantee your "survival," because they never address the actual cause of the disease (fewer pregnancies, less lactation, and aging) or try to treat it with what might be the promise of a solution—natural hormone replacement.[263]

The proof is that all of these treatments, even the ones based on the premise of prophylaxis or prevention like tamoxifen, show recurrence rates.[264-268]

Diseases that come back are not cured.

A genuine cure presupposes a restoration to a state of health (like hormone replacement) that is never again interrupted by the same disease or a different one caused by the "cure" for the original disease. Anything less is *palliative* on your way to dying from the original disease. "Palliative" is used as a verb, "to palliate," in regard to cancer and is defined in that case as "to alleviate" or "to mitigate" the symptoms produced by tumors, like pain and obstruction. However, "palliate" has another definition: "*to varnish, gloss, or sugar-coat.*"[269-270]

Breast cancer is not a localized phenomenon. It can't be removed by force or fire or toxic chemicals because if it's really malignant cancer, it's going to get you somewhere else eventually. The same forces affecting your breast to change are happening all over you simultaneously.

Fanny Burney wasn't "cured" just because she lived on after her surgery. Abigail lived through hers, too, and died. Abigail Adams Smith died because one of them had the kind of breast cancer that will kill you and the other one didn't. The point is that there is no proof that the "treatments" really had any effect on cancer in either one of them, Fanny or Abigail. The point is that the date of diagnosis or the type of treatment available through the standard of care in their time or ours doesn't dictate outcome and never has.

Then as now, it's your age and how you've lived your reproductive life that dictates sex hormone function. Without sex hormones, the environment naturally assumes you're finished, and more often than not that means cancer, heart disease, or Alzheimer's disease for you. We know that in America, it also means something disquietingly similar to medieval torture—modern medicine—until you finally succumb to nature's plan, unless you fight back with logic.

There may be a way to save your life and health with *natural hormones*. But getting them won't be easy. Even if you tell your doctor that you are not afraid of hormone replacement, that you actually *want* natural, cyclic, rhythmic hormone replacement and you want it now, and you show him the previous chapter and this one, your doctor is still going to say no. Even if he's convinced that natural hormones prescribed *naturally* won't cause cancer, he'll still say no.

He'll say no because of the old shell game that the drug companies and the NIH played with the HERS Study on hormone replacement therapy and heart disease in the Women's Health Initiative Study we've all heard about. Once again Wyeth-Ayerst tried to validate PremPro as "heart-smart," and once again, they couldn't. So now, beyond the threat of cancer, since your doctor has been led to believe that conventional HRT is the only option for hormone replacement, and the Women's Health Initiative Study, stopped in July 2002, says that PremPro is going to give you a heart attack or stroke, he'll still say no.

What else could he say?

part **three**

MENOPAUSE

seven

NINETEENTH NERVOUS BREAKDOWN

In Part Two we examined the lies we've been told about childbearing, breast-feeding, hormone replacement, and the capabilities of breast cancer screening and treatment. In Part Three we begin with the truth hidden behind the biggest lie of all: that if breast cancer doesn't get you, *you'll be fine.*[1]

The Internet site Y-Me states that breast cancer is "the overall leading cause of death in women between the ages of 40 and 55." It adds, "In the United States, 1 in 7 women will develop breast cancer in her lifetime. This year, breast cancer will be newly diagnosed every three minutes and a woman will die of breast cancer every thirteen minutes." While those numbers are accurate, it is *heart disease*,[2-3] not breast cancer, that will kill *one in two* women after menopause.

In 1999, the most recent year for which the American Heart Association provides statistics, 512,904 women died from cardiovascular disease, versus the 41,144 who died of breast cancer. Heart disease is more than ten times as big a risk.[4-5]

Truth be told, while heart disease is the leading killer of women in America, breast cancer makes a better *industry* than heart disease. After all, more female celebrities have had breast cancer than have had a heart attack. Breast cancer also has a club with pink ribbons. A heart attack just isn't as sexy or empowering as breast cancer.

But you don't have to worry *too* much about heart disease, because if you're a woman, the odds are definitive that if your first heart attack occurs before sixty, it will be your last.[6-9] Women are 50 percent more likely than men to die within a year of their first heart attack of "sudden cardiac death."[10] That is attributable to the fact that women don't always have heart attacks like men.[11]

Our heart attacks are unique.

Heart of Stone

In the case of women, until you're postmenopausal,[12] a heart attack waiting to happen is not a matter of cholesterol-clogged arteries and veins. A heart attack waiting to happen in a woman less than sixty years old is simply a matter of declining hormones.[13-16] That's why drug testing by major drug companies on lipid-lowering drugs, beta blockers, and ACE inhibitors has traditionally been done on men; even the drug companies know that those drugs are ineffectual in saving women who are not over sixty.[17] Twenty- and thirty-year-old women never have heart attacks, but by forty, some of us just can't live without our hormones anymore. Relatively young women, in their forties, just drop dead, having never had a symptom, often while exercising or just after exercise.[18-21] That's usually not how a heart attack happens to a man. He gets high blood pressure, he gets fat, or maybe he smokes, and then—bam—one day he becomes a "heart" patient. Healthy, fit women in the prime of life who have never smoked and don't have high blood pressure have very different heart attacks.

Women are susceptible to a cardiac event called *sudden vasospasm*.[22]

One day our hearts just clamp down and won't start up again. That's a sudden vasospasm. Make a fist as tight as you can and keep the pressure on in your hand. That's what happens to your heart. Those are the "first heart attacks" that women can't survive. If you make it through your forties without a sudden vasospasm, it doesn't mean you're out of the proverbial woods yet. One in five women in this country has some sort of heart or blood vessel disease.[23] Even though, if we survive a heart attack, we are twice as likely as a man to have a second one in the next six years, most of us still believe it's breast cancer we should fear.[24-25]

Now, since all the furor over the cancellation of the most recent Women's Health Initiative Study, which showed an increase in *both* breast cancer and heart disease on conventional HRT—that is, PremPro—many doctors and their confused patients have all but given up on any kind of hormone replacement.[26] Wyeth-Ayerst's stock isn't the only thing taking a nosedive;[27] so is women's health care. The cancellation of the Women's Health Initiative Study has caused a significant downturn in the number of prescriptions for all forms of HRT.[28] Both women and their doctors have been made to feel afraid of the concept of hormone "replacement," when their *hormones* were never replaced in the first place.[29-30]

Thanks to the debacle created by synthetic "hormones," a great many women will never have the chance to see and feel what the real ones could have done for them. The Sunday edition of the *New York Times* of November 10, 2002, ran a front-page article carried to the back to fill an entire page on how to wean yourself off of *dangerous* hormones,[31] even though most women reading the article have never had the chance to experience real natural hormone replacement.

I Should've Known Better

The irony here is that for most doctors, the only reason they ever felt they had for prescribing hormones in the first place—in the face of the misinformation campaign regarding HRT and cancer—was the definitive evidence of HRT's protection against heart disease. For the last thirty-five years, all randomized clinical trials and drug company studies pointed to the absolute need to prescribe estrogen (in the form of Premarin) to prevent heart disease in women at risk, which is to say all women.[32]

Back in 1995, the Post-menopausal Estrogen/Progestin Intervention (PEPI) Trials[33] used various combinations of "hormones" on the women in the trial. These various "arms" of the trial consisted of: Premarin and Progestin, no hormones at all, and the combination of Premarin and *natural* progesterone. The arm using no hormones at all showed no improvement, the arm using Premarin and Progestin (PremPro) showed minimal to no improvement. But the arm of the trial using Premarin and *natural progesterone* showed a *drastic reduction* in vascular events and heart attacks of both kinds in the long term.[34]

The arm of the trial using standard HRT (PremPro) was, unfortunately, the only one we read about in the media because they are the only ones readily available. Not surprisingly, the completely synthetic combination of HRT had far less impact on longevity. Again, the positive effects of natural hormones were overlooked.

Even so, as inaccurately reported as it was, the PEPI trials "confirmed that oral estrogen (Premarin) fibrinogen levels compared to placebo showed that the magnitude of these differences was likely to be *clinically significant*."[35] That means Premarin showed results that were the same or worse than nothing.

That was eight years ago. Did medicine pursue *natural* hormone replacement?

No. In the initial research, the PEPI trials of 1995 relied heavily on supporting numbers from a study published in 1992 in a journal called the *Annals of Internal Medicine*[36] published by the American College of Physicians–American Society of Internal Medicine. This is an arduous piece of work. Just like the breast-feeding study in Chapter Four that compiled all but about 20 percent of the world's data on breast cancer and breast-feeding, this cardiac study, which was conducted by Deborah Grady and Susan M. Rubin, reviewed all English-language scientific publications since 1970. No small job. Grady and Rubin, for all of their work, reported a solid *50 percent reduction* of cardiac death in women on hormones, *synthetic* hormones.

Remember that the tamoxifen trials were stopped early on moral grounds because the "50 percent" reduction in breast cancer they found (based on the puny statistics of a 2.7 occurrence in placebo users versus 1.4 in tamoxifen users) meant that the placebo users' lives were at great risk as long as they were being denied tamoxifen.[37] But when Grady and Rubin showed a 50 percent reduction in cardiac *death*, no action was taken to provide women with hormones.

Furthermore, a year earlier, the *New England Journal of Medicine* had published the "Ten-Year Follow-Up from the Nurses' Health Study."[38] The Ten-Year Follow-Up's evaluation of Premarin and Provera (*the* synthetic progesterone) use began in 1976. Researchers followed 48,470 postmenopausal women ages thirty to sixty-three for ten years and found that "the overall relative risk of cardiovascular disease in women taking estrogen was *significantly reduced*." The estrogen users were also "less likely to have diabetes and to be lean." Now, that's a weight loss aid.

Now these were the results on a regimen of horse urine derivatives and synthetic fake progesterone, and women were still—with all of the side effects that program would produce—better off heart- and weight-wise than women on no hormones at all.

But, most important, 71 percent of the women in the study took Premarin only—that is, without fake progesterone or progestins of any kind. Bingo. No fake progesterone, no progestins of any kind in the studies—until 1995. So we only had to look back ten years to find the red herring in the mystery of how estrogen could suddenly cause heart attacks. All you have to do is add progestins to the mix and you've got trouble.

It was only when synthetic progesterone was added directly to Premarin to prevent endometrial cancer[39-40] that the negative effects of combined conventional HRT began to show up.[41-45] This was the event that led to a contradiction to the findings by Grady and Rubin in 1992, that for the previous twenty years estrogen takers had 50 percent fewer deaths from heart attack. Users of HRT, in the past, were really just users of ERT.

It's a Heartache

The undeniable multiple benefits of any estrogen on the heart are obvious, even if they're available just as the used-up metabolites in the horse estrogen Premarin. These studies only became "confounding" when, in the HERS Trial and in the Women's Health Initiative Study, PremPro, a combination of horse estrogen and synthetic progestins, became the most used "hormone" drug. The HERS Trial report of 1998[46] actually found *more* deaths in the PremPro group than they did in the untreated group. Just as in contraceptive side effects, it looks like it's the progestin part of PremPro that's really killing women on conventional HRT.[47-62]

The Provera (synthetic progesterone) component in PremPro, in addition to negating all of the benefits of horse estrogens on the heart, caused strokes and blood clots and offered no protection against sudden vasospasm.[63]

The National Institutes of Health (NIH) and the authors of the "oh my God, we must cancel this study *now* before all of the participants drop dead of a heart attack" response,[64] however, felt no compunction about continuing the study with women who have no uterus, continuing to give them Premarin alone because they know estrogen from *any* source is better than no estrogen. And they didn't feel the need to make that salient point clear to the public or doctors who prescribe PremPro as HRT.

The disaster, healthwise, of forty-seven million women going cold turkey off Premarin and PremPro isn't going to be pretty. Even weaning off these drugs slowly for younger women may be quite hazardous. Sudden vasospasm occurs *as* we run out of estrogen[65-73] after we've lost all progesterone, somewhere between thirty-five and fifty. Without estrogen, we have no progesterone action[74-75] at all, even from our adrenals; without the hormones to be a woman, you not only risk breast cancer, you risk having a heart attack like a man. For those of us over fifty, no HRT *of any kind* is *disastrous,* because the heart attack of the younger middle-aged woman, sudden vasospasm, is a product of no progesterone, but the heart attack of the postmenopausal woman, coronary artery occlusion (men's heart attack), is really the absence of estrogen.

Listen to Your Heart

Men's heart attacks are a product of insulin and cortisol dysfunction.[76] Insulin levels report on the food supply to all of the systems inside you; cortisol is a barometer of light and fear; and good old melatonin[77-79] keeps score with the other two on where you are on the earth in relation to the spin, wobble, and tilt of our planet as it leans in toward the sun. This HPA axis (hypothalamic-pituitary-adrenal) is sort of a global positioning system, your very own GPS, to tell your systems the time of day and year based on your location on the planet.

Our hearts, men, women's, and all other living things with a cardiovascular system, evolved seasonally to survive—that is, in the summer our hearts are meant to run on glucose or blood sugar for energy, and in the winter, when all of the summer's carbohydrates are gone, our hearts would switch to free fatty acids for fuel.[80-82]

Four or five months out of the year—in summer—blood sugar and insulin are high as a result of the availability of carbohydrates in warmer weather and, simultaneously, insulin and cortisol are high from the more hours of light.[83]

In winter, when the plants are dormant and the animals have a layer of fat (just like we would from summer grazing), we'd eat the animals along with shellfish, tree bark, and any roots we could still dig until the ground was frozen solid.[84]

Our hearts have learned to run on that menu for millennia. In effect, our hearts, like the rest of the planet, should go dormant from heat-producing, hyperburning, metabolic sugar loading for seven or eight months of the year, too. That way, we could "sleep off" all of the accumulated fat in our hearts and around our middles from the previous summer's partying.[85-86]

The short light exposure in the winter always meant more melatonin and prolactin at night and less prolactin, insulin, and cortisol the next day for our hearts and brains. Only now, with year-round availability of carbohydrate energy and 24/7 light exposure, have our hearts had to deal with endless summer.[87] That's why heart disease has become the leading cause of death. In 1635, the leading cause of death in London, England, according to actuarial tables lent to us by the International Order of Foresters in Canada, was something called *King's Evil*. Your guess on that one is as good as ours, but heart attack was about tenth and cancer was nowhere.

By 1901, the leading cause of death in this country was pneumonia, which was the second leading cause of death in London two hundred and fifty years earlier. Not much had changed in two and a half centuries in public health care. In 1991, at the end of nearly a century of unprecedented progress—antibiotics, blood typing, and transfusion—the leading causes of death were heart disease, diabetes, and cancer, in that order. To a casual observer, it looks like the elimination of bacteria and the ability to replace blood might just have been a trade-off for the debilitating abundance and painful, sometimes agonizing, longevity we now "enjoy."

You're in My Heart

Before the era of medical miracles like contraception and in vitro fertilization, women were grandmothers in their late thirties or early forties. As for women over forty who would have died of pneumonia due to "weakened immune systems" in old age, they lived extra decades thanks to penicillin. *Female* disorders like excessive bleeding from uterine fibroids at menopause and rupturing ovarian cysts became survivable with the advent of anesthesia, blood transfusion, and surgery. Other possible death scenarios for women in general, like being trampled by a horse, your skirt catching fire while cooking, or tuberculosis, were all potentially treatable with surgery, antibiotics, and transfusion. But the changing environment couldn't be stopped.

In the story of human development, the trade-off for living longer is aging faster. Remember that if one summer equals one trip around the sun, then, in the world we live in, constant light, heat, and sugar for twelve months equal four trips around the sun for *man*kind, but not for womankind, *as long as we reproduce*.

The reward for going through the ordeal of childbirth, the reward for being *women*, is that we were given the catbird's seat at the table of the gods. Once women become reproductive, *women*, not men, are capable of drifting in and out of nine months (not just three) of high insulin over and over again, and of spending years and years at a time experiencing sleep deficits that actually kill men. Why? Because we're protected by estrogen and progesterone and men are not.

As women, we come equipped with the tools to do the job, and the job is reproduction. Reproduction demands that we are specially designed to escape the boundaries of space and time and, to a certain extent, of mortality for the period of time we need to make new life.

Men, on the other hand, are a transient phenomena.

They are, in evolution's terms, meant to get in, do the job, and get out. They are supposed to fight each other for the right to reproduce, most often dying in the process. One man can create, ostensibly, a new life with every sex act or, if he's really on his game, at least 365 new lives in a year in his prime, while women can only create and nurture one new life every three to seven years, depending on how long we breast-feed each offspring. Remember, there was no other food for babies but breast milk until after the turn of the century. Men's ratio to ours, reproductively, is anywhere from 1,000 to 1 to 2,500 to 1.

They are, therefore, expendable, and we're not.

A lot of them can die and there's still plenty of new life.

They *are* subject to time and space, calorically speaking. If men stay in a period of high insulin and cortisol, not only are they aging in fast forward and getting fat, but, from nature's point of view, they have eaten too much of the food supply and thereby endangered the females and their offspring.[88] This is not allowed, so fat, insulin-resistant men always have high blood pressure and coronary artery disease (cholesterol plaqueing) that in time leads to a heart attack, a man's heart attack.[89]

Thunder in My Heart

Premenopausal women have sudden vasospasm in the absence of progesterone's dampening effect on twitchy estrogen receptors.[90-91] A younger woman's heart attack, sudden vasospasm,[92-95] damages the heart because the clamping down of the heart's arteries and veins, constricting and shutting off blood flow, creating the "white knuckle effect" you see in your hand when you make a really tight fist. When the heart muscle is deprived of blood and the oxygen it carries, it dies.[96] Men's heart attacks cause oxygen deprivation to the muscle, too.[97]

In men, because they've eaten too much of the planet, a heart attack is "environmental." On their way to a heart attack, first their kidneys are affected by the constant water retention of a high-carbohydrate diet.[98] You need a lot of water to hibernate, so the more sugar you eat, the more water you retain[99-101] (that's why on a high-protein, no-carbohydrate diet, the first ten to fifteen pounds of weight loss is actually stored water). Carrying that water weight twelve months a year instead of three, and never dropping it, stresses hormone responses between the adrenal glands and the kidneys trying to control blood pressure and volume for the whole body.[102] This waterlogged state causes chronic subclinical hypertension.

High insulin from long light and too many carbohydrates also means high serotonin. Serotonin is a vasoconstrictor and controls blood clotting. During mating season, when fighting among men would be more likely, serotonin is always high perhaps to keep men from bleeding to death. Water retention, together with elevated serotonin narrowing arteries and veins, creates a disease state known as *hypertension*.[103]

The hormones from the kidney, angiotensin I and II,[104] that report to the heart how hard and fast to pump the blood[105] must alter this feedback loop when chronic subclinical hypertension damages the heart. That happens when your blood pressure doesn't fluctuate normally but instead stays high, never giving the heart a break. This heavy workload causes the left side of the heart muscle to "overdevelop" to compensate. When this happens, hypertension has led to *left ventricular hypertrophy*.[106-107] This damage is irreversible and makes the heart work even harder because its symmetry is altered.

Simultaneously, as high blood pressure is creating this scenario, the heart is also developing cholesterol plaqueing. When we eat sugar, it's turned into the factions of cholesterol—very low density lipoproteins

Carbohydrates Drive Up Insulin, Switches on HMG-CoA Reductase

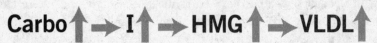

Carbo ↑ → I ↑ → HMG ↑ → VLDL ↑

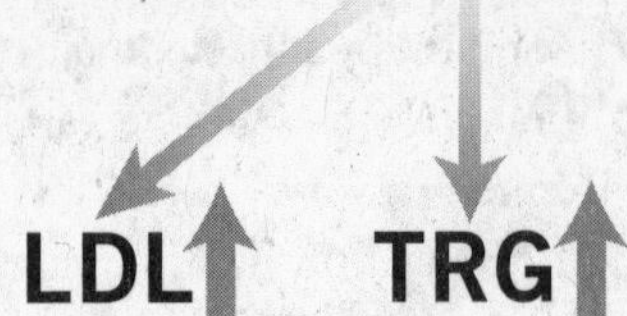

Cholesterol is the backbone of the steroid hormone production pathway. Cholesterol is so important that when it's not available from saturated fats, you make it from sugar in summer as a backup mechanism.

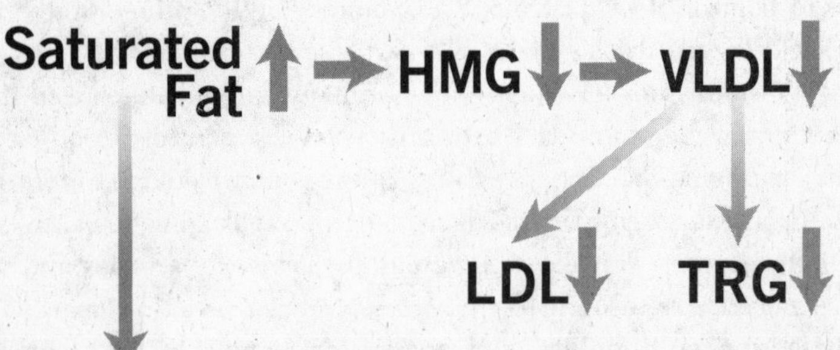

When you eat cholesterol it becomes chylomicrons and HDLs.

I	Insulin
HMG	HMG-CoA-reductase
VLDL	Very low-density lipo
LDL	Low-density lipo
TRG	Triglyceride
HDL	High-density lipo

(VLDLs)—in the liver by the enzyme HMG CoA-reductase.[108] VLDLs become intermediate-density lipoproteins (IDLs) and then low-density lipoproteins (LDLs) or triglycerides. VLDLs, IDLs, and LDLs constitute the cholesterol "number" that all of America lives in fear of.[109] High-density lipoproteins (HDL) scoop up VLDLs, IDLs, and LDLs and take them back to the liver for recycling.[110] That's why doctors refer to HDLs as the "good cholesterol." These factions of cholesterol are the components of the cholesterol plaqueing found in the arteries of men's hearts as they age.[111-112] They're primarily found in the arteries of women *after* menopause.[113-116]

Heart of Gold

Triglycerides, which are high in all of us any time we eat sugar, are the part of the sugar you've consumed that sticks to your backside to "insulate" you from cold and starvation.[117] The insulin weight that accumulates around the middle in men and, later, in women as they age is the other half of the cholesterol equation and the reason that the cholesterol-lowering drug Lipitor is not a weight-loss aid. The drugs invented to lower cholesterol knockout the enzyme HMG CoA-reductase, the enzyme that makes VLDLs, not triglycerides.[118] "Good" cholesterol, high-density lipoprotein or HDL, is made in men's and women's guts under the control of estrogen. There are no drugs to raise HDLs. As a man's testosterone drops with aging, he has less to convert to estrogen and his lipid profile gets skewed, even if he's not fat and hypertensive.

High blood pressure causes your blood to rush through narrowed veins and arteries harder and faster. The rush of the blood, the velocity of the push and pull, is called *shear stress*.[119] Your arteries actually *feel* the blood flowing through them. The sensors that read how hard your blood pushes and pulls are called *endothelial cells*,[120] and the endothelial cells lining your heart and vascular system are called the *intima*. That makes sense because they are the *intimate* control between life and death in you. In response to blood pressure, velocity, and the hormones that they detect in the blood, endothelial cells control the fluid dynamics of your circulatory system.[121] As well as keeping you standing, these cells are alive in their own right, too. They actually "decide" how and when to spread out the forces of flow to avoid dangerous extremes[122-124] of pressure.

They also control how the free fatty acids that are floating in your blood are eventually metabolized in response to sex hormones.[125-133] The floating cholesterol from the sugar you've eaten is too abundant when summer continues all year just to be used as fuel.[134] Besides, the system is designed for you to use cholesterol or free fatty acids as fuel in the *absence* of carbohydrates, not while you are still consuming them. The higher-than-normal serotonin you make when your insulin is always up[135] makes your blood platelets sticky enough to clot. Then the expanded volume and velocity of subclinical hypertension alone causes your blood to rush into your heart and slam around the corners. This abrupt change in shear stress, which is the mechanical effect of the blood rushing against the walls lining your arteries, will cause endothelial "migration."[136-137]

Piece of My Heart

Under shear stress, endothelial cells "migrate" with their little feet, called *pseudopodia*, which leaves a bare spot on the artery wall.[138-140] Free-floating cholesterol will then collect in the bare spot—thanks to "adhesion factors" also controlled by sex hormones[141-143]—to form a Band-Aid.

This is known as cholesterol plaqueing, which causes the recruitment of inflammatory factors, like macrophages and lymphocytes, to the area.[144-145] The "healing" of the bare spot by the cholesterol makes a huge mess of scar tissue called *foam cells*.[146] These lumpy bumps close off the flow space in your already narrowed artery, and when a blood clot finally sticks, as eventually it will, you have a completely blocked artery. That's a heart attack. A stroke is the same process, and is also caused by high blood pressure, but it happens in your brain.

These events never happen to real women, hormonally speaking.

They only happen to women with the hormonal profile of a man.[147] That is, to old women, which is how nature views us when we're out of estrogen and progesterone.

Estrogen and progesterone, *in tandem* control:

- cholesterol metabolism (how much and how long it hangs around)[148]
- homocysteine levels[149-150]

- nitric oxide action (vasodialation)[151-152]
- clotting factors, endothelin 1, thromboxin A2, fibrogen
- inflammatory reactions to abrasion
- shear stress involving C-reactive protein
- fibrinolysis (dissolving of blood clots)[153-154]
- atrial naturetic peptide (ANP) and nerve growth factor[155]

in a normal, natural way that no drug can ever hope to match. Estrogen is actually antiproliforative in studies on increased left ventricular mass (thanks to ANP), *meaning high blood pressure can be normalized by natural hormone replacement, and left ventricular hypertrophy can be avoided.*[156-158]

It only makes sense that this truth is the case, because young women are full of naturally produced hormones and they don't have heart attacks.

Unchain My Heart

How your heart beats matters, too. It's called *cardiac coherence*. The beating mechanism slides into dysfunction in sudden vasospasm. Estrogen and progesterone are in control of the wiring. The electricity for your "body electric" comes from the ion fluxes between the outside and inside of each cell. Just like the batteries in your flashlight, salts like potassium, sodium, and calcium trade places through channels in the cell's membrane to make the spark. These ion fluxes determine the cell membrane *potential* of each and every cell, minute to minute, second to second. Membrane potential is the ability of the cell to conduct electricity—that is, do we spark? Too much firing, erratic firing, or too little firing are states known as tachycardia, bradycardia, and cardiomyopathy, respectively.

These misfires, or arrhythmias, are seen in women as a fundamental gender difference because women have more difficulty with repolarization than men do under the same circumstances. That means women can't pick up the beat as well as men can. Estrogen controls calcium release and modulates calcium channels; as your estrogen falls off, your heart muscle gets "twitchy" or hyperreactive because calcium flux can become dysfunctional. Progesterone blocks the estrogen receptors in your heart muscle to calm down hyperreactivity.

Hyperreactivity was examined by researchers at the Division of Reproductive Sciences at the Oregon Regional Primate Research Center in rhesus monkeys whose hearts were young and healthy. R. Minshall and colleagues reported in the *Journal of Clinical Endocrinology and Metabolism* in 1998 that they ovariectomized (they took out their ovaries) the monkeys and made up cocktails of vasospasm-inducing substances identified from the blood of women who had experienced vasospasm.[159]

The researchers injected the monkeys with this prescription for death—serotonin, thromboxin A2, endothelin 1, or angiotensin II. Although no one agent alone caused vasospasm, the combination was pathophysiologic in five out of the seven monkeys—they died. When they went on logically to use HRT in the same set of circumstances, they found that estrogen plus progestins did not protect from coronary vasospasm, but natural estrogen (17-beta estradiol) plus natural progesterone did.[160]

They concluded that "vascular hyper-reactivity, which may be the critical factor involved in the increased incidence of coronary artery vasospasm and ischemic heart disease [regular heart attack, too] in post-menopausal women, can be normalized by E2 [17-beta estradiol] and/or P [natural progesterone] through direct actions on the coronary artery vascular muscle cells."[161] No surprises here. Natural progesterone *with* natural 17-beta estradiol (the estrogen in your body) works, but synthetic progestins not only don't protect, they *cause* stroke and heart attack, and studies[162-163] supporting this premise have been around long enough to be included in the historical report by Grady and Rubin.

Shot Through the Heart

Beyond their ability to negate all of the positive effects of estrogen, horse or otherwise, progestins completely interfere with vascularization, clotting factors, how cholesterol is metabolized by the endothelial cells lining your heart,[164-165] and the calcium exchange that controls polarization,[166] or firing, in the muscle cells of your heart. And we're sure it interferes with at least a thousand other things.[167-173] They do that by blocking your estrogen receptors. Natural progesterone blocks estrogen receptors, too, but in a normal rhythmic cycle with a molecule evolved for the job.[174] Progestins are drugs, not hormones.

Blocking estrogen changes how your arteries dilate and respond to any and all stimuli. Estrogen receptors come in at least two flavors, alpha and beta. There is new and significant research implicating estrogen in blood pressure control through estrogen receptor beta. This news implies that if you can't receive estrogen cyclically, your blood pressure is not under tight control. Rats bred to have genetically inactivated beta receptors all developed moderate hypertension.

You should know that genetically inactivated estrogen receptors in rats aren't really much different than continuously (or chronically) blocked estrogen receptors by natural progesterone or progestins.[175] Taking natural progesterone continuously, without making a cycle, will wipe out the action all of your estrogen response, which will eventually keep you from receiving progesterone, too.

The "cancer-fighting" drug Herceptin, considered a boon to womankind when it was invented, uses a lab-derived antigen (antibody) that fits into the epidermal growth factor receptor (EGFR) to slow the tumor growth in HER-2 breast cancer.[176] There are more than a few things wrong with this drug. The first thing is, it was invented to fill a growth factor receptor that is already known by science to be turned off by estrogen.[177] Instead of losing profit margin on 17-beta estradiol, which could do the job naturally, the pharmaceutical company Genentech, Inc., invented a man-made antibody to fit into the EGFR to do the same thing.

Herceptin, their drug, will turn off EGFR successfully (slowing the growth of HER-2 breast cancer) until your immune system identifies Herceptin as "nonself"—that is, not you—and creates a string of antibodies to counter Genentech's antibody. The third or fourth antibody generated down the line acts exactly like the *herculin* molecule. Herculin is the natural switch that turns on the EGFR made in your own body. So, eventually, Herceptin by Genentech creates the same effect that it was designed to block.[178-179] One of the reasons this matters to your heart is that nature creates this rebound effect because EGFR is a major player in heart muscle tone.

There's worse news for takers of tamoxifen: the epidermal growth factor receptor, in tandem with estrogen and progesterone, creates the muscle tone in your heart. Muscle tone is the indicator of a strong steady beat. The exercise gurus promise that a hard workout will strengthen heart muscle when in fact only hormones can do that. If you turn off EGFR for too long with Herceptin or turn off estrogen reception for too long with tamoxifen, you lose muscle tone in your heart, a clinical sign of old age called *cardiomyopathy*. Treatment with Herceptin causes cardiomyopathy.

Cardiomyopathy is not curable. Women on these drugs can die from the treatment, not from their breast cancer. Women on Herceptin can also die from cardiac arrest.[180]

The interaction of estrogen on the EGFR happens not just in your breast and heart, but all over the body, naturally. Estrogen and progesterone are reciprocal hormones. Insulin and thyroid hormone create estrogen receptors. When estrogen meets its receptor at a high enough level, a progesterone receptor is created. When progesterone finds its receptor, estrogen activity is halted. This *negative* feedback loop stops insulin and estrogen from permanently stimulating growth factor receptors like EGFR. But when progesterone is gone because ovulation has stopped because estrogen is too low and too chronic to make a preovulatory peak, medical science proposes blocking what little estrogen reception you have without ever investigating the effects of estrogen deprivation on your heart and brain.

Estrogen receptors were shown to be responsible for a reduction of blood levels of cholesterol and less invasive plaque lesions when estradiol was in place. Cholesterol and plaqueing are the key elements in the postmenopausal heart attack, also known as a "man's heart attack," because without estrogen, we can't deal with aging any better than men can.

The big news is a new drug trial using the SERM raloxifene, tamoxifen's closest cousin, in coronary heart disease. Yes, that means they're trying to find a new "off-label" use for their drug, which is now prescribed for breast cancer and osteoporosis. "Off-label" just means any use for which the drug was not intentionally created. They actually intend to shut down what estrogen reception is left in forty- to sixty-year-old women in their hearts on purpose. The recruitment goal of this study is ten thousand women.

Our goal is to make sure you aren't one of them.

My Heart Will Go On

When you have a purpose in nature, better yet, when you have *the* purpose in nature—being reproductive—sex hormones do double duty in your heart. As long as you continue to mate, give birth, and breast-feed, it seems that you are protected from the ravages of sleep loss, high insulin, and high cortisol in a way that men are not.

Women's hearts are not men's hearts until after menopause.

If there's no money in the actual cure for cancer, natural hormones, and if they also cure heart disease, then there is certainly no money in the eradication of heart disease in women. There is, however, an extraordinary amount of money in the treatment of heart disease. It's almost as big a bonanza as Type II diabetes.

Because going to sleep when it's dark outside and eating no carbohydrates in the winter is too hard for us as individuals and remarkably unprofitable for the industry of medicine as a whole, we have been sold a class of drugs called *statins.* Lipitor is probably the one familiar to most of us because of the relentless advertising campaigns.

One ad shows a woman jumping into her waiting husband's car after her doctor's appointment. The mood of the ad is dark and rainy, even stormy. She turns and says to him, "The doctor says my numbers aren't good."

They drive off, both looking terrified. Cut.

Next we see the same scene in bright sunlight with birds singing.

She turns and smiles and says, "Honey, he says my numbers are great, now." They drive away into the sunset, giggling with relief.

Not too subtle.

Her numbers weren't good because she's a woman of "a certain age," as the French say—insulin-resistant, chronic low estrogen, no progesterone, prolactin up, melatonin down, testosterone approaching low male levels, and no cortisol to speak of. She could be pre- or postmenopausal. If her doctor had thought to offer her hormones, she might have said no after the last canceled heart trial. Or perhaps she asked for them and he told her she was safer on Lipitor.

He would have told her this because of the Scandinavian Simvastatin Survival Study[181] back in the early 1990s, which reported a reduction of total mortality of 30 percent in 4,444 patients (mostly men) who were treated with HMG CoA-reductase–lowering drugs. We've already explained about the ninety different ways that the researchers can "cook" the numbers in any study. This one was no different. They claimed a 30 percent reduction in mortality on the difference between 9.5 percent death from cardiac arrest in the placebo group versus 5.4 percent in the Simvastatin group *in men*. Of

4,444 people in the study, 3,617 were men. The 30 percent reduction is really only 145 people, or 4 percent of 3,617.

This is a quote from the authors of this famous study that underpins all clinical use of statin drugs: "There was no significant effect on non-MI acute events." That means there was no improvement at all in the statistics of any pathological cardiac event except heart attack or myocardial infarction (MI). More important, to us as women, there were only 827 of us included in the 4,444 study participants. The authors also admit that "mortality in women as a group was not decreased." A study done by the University of Illinois on 506 men who had bypass surgery found that only 14 percent had cholesterol levels above 240. Fifty percent of the men had levels below the danger zone of 200.[182-183] No wonder the Scandinavian Simvastatin Study needed to portray the results as much better than they were, because your cholesterol number, even if you are a man, has very little to do with the potential of cardiac arrest.[184]

The doctor of our woman in the commercial also may have cited the National Cholesterol Education Program guidelines, which include aging, no hormones, obesity, and diet as risk factors. If you have a high-fat diet (higher than 20 percent ten years ago; today a 10 percent fat diet is encouraged), your estimate of risk skyrockets. This metabolic misinformation has been sold to the public since the 1980s, when the factions of cholesterol were identified. When it was discovered that the cholesterol in an egg had the same chemical constituents as the plaque in your heart, medical science made the impossible leap to the notion that "if you eat it, you wear it," arterially speaking. Not so.

In 1997, the *American Journal of the College of Nutrition* said as much: "Many studies reported over the past 2 years have shown that dietary cholesterol is not a significant factor in an individual's plasma cholesterol level or in cardiovascular disease risk. Reports from the Lipid Research Clinics Research Prevalence Study and the Framingham Heart Study have shown that dietary cholesterol is not related to either blood cholesterol levels or heart disease deaths."

In fact, through the method of "competitive inhibition," the reverse is actually true—if you eat enough *saturated* fat in meat, eggs, butter, and whole milk, you will down regulate HMG CoA-reductase and make less cholesterol out of carbohydrates.[185] This fact has never stopped the drug companies.

Faced with the scientific evidence that “diet,” in this ca[illegible] could not contain the epidemic of heart disease in Am[illegible] tinued to prescribe lower and lower percentages of fat in [illegible] restricting two of the three available food groups—protein and fa[illegible] encouraged the overconsumption of carbohydrates, furthering the insulin resistance needed to clog everyone’s arteries. Since low-fat living was clearly not going to help, because the principle was flawed, the only path left (other than to recant) was to invent the “statins.” Which they did, with little or no forethought about what disasters might occur in *other* parts of your body deprived of an essential enzyme like HMG CoA-reductase.

Hungry Heart

The statins stop cholesterol production all over the body and brain. Chole-*sterol* is a precursor to *steroid* hormones. Cholesterol becomes pregnelonone, which becomes progesterone, which becomes testosterone and cortisol, which become estrogen and dihydrotestosterone (DHT), and so on and so on. Reproductive girls have consistently higher absolute cholesterol values than boys because of cholesterol’s importance in reproduction.[186] Cholesterol esters are converted to progesterone in human granulosa cells in the ovary and the testes; HMG CoA-reductase converts cholesterol to make sperm. The same process goes on in the brain.[187] You can’t make enough neurosteroids (estrogen and progesterone used as neurotransmitters) locally in the brain[188] when you’re on statins.[189-191] Rapid brain growth in babies and liver and immune function in all of us depends on having available HMG CoA-reductase.

If you take Lipitor, you don’t have this enzyme available.

Cholesterol is inhibited by as much as 70 percent by statin drugs like Lipitor. Different variations of these drugs inhibit cholesterol tissue *selectively*, meaning, in your eyes, that some will cause cataracts, while those in other places in your body will cause infertility or cancer.[192-193] The *Journal of the American Medical Association* published an article in 1996 entitled “Carcinogenicity of Lipid-Lowering Drugs.”[194] This article reported that “All members of the two most popular classes of lipid-lowering drugs (fibrates and statins) cause cancer in rodents, in some cases at levels of animal exposure close to those prescribed to humans. Evidence of carcinogenicity of ı-lowering drugs from clinical trials in humans is inconclusive because . inconsistent results and insufficient duration of follow-up."

In other words, they'd rather not know. Or know about the evidence connecting statins to Alzheimer's, blindness, joint pain, erectile dysfunction, weight gain, diabetes, brain damage, depression, and an excess of death by suicide.[195-196] The only side effects connected with statin use published by the drug company are constipation, flatulence, dyspepsia, frank abdominal pain, and liver failure.

What is dangerous is what Lipitor really does to your artery wall while it makes your "numbers" look *good*. After a first heart attack, people on HMG CoA-reductase inhibitors were far less likely to survive a second one than people not taking these drugs.

Many women on Premarin have been prescribed these lipid-lowering drugs. The interaction between these two drugs has never been addressed. Although Premarin has estrogenic effects, it is not the estrogen produced in your body, so it has side effects. The most pertinent one to the discussion of conventional HRT and heart disease is Premarin's power to raise C-reactive protein,[197] the one absolute marker for heart attack. As a result, cardiologists who routinely check this marker in a woman on Premarin would find it high and offer her Lipitor. Doctors will prescribe Premarin and Lipitor together instead of natural estrogen for patients. Natural transdermal estrogen—17-beta estradiol—never raises C-reactive protein and keeps arteries clear, eliminating two risk factors for heart disease and two for Alzheimer's.

How Can You Mend a Broken Heart?

Since C-reactive protein is also a marker for subclinical infection in pregnant women, obstetricians in France looked at the C-reactive protein levels in eighty-five pregnant women admitted to the hospital for normal labor and delivery. The control group was twelve *not*-pregnant young women. C-reactive protein was normal until the onset of labor, when "dramatic increases" were seen that continued postpartum.[198]

The sharp fall of estrogen and progesterone at labor and delivery is not just the trigger for prolactin production to breast-feed; this drop is also the trigger for the entire immune system to kick into overdrive to program the baby's immune system.

C-reactive protein is part and parcel of that cascade.

When your hormones are finally gone and you're completely autoimmune and swimming in prolactin, it just so happens that the C-reactive protein elevation seen in heart disease is no higher than it is postpartum. The problem is that it just goes on too long. The postpartum period is a transient state—estrogen comes back and prolactin drops, eventually you ovulate, and then in the real world you'd become pregnant again.

That's not going to happen in our lives anymore.

But we can put back 17-beta estradiol and real natural progesterone, we can make a cycle to fool Mother Nature into thinking we can still reproduce, that we are still viable. Without this hormonal sleight of hand, the falloff of estrogen and progesterone, which triggers lactation and its attendant heightened autoimmune state at labor and delivery and for months afterward, may, as we elucidated in Chapter Four, cause breast cancer, and now, you can see, a heart attack as well.

Unfortunately, the inflammation, due to the lack of rhythmic estrogen and progesterone, forming around the sites of plaqueing in your heart is also forming around the buildup (plaqueing) of a protein called *beta-amyloid* in your brain, which would normally be disposed of by estrogen.

While a stroke is occasionally referred to as a "brain attack," in the same vein as a heart attack, the inflammatory state of affairs roiling in your brain, in the absence of hormones, is most often called *senile dementia*, or Alzheimer's disease.

eight

PAINT IT BLACK

Dying of cancer is something we all fear. Having a heart attack, although it seems more remote, because we don't hear about it on television every day, would probably kill us where we stand. But the possibility of losing our minds and independence and not even really knowing it is truly the most dreaded potential out there ahead of us.

Every day, we're all one day closer to Alzheimer's disease.[1-3]

And it's preventable, according to the gold standard of research at hand. Dementia, memory loss, and Alzheimer's are preventable with natural hormones prescribed in a cycle that mimics the rhythmic, escalating, and descending doses your body naturally produced when you were young; this is *not* the case with conventional HRT. Over four million people suffer from Alzheimer's disease, which affects one in two people over the age of eighty.[4] That means if you're in a room with one other person right now, it will, sooner or later, down the line, be you or him.

Fifty Thousand Miles Beneath My Brain

Hormones produced in your brain like estrogen and progesterone orchestrate, directly and indirectly, your entire nervous system.[5-29] Your nervous system, under the control of directives from the brain,[30] includes your heart, stomach, liver, pancreas, and immune system. All of these organs were created from the neural crest[31] when you were an embryo. The neural crest is the visible backbone of the tadpole fetus in the pictures of life in utero.[32-34]

The cells of the neural crest divide and differentiate into your brai stomach, liver, and pancreas, all connected by your spinal cord to t side world by your immune system.

All of these organs respond not only to hormones fitting into their receptors directly, but to proteins called *neurotransmitters*, such as serotoni dopamine, and acetylcholine. These neurotransmitters are the stop/star currency of cells called neurons in your brain and in target organs and muscles. All of the firing, the snap-crackle-and-pop of thinking, moving, and even autonomic functions like lungs breathing and hearts beating, happens because of neurotransmitters and thereby indirectly because of hormones.[35-37]

Hormones made in the brain can act too locally as neurotransmitters,[38] effecting the other neurotransmitters[39] or the axons, which are the cables and wiring along which firing happens.[40-42] That fact is the reason that synthetic hormones and derivatives of hormones from another species like the horse cause such havoc in your body and brain. You are hardwired for the radio frequency of sex hormones, insulin, and prolactin to read the environment and, literally, throw the switches on your behavior and thinking. The main mechanism of destruction that ensues when you take Premarin isn't caused by its weak estrogenic action.[43] It's caused by an immune response to Premarin due to a cross-species reaction, because, for your body, it's a foreign substance that actually puts your immune system on alert.[44-46]

Progestins, on the other hand, also confuse all your neurological systems because they have the power to affect estrogen, progesterone, and testosterone receptors, but not in any natural or known template, because they are *invented*. They *do not* occur in nature.[47]

Since all of the cells in your brain produce sex hormones from cholesterol, the entire nervous system from your head to your toes and fingers is really itself an *endocrine* system. And why estrogen and progesterone are also classified as *neuro*steroids.[48-50]

The *Journal of Clinical Endocrinology and Metabolism*,[51] in a review article sponsored by the Endocrine Society, reported that "estrogen maintains function of key neural structures, such as the hippocampus and basal forebrain, and the widely projecting dopaminergic, serotogenic, and noradrenergic systems." That's pretty much *all* of your brain. "As estrogen levels decline over the menopause, these systems and the cognitive and other t depend on them also decline, at least functionally; *to estrogen replacement*."[52] That means that run- akes you display the behaviors that we all identify as estrogen back can reverse that. Insulin resistance and terol levels in old age are a compensitory mechanism to pro- e estrogen in the brain.

holesterol becomes pregnelanone, then progesterone, then testos- terone, and finally testosterone converts through aromatase[53-56] to the most active sex steroid in the brain—estrogen. The irony here is that the drugs for high cholesterol, osteoporosis, or cancer that will be prescribed to you as you age *naturally* can cause brain injury in a myriad of other ways[57-58] that can only exacerbate aging even further.

Accidents Will Happen

In fact, taking Lipitor, tamoxifen, raloxifene, or Arimidex will increase your chances of developing brain disease.[59-70] Cholesterol-inhibiting drugs, by inhibiting the enzyme HMG-CoA-reductase locally in the brain, can cause dementia[71] faster than normal aging can without drugs, because cholesterol is the precursor needed to make estrogen and progesterone in the brain.[72-76] Tamoxifen, too, is well documented to cause brain damage and memory loss by blocking estrogen reception in the brain.[77-78]

When doctors misuse testosterone as hormone replacement for women, it seems to make you better because it converts to estrogen in the brain, just as our own adrenal testosterone does as long as we have aromatase around. Remember, it takes some body fat to have aromatase,[79] being thin is a deficit. The trendy new aromatase inhibitors like Arimidex now being used to block estrogen production in breast cancer must cause dementia in the long run—because testosterone converts to estrogen by way of aromatase, and it's estrogen that controls brain function primarily on its own and also through the generation of progesterone receptors.[80]

Here, There, and Everywhere

Both insulin and thyroid hormone foster the creation of estrogen receptors in the body and brain. Just as elsewhere in the body, when estrogen (17-beta estradiol) is received, either through its receptor or on a gene's estrogen response element (ERE), progesterone receptors appear all over the brain, too. Thyroid hormone is a peptide hormone like insulin, but acts like sex hormones (steroids) in the brain. All of these hormones control the expression of genes that make growth factors and neurotransmitters at the behest of estrogen and progesterone and their effect on their own receptors.[81-83]

One of the best-documented effects of steroid hormones in the brain is the action of the metabolite or end product of progesterone on the receptor for a neurotransmitter called *g-aminobutyric acid* (GABA).[84] GABA's effect on your circuitry is to smooth you out and calm you down. Gabanergic effects are well known to be soporific. Escalating progesterone turns on GABA; that's why we're so very sleepy in early pregnancy and so tired right before a menstrual period. Estrogen, through a much different route, is in charge of serotonin transport and is the facilitator of antidepressant effects from selective serotonin reuptake inhibitors (SSRIs) by way of the progesterone effect on GABA. Estrogen receptors go up when insulin crosses the blood-brain barrier; at the same time, so does serotonin. Estrogen, through the generation of progesterone receptors, is the tail end of the whip, so to speak, of antidepressant action through GABA.[85-86]

In the brain, the high levels of escalating estrogen and progesterone in pregnancy have also been found to change the brain in some permanent fashion, too, just like p53 in the nucleus of all cells. That means pregnancy and lactation serve to developmentally design continuing brain health. University of Richmond professor Craig Kinsley reported that[87] "Our research shows that the hormones of pregnancy are *protective* in the brain." His group's tests on rats show that those who raise two or more litters of pups do significantly better in tests of memory and skills than rats who have no babies, and their brains show changes that suggest they may be protected against such diseases as Alzheimer's, too. Kinsley concluded his report with, "It's rat data, but humans are mammals just like these animals are mammals."

From the vantage point of our research, it only makes sense that moms get smarter—they have to. The problem-solving requirements of child rearing would presuppose that the high hormones of pregnancy would "condition" and prepare mom's brain for the upcoming more complicated tasks of keeping two people alive.

FM (No Static At All)

The brain's architecture is constantly being modified and remodeled, depending on the demands that it must meet. In order to retain the same plasticity of youth, your brain must be soaked in hormones that control all of the on and off switches as well as the maintenance routines. The brain really is a yin and yang like every other system in the body, but in this case, it consists of white and gray matter made up of cells called *neurons* and *glia.*

Glia cells are both big and small—*macro*glia and *micro*glia.

Macroglia take the shape of *Schwann cells* and *astrocytes*. These macroglia affect all aspects of neuron migration (where and how neurons travel) and maturation, survival, and differentiation—that is, what *kind* of nerve impulse the neuron carries. Schwann cells are macroglia that "myelinate" *axons*. Axons are the "wiring" between neurons. Myelin is the pretty plastic coating insulating and feeding the wires. Schwann cells morph octopuslike and wrap around axions.[88-90] How many times they wrap or how thick the coating on the wire is determines the speed of communication the axon can handle.

When this coating is missing or thinning, because your immune system isn't suppressed by progesterone, the neuron demyelinates. Progestins and Premarin actually cause demyelination and an inflammatory brain state, whereas natural estrogen makes progesterone receptors happen and natural progesterone suppresses immune reactions that degrade and deteriorate the myelin sheath.

Not only the speed of the transmission and the heat it generates matters, but the distance the communication must travel matters, too. If one axon must reach from your head to your toe—and they do—the myelin must be very thick so the axon can stand the molecular heat and chemoelectrical stress of rapid-fire communication. That's why peripheral nerves farthest from the brain are often the first affected by the demyelination of multiple sclerosis (MS) or amyotrophic lateral sclerosis (ALS).[91-92] Your legs fail first because they're farthest away.

Free Fallin'

All of these brain cells, the neurons and the different forms of the glia, are capable of receiving and reacting to estrogen, progesterone, and testosterone, as well as thyroid hormone and cortisol. The small glia in the brain have a function comparable to immune cells like *macrophages*, or white cells, in the rest of the body. *Microglia* serve as the immune system of the brain. They occur more densely in gray matter and near blood vessels.

These microglia change shape and become mobile to travel to injury sites and assault debris by eating away dead tissue through inflammatory response, including the recruitment of immune factors called *cytokines*. Any metabolic dysfunction like high blood sugar, insulin resistance, or hormone deprivation is seen as an injury as well, because as the cells die, they provoke the same kind of inflammatory reaction as germs, viruses, or the violence of Alzheimer's, MS, ALS, and AIDS brain syndrome.[93-94] So running out of hormones—estrogen and progesterone—can spike an immune response. Sex hormones actually "activate and deactivate" the nervous system. In adults, the effects of sex hormones are reversible, meaning the effects only last as long as the hormone is around. Exactly the same ups and downs of FSH, estrogen, LH, and progesterone that we traveled through as we discussed *ovulation*, control myelination of neurons simultaneously.[95-112] The *natural* fluctuations in estrogen levels stimulate a coordinated and *dramatic* reorganization of synapses and glia on a monthly basis. The rhythm of hormones, cyclically, unsheath and resheath axions and retracted neurons. The preovulatory surge in estrogen literally remyelinates the brain and body (spinal cord included) every month.[113-129]

Flirtin' with Disaster

Taking these facts into consideration, you can see why losing your menstrual cycle affects your mind in such an elaborate way.[130] An article published in the *Journal of Neurobiology* by Cynthia L. Jordan[131] at Berkeley states, "It is clear that estrogen can promote synapse formation in the brain." And she concludes, "Exogenous estrogen produces the same effects." That means we should be able to get our minds and memories back with the correct hormone replacement. Bio-identical estradiol and progesterone replacement should successfully replace lost youth in the brain.

Progesterone modulates, among others, nicotinic receptors in the brain. *Nicotine* was so named because it affects these receptors. Nicotinic receptors use a neurotransmitter called *acetylcholine*, too.[132] Acetylcholine is the neurotransmitter that enhances the flow of information from one neuron to another through synapses. This synaptic activity is the snap, crackle, pop of thinking. Cigarettes really do help you to think more clearly.[133] Synaptic function between neurons depends on cell adhesion molecules called *e-cadherins* that are controlled by estrogen.[134] Estrogen is the "glue" between neurons that fosters synaptic plasticity (flexibility) and dendritic growth (branching out of neurons).[135-136]

The big point here is that your brain, too, must have rhythmic blasts of estrogen and then progesterone repeatedly in different harmonies with other hormones—like thyroid, prolactin, and human growth hormone, just like your breasts, ovaries, and heart—to be healthy.[137-141]

I Go to Extremes

These facts also mean that natural hormone replacement *must* be prescribed in a rhythmic cycle, mimicking the preovulatory surge. It's the rhythm that should restore brain function, with regard to firing, memory, and synaptic activity, to peak capacity.[142-144] Scientists have proven as much.

I. Barakat-Walter published evidence[145] that thyroid hormone replacement, along with rhythmic estrogen and progesterone, regenerated nerves damaged by the immune system. This hormone replacement worked in disease states such as injury, MS, or diabetic neuropathy by preventing injured neurons from dying. Normal myelination and continued brain development throughout adulthood depends on constant rhythmic pulses of estrogen and progesterone.[146]

This mechanism of action is enacted through *estrogen and progesterone response elements*. These areas on genes allow progesterone to control the output[147] of myelin sheath *genetically* from Schwann cells, a type of glia. But without a progesterone receptor, remyelination can't happen. The timed rhythm of a peak dose of estradiol prescribed by nature on Days 11 and 12 of a normal menstrual cycle causes progesterone receptors to appear in every hormone-responsive cell in your body,[148] not just in your breasts or the lining of your uterus. Neurons, too, require estrogen, in the form of 17-beta estradiol only, to make progesterone receptors appear.

The *Journal of Steroid Biochemistry and Molecular Biology* reports that natural progesterone enhanced myelination by 65 percent (thicker myelin) and synthetic steroids had almost no effect.[149] It's clear that remyelination can't happen on synthetic progestins like MPA or the Pro in PremPro, either.

Head Games

The diminishing hormones are the cause of the classic lower back pain common in middle-aged people. If you just turn the wrong way, a normal case of nerve injury that would heal quickly and easily in someone younger, doesn't. The backache of old age is really just a case of threadbare sciatic nerves.

That's why young people aren't walking around saying "Oh, my aching back!"

In the sciatic nerves of aged rats, scientists found that natural progesterone increased the expression of the gene that remyelinates the nerves in the rat's "lower back." At main nerve junctions of communication, like the heart and brain stem, wires start to fray when hormones levels fall off. Without estrogen to peak and cause ovulation, there's no progesterone. Without progesterone to remyelinate nerves, peripheral nerve bundles that are farthest from the brain fray first. The biggest one, farthest down, after the one in the base of your neck, is at your tailbone area in your lower back.[150]

Sometimes low back pain *unaccompanied* by that familiar twinge down one leg can also be vascular, just like a migraine. In your head and heart, the neurotransmitter serotonin controls vaso*constriction*. Estrogen, in your brain, is in charge of serotonin transport. When we experience the falling estrogen of perimenopause and menopause, some of us get migraines because serotonin effects also drop.[151-152] When vaso*dilation* occurs in the absence of serotonin's vaso*constricting* effect, the vascular bundles press on nerves to cause neuralgia (face pain) or migraine or *backache*. In other words, you can have a headache in your back.[153]

The pain of weak knees in women runners are different from the wear-and-tear injuries experienced by men. Weak knees in women are the end effect of demyelination and are vascular,[154] too. All the knee surgery in the world won't get you back on track, so to speak, without natural hormone replacement.

Breakdown

Free radicals are the by-product of your breathing in every cell. Oxidation, or the breakdown of oxygen, is a chemical reaction that uses oxygen to burn with nutrients and release energy adenosine triphosphate (ATP). The by-products of the release of ATP are referred to as "free radicals." Free radicals are really loose electrons that bounce around in the mitochondria (ATP generators) of all cells. Each cell, be it brain, skin, heart, or bone, has about 10,000 mitochondria when you're young.

The ring shape of the estrogen molecule appears to have special properties with respect to the formation of free radicals, and special protective effects on cells in culture that are deprived of blood or exposed to free radical generators.[155] Every day that you live, you breathe or dissipate (remember entropy), leaving free radicals free to break down the DNA in your mitochondria, literally knocking out the lights in your cells, until they go dark and cold, and die.[156]

Free radicals are the predominant mechanism of aging in every cell in your body. Any cell that doesn't die on purpose from apoptosis or the necrosis of infection dies from "natural causes," or free radicals. In the brain, this kind of aging leads to an irreversible brain state called *dementia*. Dementia is, of course, really a complement of behaviors recognizable in mentally ill people. It just so happens that the brain shrinkage (cell death) of Alzheimer's is also seen in mentally ill people.[157]

Don't You Forget About Me

There are two major physical kinds of dementia. One, *multi-infarct* dementia, is caused by little strokes and broken blood vessels in the brain that ultimately deprive the tissue of oxygen. The other, Alzheimer's disease, was identified in 1906 by Dr. Alois Alzheimer,[158-159] who first saw the changes we call "tangles and plaqueing" in the brain tissue of a woman who had died of unusually severe mental illness. The tangled bundles of nerve fibers (called *neurofibrillary tangles*) and plaques that Dr. Alzheimer found have become the definitive diagnostic finding to distinguish Alzheimer's disease from multi-infarct dementia.[160]

As of this writing, medical literature insists that there is "no treatment that can stop Alzheimer's disease." Alzheimer's disease is, in fact, the most common cause of dementia and memory loss in older adults. One in ten of us will be diagnosed with Alzheimer's by age sixty-five, which is right around the corner for some of us. By age eighty-five, the numbers show it to be five in ten, or half of all of us. The death rate annually from Alzheimer's disease is the same as that from breast cancer at about 50,000 people a year, every year.[161-164] But now it's building.

Because of the baby boom, the total number of Americans with Alzheimer's disease, which stands at about four million now, will skyrocket to fourteen million by 2050.[165] It is a slow disease, starting with mild memory problems and ending with severe brain damage due to the tangles and plaqueing unique to the disease. Death from Alzheimer's comes eventually from the destruction to the brain stem. Breathing, heart function, gut motility, and a myriad of other unconscious, "automatic" bodily functions stop in the end stages of Alzheimer's, resulting in death to the victim.

Doctors currently say they have very little to help the Alzheimer's patient. Mostly doctors prescribe various medications to reduce the incidence of troublesome behaviors like memory loss, agitation, anxiety, depression, aggression, and sleeping problems. It bears noting that these states are also, in kind but not degree, the garden-variety behavioral symptoms of menopause.

In 1987, A. F. Jorm and colleagues reviewed forty-seven studies of the prevalence of dementia published between 1945 and 1985. Across all of the studies[166-167] the most obvious finding was that the incidence of dementia rose with increasing age, doubling with every five-year increase in age, just like cancer and heart disease. Prevalence estimates have been remarkably stable.

It's Money That Matters

Direct or indirect costs of this disease to the American public are more than $100 billion in a year. In two years, by 2005, our not-so-good friends the drug companies expect the market for a drug or drugs for Alzheimer's disease to exceed $8 billion in revenue. That means that whoever comes up with something patentable will virtually "win the lottery," just as the makers of tamoxifen thought they had.

There are two schools of thought within the drug company research on the tangles and plaques unique to the disease. In the mid-1980s, scientists determined that the tangles consisted of a protein called *tau*,[168] and the plaques contained another small protein fragment, or peptide, called *beta-*

amyloid,[169] which was one of the end pieces of the larger "amyloid precursor proteins." The researchers looking at the trees, not at the forest, are in a hot debate as to which causes the devastation of Alzheimer's, tau or beta-amyloid protein (BAP). For our purposes, we'll refer to those researchers as Tauists and BAPtists.

Losing My Religion

The Tauists are, at this writing, losing this academic debate and the BAPtists have about 80 percent of the vote. The BAPtists are convinced that beta-amyloid protein is either directly toxic (which we think is impossible in the framework of biology), or constitutes the plaque that provokes the inflammation that eventually kills the neurons,[170] or both. Beta-amyloid protein grows like a blade of grass out of the membranous cells that cover the neuron.

In young healthy brain function two scissorlike enzymes called *alpha-secretase* and *gamma-secretase*[171-172] work in a series action to clip the amyloid precursor protein twice, first near its base and then right at the base. As we age, rather than the alpha enzyme making the first cut, sometimes the errant beta makes it instead, in a slightly different place. When the gamma enzyme comes along and makes the second cut, the resulting fragment is called *beta-amyloid*. In *their* Alzheimer's theory, the protein piles up between brain cells, forming the plaques and killing the surrounding cells.[173-174] We think that's a reasonable observation, but it may not be what's actually happening *behind the scenes*.

Given the BAPtists' premise, they have set about searching for secretase *inhibitors*.[175] Remember, Alzheimer's disease is worth $8 billion. But this plan to inhibit secretase is a really bad idea because the precursor protein for secretase occurs in very normal cells, too, including the neurons next to the plaque that the drug companies would like to save.

So, really, it's get rid of the plaque, get rid of the neurons.

It's not just the neurons, either, because since secretase occurs in a variety of cells, an invented inhibitor could cause far-ranging side effects from hair loss to psychosis. But, as one drug company researcher confided, "My CEO says it's costing us $150,000 a day not to have an Alzheimer's drug on the market."[176] So the urgency to find the "cure" is obvious in the potential profit.

Brain Damage/Eclipse

Bristol-Myers Squibb, DuPont, Merck & Co., Glaxo Wellcome, and Eli Lilly and Co. are all still working on it. But the Irish company Elan, in conjunction with the makers of conventional HRT, Wyeth-Ayerst, decided it was a better idea to *vaccinate* against the protein beta-amyloid. They were hoping that this would be a drug that we would all take *for life* in the form of regular injections. Recently it was announced that Elan of Ireland and their American partner, Wyeth-Ayerst, had just canceled a 360-person trial of their new vaccine after four patients,[177] which soon blossomed to eleven, showed "clinical signs consistent with inflammation of the central nervous system."

The problem was that Elan's vaccine contained a synthetic version of the beta-amyloid protein and was intended to cause the body's own immune system to attack the real beta-amyloid being produced by the aging metabolically dysfunctional brain—and it did.

But, again, not a good idea.

This was a bad idea because inflammation is the most destructive part of the degenerative aspect of the Alzheimer's process—and they created it on purpose.

The only natural way to stop the onset of either dementia—multi-infarct or Alzheimer's—is to turn back time by taking natural, rhythmic hormone replacement *for life* when yours start to diminish.

She's Not There

A new finding further defining predisposition necessary for and the severity of damage in Alzheimer's came out of *The Nun Study*,[178-181] created by University of Kentucky researcher David Snowdon. In 1986, Snowdon discovered an ideal study population in the School Sisters of Notre Dame. The nuns made a good study group because they didn't drink or smoke and shared a similar lifestyle. From our perspective, we can also cite no childbirth, no nursing, no birth control pills, and a reasonable amount of sleep and meditation. Their diet is up for grabs, but we know the approach was, at least, "everything in moderation."

In 1987, 678 nuns[182] at six different convents eventually agreed to donate their brains to science. In 1991, Snowdon and his team in the Nun

Study received their first donated brain from the sisters. Snowdon, at the University of Kentucky's Sanders-Brown Center on Aging, had already devised a battery of tests for assessing the sisters' mental and physical abilities—tests that would later be correlated with the results of the tissue examinations. All was already going incredibly well when Snowdon hit the mother lode.

Wavelength

He found the autobiographical essays of sixteen of the nuns required for admittance to the convent in 1930. Snowdon and his colleagues knew that the "ideas density," or the number of discrete ideas per ten written words, was a good marker of cognitive function, while grammar usage was a better marker of working memory. With the essays in hand, Snowdon found that by reading their early writings he could predict with 85 to 90 percent accuracy which ones would show the physical brain damage typical of Alzheimer's disease sixty years later.

"When we first looked at the findings," Snowdon said, "we thought, Oh my God, it's in the bag by the time you're in your twenties."[183] What Dr. Snowdon means is that whether or not you will get Alzheimer's can be definitively estimated by a writing sample done in your twenties.

In one part of their study, selecting only the brains of sisters who had earned a bachelor's degree—to eliminate any differences attributable to education—they found that among nuns with physical evidence of Alzheimer's in the brain, those *who also had evidence of strokes* inevitably had the outward signs of dementia.

Snowdon's Nun Study is one of the first to look at the *cardiovascular* component of Alzheimer's disease. Simultaneously, as Snowdon was examining the vascular component of Alzheimer's, British researchers announced that Alzheimer's victims have very low blood concentrations of folic acid, a B vitamin known to speed the elimination of homocysteine in cardiac studies.[184] Folic acid deficiency is also known to play a role in some forms of mental retardation in children and in cognitive problems in adults.

One especially telling case Snowdon examined, a Sister Bernadette, who had, even at the end, never shown outward signs of Alzheimer's and whose youthful autobiography was rich with ideas and grammatical complexity, turned out, at death, to be riddled with plaques and tangles, *but very little stroking*.[185-186] That means that the same controls on vascular disease and heart disease—insulin, estrogen, and progesterone[187-192]—are at stake in brain health, as well, because it's the strokes, not the plaque and tangles, that really cause the brain to die.

Radar Love

Estrogen has long been investigated as the confounding factor in the blatant sex differences found in the *verbal* abilities between men and women. It was the verbal abilites, Snowdon concluded, that were the tip-off in the nuns' writing samples. Since estrogen has been established as the bedrock of memory, if the ability to produce grammatical complexity in youth correlates to better memory in old age, it could be concluded that the more estrogen one has in youth, the more slowly the falloff occurs in old age. Or perhaps that higher estrogen levels permanently "season" brain systems in the very same way early-in-life pregnancy permanently changes apoptosis rates in the breast and whole body, and estrogen protects the heart in cardiac studies.

Since sex hormones act as the control on all major physiological systems for survival—reproduction, heart, brain, and nervous system function—the "falling apart" of those systems in aging really starts at the end of perimenopause, when you've been out of hormonal balance for at least ten years, unless you've spent the major portion of your adult life replacing those rhythmic hormones with long escalating expanses of time consumed by multiple pregnancies and bouts of nursing. Then you'd be healthier in old age as a "reward" in nature for doing your part. The relationship between the physical and emotional is through neural and immune pathways which are controlled by hormones that cause you to nurture and love. That's really *how* hearts and brains are connected, by nerves and hormones. And *why* things that occur in your mind, like love, seem to come from your heart.

Manic Depression

Both Snowden's Nun Study and the epidemiology of Alzheimer's, then, speak to the benefit of a life lived in simpler, more recognizable rhythms[193]—less electricity, less food, less medical intervention and drugs, and more children and more breast-feeding. Short of starting to live in the dark and eat dirt tomorrow, meditate in between, and, of course, somehow turn back the clock and have a bunch of kids, what's there to do? Well, if, in fact, sex hormones control the neurotransmitters, like dopamine for memory, serotonin for impulse control,[194] GABA to calm us down, and acetylcholine for the flow from one neuron to another, we might just have a chance by putting estrogen and progesterone back in the form of natural transdermal hormone replacement.[195]

Of the forty studies published and subsequently reviewed by Jorm and others, eleven were from the United States, six were Japanese, three were from developed Asian economies, and two were from Australia. The rest were from developing parts of the world—for instance, Nigeria, Kashmir, sub-Saharan Africa, and the Cree Native American Indians. To the surprise of most of the researchers, the studies overall reported unusually *low* prevalence rates for dementia.[196]

So if doing crossword puzzles, memorizing names, or as Snowdon hoped, advanced education could stave off dementia, developed nations with educated populations bombarded with the stimulus of technology should fare better than our more simply living brothers—but that's not the case. The underdeveloped nations, when they have elderly people, do not show the great rates of dementia that we do. Since the prevalence studies compared *living* elderly in developed nations to living elderly in undeveloped nations, the numbers were not skewed by shortened life expectancy in undeveloped nations.

Can't Get It Out of My Head

The drug companies have their own agenda—to patent substances that they can sell exclusively—but even if they didn't, they could make a decent living just selling estrogen to eradicate Alzheimer's. Multiple studies using the real stuff—estradiol and natural progesterone—prove the point. Researchers in a study presented in the *Journal of Nature Medicine*[197] in April 1998 stated, "Here we present evidence that *physiological* levels of 17-beta estradiol reduce the generation of beta-amyloid plaques in human embryonic cerebrocortical neurons."

According to the *Journal of Biological Chemistry*[198] in April 2002,

Rockefeller University researchers found that "17-beta estradiol lowers Alzheimer's beta-amyloid generation by stimulating the trans-golgi network vesicle biogenesis." That's just one of the mechanisms by which estrogen, when it's around, controls the plaqueing of Alzheimer's.

Cornell University researchers reported in 1994, in the *Journal of Biological Chemistry*,[199] that "We found that physiological levels of 17-beta-estradiol regulates the metabolism of Alzheimer's beta-amyloid precursor protein." Again, natural estrogen, estradiol, stops the beta-amyloid plaqueing of Alzheimer's.

But what about the tangles and brain damage from free radical oxidation?

The tangle formation and the disruption of neurons' stores of calcium ions that are critical to nerve firing (remember membrane potentiation) are the devastating *aftermath* of beta-amyloid plaqueing. The same mechanisms are evident in the progression of heart disease and the treatment doctors employ when they prescribe the drugs called *calcium-channel blockers*. The excessive loss of calcium ions from cardiac cells changes firing or "beat" patterns, just as the loss of ions interferes with neuronal competence.

The *Journal of Cellular Molecular Neurobiology*[200] in February 2001 concludes that "pre-administration of 17-beta estradiol significantly decreased the rise of calcium. These findings support the idea that the disruption of calcium homeostasis by beta-*amyloid* protein channels may be the molecular basis of the neurotoxicity and pathogenesis of Alzheimer's disease." If plaqueing has already occurred, the *Journal of Brain Research*[201] of December 1997 says, "physiological doses of 17-beta-estradiol was found to be neuroprotective, as the severity of insult on cell viability was decreased by 40% at 15 hours and up to 71% at 72 hours."

Take the Long Way Home

Beta-amyloid plaqueing causes an increase in free radical production in the surrounding cells, which is one way brain cells die in Alzheimer's disease. That fact and the numbers—by eighty-five years of age, one out of two of us will have Alzheimer's—makes it obvious that it's a disease of aging, not genetics. Families have inherited *genetic* thresholds of hormonal falloff, but the media- and medically propagated idea of the "gene for Alzheimer's" is as ludicrous as a gene for heart disease or a gene for osteoporosis or for menopause.

We will all most likely experience all of those disease states to some degree without hormone repacement. Estrogen replacement, cyclically, in high, rhythmic doses, seems to stop brain cell death, calcium loss, and as mentioned in the previous chapter, the production of homocysteine, while making progesterone receptors appear. A study in the *New England Journal of Medicine*[202] found that people who have Alzheimer's also have high levels of homocysteine and C-reactive protein just as heart patients do.

In Chapter Seven, when we dissected heart disease, we described how natural estrogen lowers C-reactive protein by creating an avenue for natural progesterone to suppress your immune system's overreaction, but the horse estrogen in Premarin *dramatically* upregulated C-reactive protein.[203] This also happens in the brain.

We think Premarin and PremPro do this because an immune response to the molecules of another species circulating in you is a fairly reasonable reaction by your body. It's interesting to remember here that Wyeth-Ayerst, the maker of Premarin, tried to invent, by way of Ireland, a vaccine to destroy the plaques of Alzheimer's.[204] Here is a sterling example of the win/win situation for the drug company that makes both drugs.

If we can find all of this evidence showing that replacing your diminishing natural hormones with bio-identical natural hormones derived from plants will save your mind and body, why is it that the most recent—October 28, 2002—headline on WebMD,[205] an Internet website run by doctors, is "Long-term HRT Worsens Memory"?

Because they used Premarin in the study, that's why.[206]

This Internet posting was picked up from the *Journal of Behavioral Neuroscience*. This is a classic case of the old shell game that we referred to in Chapter Five being perpetrated on us and our doctors by the bought-and-paid-for system of research that has a stranglehold on medicine in this country. The paper referenced on the WebMD website is titled "Long-term estrogen therapy worsens the behavioral and neuropathological consequences of chronic brain inflammation."

In the study[207] on forty female rats, the researchers infused half with lipopolysaccharide (LPS), a by-product of bacteria activity, a sort of bacterial "sweat." It's often used in lab scenarios to cause inflammation or an immune reaction in the cells being tested because we, as mammals, have that response to germs hardwired into us from our evolutionary history with them.

LPS from the symbiotic bacteria growing in our guts produces the same inflammatory responses seen in the blood after sleep loss.[208] That means that sleep loss over the course of your life can actually cause neuroinflammation akin to Alzheimer's. One of the reasons you wake up with a headache after a late night is that your brain swells.

Along with a headache, the researchers gave the rats Premarin in a steady-state dose equivalent to chronic levels of Premarin seen in women on the drug as it's taken seven days a week for about a decade, exactly the dose that women are prescribed in conventional HRT.

All of the rats' memories got much worse.[209]

WebMD says, "The study may point toward beneficial effects from short-term ERT—perhaps women should take estrogen pills two or three days every month."

Dr. G. L. Wenk, one of the doctors on the study, said, "Chronic estrogen (Premarin) is not a good thing. Maybe it would be a more natural estrogen surge that would have a protective effect."

We say, yes, surging would be a good idea.

That premise really could work if you added progesterone for two weeks out of the month to the mix and gave it a high dose peak, too.

But if you really want it to work, the estrogen can't come from a horse and be prescribed in a pill called Premarin.

nine

NOT FADE AWAY

The point of this examination of facts and myth is to ascertain why *so many* of us in our culture die of breast cancer and heart attack at such a *relatively* young age. The answer we've found to that question is that women at midlife, women in their forties and fifties, women who are perceived as relatively young in our culture, are not really young *reproductively*.[1-15]

Furthermore, it is the falloff of estrogen and progesterone at midlife, along with increasingly absent developmental milestones of pregnancies and subsequent long periods of lactation, that has made us vulnerable to breast cancer. We become vulnerable through the loss of hormones and their control on regulatory genes in charge of normal patterns of growth and death in cells.[16]

That's the "why" and "how" of breast cancer, as evidenced by the research we've presented. But, conversely, if the falloff of estrogen[17] and progesterone[18] are the cause of cancer and if, universally, women over forty will experience this rapid decline in the hormones that control cell cycles, *why don't we all get cancer*? After all, we can no more escape menopause than we can escape death and taxes. Certainly more of us will have a heart attack than will be diagnosed with breast cancer. That's in the statistics.[19] But many others of us who haven't spent our reproductive years childbearing and breast-feeding won't die of cancer, either.

If all of the research that we've examined is true, how can that be?

There must be some other fallback mechanism of control on overgrowth of cells, some other *apoptotic* intracellular pathways that nature employs.

There is one striking shared characteristic of the “old of who don’t die of cancer in our forties and fifties or hear ties—autoimmunity. The hallmark of being old is stiff arthritic sis, macular degeneration, and every other autoimmune state y name. Could autoimmunity in some *compensatory* way save us from canc in the long run when our hormones are gone?

Please Don’t Let Me Be Misunderstood

Strangely enough, the answer to this question lies somewhere in the effects of the synthetic ERT Premarin. Premarin is a “conjugated” estrogen.[20] That means it’s a drug made up of *various* kinds of estrogens, ten to be specific.[21] The “estrogens” in the drug Premarin, except for the metabolites of horse estrogen called *equilin*,[22] are bio-identical to our own endogenously produced estrone and estradiol. The estrogenic effects of Premarin consist primarily of lessening the severity of hot flashes, causing the lining of your uterus to *over*grow,[23] and increasing vaginal moisture.

But the broad-spectrum hormone replacement effects of Premarin are really pretty minor compared to those of transdermal 17-beta estradiol used alone. For us the question has always been, why has Premarin been so successful at masquerading as hormone replacement if it has such diminished potential compared to natural—and more effective—hormone replacement? This is due, in part, to the fact that Premarin is a pill, instead of a transdermal preparation that goes through your skin.

“First pass,” the liver function that screens your blood the minute you swallow anything questionable to keep toxins[24] out of your bloodstream, concentrates the horse estrogens of Premarin in your liver, keeping their action on estrogen receptors to a minimum.[25-26] This toxin also alerts your liver to produce large quantities of C-reactive protein, as we’ve seen in heart disease and Alzheimer’s disease in Chapters Seven and Eight respectively.[27] Interestingly, it seems that Premarin’s effect on C-reactive protein[28-30] (the “inflammatory marker” for heart disease and Alzheimer’s) is the real basis of its hormonelike effect, that and, of course, the fact that it’s 80 percent estrone, the weakest estrogen metabolite in your body. Premarin administration, at normal doses, causes a dramatic increase in C-reactive protein.

ɔon't Come Easy

ɿe immune system divides the world inside and outside your body into self" and "nonself"; when human beings swallow the hormones of another species, like a horse, our immune system declares the substance to be definitely *nonself* and react to it. This reaction occurs anytime we ingest molecules that aren't recognizable as food or hormones.

In Chapter Seven we presented a French study in which researchers gave women 17-beta estradiol in huge amounts, akin to third-trimester pregnancy levels; this caused no increase in C-reactive protein, but that wasn't the case with Premarin. *Any* increase in C-reactive protein in response to Premarin would have constituted an immune reaction, but a dramatic one indicates that a whole suite of immunological events are occurring.[31-33]

The whole suite of "allergic" reactions to Premarin causes your liver to pour C-reactive protein and causes immune system cells, called *B-lymphocytes,* to make antibodies, which is the same response seen during infection. C-reactive protein always dramatically increases in the absence of estrogen and progesterone, as evidenced by the steep rise in prolactin during labor and in C-reactive protein postpartum.[34] But it's the antibodies that matter in our discussion of hormone replacement. Both antibody production and C-reactive protein are evidence of the two arms of global immune responses called *immunity* and *autoimmunity*.

Autoimmunity[35] is when your body reacts to your own tissues as *non*-self. Antibodies can fight the infection of disease by killing cells that have been invaded by nonself germs, but they can also attack your body's own tissues. This is how your immune system functions, both to defend you and defend against you when your useful time on this earth is over.

It's also well known in medicine that the very young and the very old have "weakened" immune systems, meaning they have lesser defensive capabilities in terms of germ-induced disease and infection. This is because the very young[36-37] and the very old have no sex hormones. Sex hormones not only serve to enhance the defensive arm of the immune system, they also suppress autoimmunity,[38-46] *simultaneously*. Just as in pregnancy, when escalating progesterone immunosuppresses mom to keep her from rejecting the fetus[47]—which has genes that are not hers, that is, nonself—regular menstrual cycles producing both estrogen and progesterone can strengthen *both* arms of your immune system.

It is in between fertile periods and ensuing pregnancies that women are intensely autoimmune and in an antibody-producing state expressly for the purpose of breast-feeding. When your sex hormones read to your systems as having "flatlined," your immune system then switches into *high* gear in preparation for delivery and breast-feeding.

Remember, we have evolved *biologically* to re-enact *only* those templates over and over again.

That's why your immune system turns on in the wake of menopause. When your estrogen and progesterone are gone, as they are in lactation, your immune system steps in, as it does during lactation, to control cell growth and death until estrogen comes back up a year or so later to prime ovulation to precipitate progesterone's return.

At the end of menopause, this scenario is hormonally reenacted all over again, but this time estrogen and progesterone won't be returning ever again.

In Chapter Three we explained how a mistaken trigger sets the scene for breast cancer after fifty. Chronic pouring prolactin, in the absence of estrogen and progesterone, turns on the machinery of lactation, which includes growth factors of all kinds, like HER-2, and fetal oncogenes like BCL2, factors also turned on during breast *cancer.* This is because lactation is a cancerous state that, just like any other hormonal state, peaks and then resolves itself again if it continues long enough.

The rhythm of growth *and* death, the same rhythm in a monthly fertile cycle and the same rhythm in pregnancy and lactation, is the rhythm of life. If you get stuck in *growth,* you're in big trouble. But those of us who become *more* autoimmune very suddenly after perimenopause may escape cancer for just that reason. In the state of pregnancy or nursing or having regular cycles, we are protected by this backup system, so if we don't succumb in our forties and fifties to breast cancer, or any cancer, for that matter, the pendulum in nature saves us by making our "declining years" extravagantly autoimmune. Those of us who die of cancer maybe didn't become autoimmune enough, quickly enough.

High-volume antibody production can control the overgrowth of cells by sitting near growth factor receptors and turning them off. Other immune cells, called *T-cells*, can provoke apoptosis. It's the Herceptin effect. Herceptin is a synthetic antibody that was invented to turn off the epidermal growth factor receptor in cases of HER-2 breast cancer.[48]

The secret that the inventors of Herceptin were working from is this: Antibodies can control growth factor receptors like epidermal growth factor receptor (EGFR), fibroblast growth factor (FGF), leukemia inhibitory factor (LIF), and others.[49]

This is a backup system for old people without hormones.

It's also why it's so miserably uncomfortable to be old

After age fifty, medicine treats autoimmunity because of the pain and discomfort, but intervention will also turn off nature's backup system on control of new growth in cells by suppressing antibody and T-cell reactions. The incredibly high antibody output of over-the-top autoimmunity of old age—dry eyes, arthritis, lupus, macular degeneration, eczema, Hashimoto's thyroiditis, Graves' disease, psoriasis, obesity, Type II diabetes, acid reflux, irritable bowel syndrome, and asthma—actually serves to protect us from cancer through the Herceptin effect of antibody control of growth factor receptors. However, the biggest killer of women, heart disease, and, of course, occurring later in life, senile dementia, are most likely the product of massive C-reactive protein activity, which makes these disease states—Alzheimer's and heart disease just *common side effects* of the compensatory mechanism for the falloff of estrogen and progesterone—autoimmunity.[50]

The classic autoimmunity of aging also means that T-cells from the thymus handle a lot of the apoptotic—cell-killing—work of your missing progesterone.[51] The problem is that these cells aren't very discriminating in high gear; that's why joints, bones, eyes, skin, kidneys, and thyroids are undergoing steady degradation at the same time as the antibodies and T-cells free us from cancer.[52-53] Not only do they kill the overgrowth of cancer, they kill other cells as well.

Farther Up the Road

This is what happens to the other seven of us in the statistic "one in eight women will die of breast cancer in America in their lifetime." Those of us who aren't stricken with cancer grow old painfully,[54] and take a lot of Vioxx, Celebrex, Liquid Tears, calcium supplements, Fosamax, hydrocortisone cream, Advil, Tylenol PM, and antihistamines. This doesn't mean we will all get to be old, because autoimmunity is also at the foundation of how most women over fifty really die—heart disease and hypertension.[55-62] It just means that those of us who didn't have a heart attack are in pain waiting for Alzheimer's to occur.

The relationship between allergies and the risk of brain tumors in adults illustrates our premise. There is a clear *inverse* association between autoimmunity and meningioma, neuroma, and glioma.[63-64] The only autoimmune state that seems to break the rule actually proves it—arthritis. This is complicated, but important.

At first glance, it seems that having rheumatoid arthritis, a condition of autoreactivity in B- and T-cells,[65-70] predicts a *sixfold* greater likelihood of developing lymphoma down the line of disease progression.[71] That doesn't fit our model. So we ask, Why? Whenever there is clear evidence for a pattern in nature and one example doesn't fit, human intervention is the likeliest culprit. It may be that the cure for arthritis kills you a different way. The standard of care when you display excessive autoimmunity is for the doctor to prescribe steroid drugs like cortisone (synthetic cortisol) or prednisone (synthetic progesterone) to suppress your immune system and stop the degradation of bone and collagen.

But what do these over-the-counter and stronger prescriptive immunosuppressants really do to us over time? Certainly they stop some of the apoptotic effects and ease the pain caused by the constant inflammatory state. But there must be a price. There is always a price. Huisman and associates[72] reported that *lymphocytes* (the cells growing out of control in lymphoma) from arthritis sufferers have *decreased* numbers of cortisol receptors. There's a clue.

The common perception in research today is that arthritis is a result of this low cortisol action,[73] but are the decreased number of cortisol receptors really the basis as we age for rheumatoid arthritis, or does the treatment down-regulate your cortisol receptors? Is it really that cortisol can't be received, so immune reactivity never turns off? The premise from which they are working is that you can't suppress your immune system with your own cortisol without enough cortisol receptors. That's a fair assumption, but then one must wonder, is this a truly inherited condition of threshold entropy or are the receptor numbers down for another reason?

Could treatment of the arthritis with prednisone or cortisone over the long haul cause cortisol receptors to *retreat,* simultaneously turning off antibody production?[74]

The answer is yes.

Corticosteroid drugs can create *cortisol receptor resistance* and, of course, they stop antibody production. That's what they were designed to do—suppress your immune response. We'd like to see if rheumatoid arthritis caused lymphoma sixty years ago, before cortisone and prednisone were the standard-of-care treatment for autoimmune diseases, because we think that the treatment might be the cause of the cancers. We think that the arthritis patients would not have developed lymphoma if they were allowed to continue producing the antibodies of autoimmunity that *prevent* cancer, or if they received complete rhythmic cyclical natural bio-identical hormone replacement. Estrogen would make progesterone receptors and progesterone would result in immunosuppression.

Comfortably Numb

Does it really matter if in old age we take drugs to immunosuppress? After all, when we were young, progesterone did the same thing. But the difference is that when we were young, we *had* progesterone.[75-76]

Now we don't.

Progesterone was a timed body-wide phenomenon, not a chronic "point-solution" with side effects. Fooling with your immune system is really toying with Mother Nature.

Past menopause, without sex hormones, all we have are antibodies and the arthritis pain or corticosteroid drugs that can't even reliably stop autoimmunity anyway, because of the phenomenon of receptor resistance[77] that causes them to stop working. That's why the drug companies have invented Vioxx and Celebrex to effect other pathways, but these drugs are known to cause side effects like intestinal bleeding and heart attacks.

Would the Herceptin effect of an antibody stopping cancer apply to lymphoma? Yes, an antibody can stop cancer in this case. One of the most successful cancer treatments used today is called *monoclonal antibody therapy* for non-Hodgkin's lymphoma. The most recent incarnation of this drug is called Rituxan.[78-79] The same way that rheumatoid arthritis might not become lymphoma if left untreated by steroid drugs, lymphoma itself can become a different cancer when treated with the fake antibody Rituxan. While Rituxan is effective at causing remission by acting like estrogen on the growth factor receptor,[80] the tumor can rearrange its DNA and become not only resistant to Rituxan but a different animal altogether.

It's the same story of compensation and receptor resistance that we saw in Chapter Six. When breast cancer was treated with tamoxifen and the cancer reoccurred in the other breast, the new cancer was virtually always estrogen receptor negative, a much more virulent form of the original cancer. The same sort of thing can happen when lymphoma is treated with the invented antibody Rituxan. The lymphoma can evolve further along the spectrum of disease[81] to a large B-cell carcinoma, again a much more virulent type. There is no free lunch. These drugs almost always cause a far worse effect down the line.

Do It Again

Synthetic antibodies can't really stop cancer for very long because of the "ripple effect" of immune function when it comes to antibody production. This is because the body perceives the invented antibody as an antigen, or nonself.[82] Our defense system is set up to have one antibody for every possible antigen (nonself) out there in the whole world. That number, 10^{12}, is too big to contemplate. The immune system learns by its first contact with the antigen and then extrapolates. When B-cells are stimulated to divide and mature, its descendants will end up secreting about two thousand antibody molecules a second, all of which will then make more and more and more.

The famous Danish Nobel Laureate Niels Jerne described[83] a region of variability on all of these antibodies that can invoke the production of *anti*-antibodies. So antibodies not only kill germs or fight viruses, they can create antibodies to themselves, called an *idiotype*. They are themselves perceived, or nonself. That means that after your immune system has produced an antibody, it continues to produce antibodies to the idiotypes of the antibody that it has itself made. These antibodies, likewise, do the same and on and on. So that the possible strategies in nature are endless.

That's why we said in Chapter Seven that Herceptin's effect on the regression of tumor growth can't last. Your body kicks into a chain reaction, making antibodies to "fight" the invented antibody. The fourth or fifth antibody down the line, unfortunately, actually turns the epidermal growth factor receptor (EGRF) back on. That can happen with Rituxan. The anti-anti-

anti-anti-idiotype of Rituxan can eventually turn lymphoma on again, because Rituxan is a synthetic antibody and does not occur in nature.

Your own immune system was designed to compensate for sex hormone action. As in the example of: protection from germs at the site of the wound of childbirth or the needs of lactation to program the baby's immune system, these events all dovetail with the dramatic decline in estradiol and progesterone at birth.

Find Your Way Back Home

The Western medical system never accounts for the balance intended by homeostasis; if it did, we would never have side effects from prescribed medications. Eastern medicine, on the other hand, views dysfunction and disease very differently. In Sanskrit, the word *tantras* means "to weave." It refers to the interwovenness and interdependence of all things and events. *Tantric* medicine would follow the "path" of a disease like cancer. For example, it would look to pregnancy as a template to understanding the growth and death of tumor cells, since a baby and a placenta are two kinds of tumors we actually live through and benefit from. It's apparent that at the level of molecular genetics, the system is preordained to control itself at the behest of the environment toward the goal of our survival. That's where hormones come in. At the directives of the environment—light, food, crowding, and temperature—hormones not only flip genes on and off, they simultaneously affect your consciousness to make you behave in a way that should ensure your survival.[84-85]

But always remember that "your" doesn't necessarily mean "you"—it can also just mean your species.

The confusion created in our brains and bodies by advances in technology in the last 150 years are what we know as the diseases of civilization. Nature had our existence all wrapped up, in the bag, so to speak, until we invented agriculture and electricity. Life moves like the child's toy in which a marble drops and keeps dropping, tripping one new action after another all the way down. In other words, biological life is a complex, dynamic, and, most importantly, nonlinear system (many things happen simultaneously) of variables resting on variables resting on variables resting on variables all the way down. "Complex" in this instance means groups of genes controlling groups of genes—*epigenetics* or antibodies making anti-anti-anti-anti-idiotypes.

These groups control each other in a "dynamic" or interactive way that is never linear or one-to-one in action. This multiplicity of layers of interactive potential gives us as many possible outcomes as there are stars in the sky, as is evidenced in the immune system's actions of defense and internal maintenance after hormone falloff. This also means that any drug invented as a "point solution" has to make you sick somewhere else.

The controls on the homeostatic system are the Sun, the moon, the climate, food abundance, and mating cycles. These are the initial variables. The system self-regulates constantly, because until you run out of hormones, it's energetically *homeostatic*. If the variables affected by the initial variables are supported with the raw materials, every function resets the others, and life runs like a well-oiled machine.

Domino

To "see" this premise, imagine a clear glass vase filled with clear marbles. If you could reach into the middle and pluck out a marble, all the other marbles would move, would re-adjust themselves to compensate for the missing one. The marbles or variables that control the positioning of all the other marbles—*sleeping, eating,* and *reproducing*—we will call *1, 2,* and *3,* respectively.

How much you sleep (1) is reported by melatonin to cortisol and prolactin; (2) or how much carbohydrates you eat is determined by (1) and reported by insulin levels to (3); (3) is how fast you age or your reproductive status in terms of estrogen, progesterone, and testosterone levels. The formula for existence is, then, 1+2=3. Sleeping and eating equal how fast time passes metabolically.

The rate at which you age determines how fast you reach menopause, since menopause is a function of time passing internally, because time and materials are the same thing.

This view of life as it truly exists is necessary to understanding physician-caused, or iatrogenic, disease that we all incur when we seek medical care.

Iatrogenic disease can be caused by any medicine, any drug at all, because the addition of any foreign (not food, not plant, not animal) substance into a self-regulating system is, in effect, like plucking out a marble at random. Iatrogenic disease is any dysfunction or disease state caused by the rest of the marbles *moving*. The less life-threatening slips and slides are called *side effects*. The worst possible iatrogenic effect is death.[86] Most physicians and scientists agree that death is an unacceptable side effect. If we assume that the environment controls the cues for sleep through light and dark cycles that time our behavior with respect to eating, mating, and reproducing, then it becomes obvious that artificial triggers like recent-in-human-history light-after-dark year-round availability of carbohydrates will, in fact, cause disease, in and of themselves.

If changing a variable, or moving the marble, for food and light is enough to cause diabetes, infertility, and mental illness, then taking a beta blocker for heart disease or Prozac for depression is like moving more than a few marbles. Many other systems connected to the one that just changed go sideways because biology—life—is based on an interactive, self-regulating system of variables resting on variables controlled by the light, the food supply, temperature, and gravity. There's no changing the rules, ever.

But, Western medicine just keeps moving the marbles, anyway.

Blinded by the Light

"Point solutions" like Lipitor for cholesterol, Vioxx for arthritis, or Fosamax for osteoporosis can never address the real dysfunction; they can only halt a symptom for a while until, downstream, they create many more problems than they ever addressed in the first place.

The world we live in has antibiotics, surgery, and blood transfusion, so while we're unlikely to die from "natural causes," we probably will die from the side effects of a misguided treatment intended to save our lives. There is no way to affect any part of your health *positively* by moving marbles. The realistic way to achieve recovery from being dysrhythmic is to fall back into sync with normal planetary rhythms—that is, to sleep and eat in season and so restore chronobiological homeostasis. The only hope of a return to well-being is to go back and effect the effectors we called 1, 2, and 3. That means sleeping when it's dark if at all possible, eating carbohydrates only in season, and replacing diminishing raw materials like sex hormones with the real thing found in nature.

The old saw that reminds us that "you can't fool Mother Nature" refers to the "marbles," which are a combination of DNA, genes, and consciousness that come together to form your immune system. The immune system, in total, isn't just organs that produce immune cells—like bone marrow or the thymus, which turns out T-cells—but a mind-body entity, a biochemical self of neuropeptides (hormones, neurotransmitters, and cytokines produced by immune cells) and their receptors that join the brain, body, and environment through the network of communication. The immune system is a "free-form brain" in which nerve cells communicate with immune cells through hormones by the same snap, crackle, pop of "mobile" synapses.[87] That's why you can have a headache in your lower back or why you get a stomachache when you're anxious. Our anxiety about aging is not all in our heads; our bodies are *worrying*, too.

Anxiety is an early warning system that gives us a heads-up on the internal landscape, and the report says things are beginning to fall apart. We're told to ignore the obvious and join a gym, eat health food, take supplements, and visit our doctors regularly. We are devoted to the notion that the American medical system is the most advanced in the world, but maybe that's what's killing us.

Canary in a Coal Mine

Cancer, heart disease, and Alzheimer's are often referred to as the "diseases of civilization" because their natural incidence in developing nations and technoenvironmentally challenged peoples is low to nonexistent.[88] The most popular theory condemns "toxins," any by-products of modern life, as the culprits in cancer (xeno-estrogens) and Alzheimer's (cooking foods in aluminum cookware). It's certainly not the toxins, but maybe our medical system, itself.

In order to truly manipulate our fate in the course of any of the diseases of civilization successfully, medicine would have to examine the pathways of natural dynamics in and among the organisms in the environment we inhabit. The pathway is the route a disease takes in context, the "disease process." Doctors and scientists call this the *etiology* of the disease. Scientists are very fond of looking for the tiniest clues first, like the relationships between atoms and molecules. They spend, quite literally, billions of dollars on research into the *molecular* mechanisms involved in only one small part of a disease process without ever considering the entire picture.

We illustrate this point of view with the "broken vase model." When you break a vase you love and you would like to have it back, you pick up the pieces and try to glue them back together. It's safe to say that all of us start with the big pieces first—fitting them together, gluing one to another as the pieces get smaller and smaller, until all that's left is the point of impact, the place where it hit the floor. Most of the time you just have to turn the hole to the wall the next time you use it because all that's left to glue is too small to be organized; it's just powder.

Science and medicine keep trying to unravel the pathology of a disease by starting with the powder, identifying and naming the dust. The big pieces never really come into play because they have nothing solid to adhere to. That's why no real progress is ever made toward a cure for anything that an antibiotic won't eradicate. If researchers started with "health" and examined normalcy in context as, say, in the case of breast cancer, and looked at life in a time when it occurred in women at the rate of one in ninety-one instead of one in seven as it is now, the answer would be easier to find. Approached in this manner, medicine and the treatment of disease can become a lot simpler, especially if you find a way to remove *profit* from the equation.

ten

SATISFACTION

There is a certain faction of the women's movement that feels that no hormones at all are your best bet for a natural adjustment to aging. They frequently quote the venerable anthropologist Dr. Margaret Mead when describing the "joy" of unmedicated, *natural* menopause and the thrill of entering the second half of life *unencumbered* by the responsibilities of children or a career.[1-3] This has become feminist "gospel" and their credo is best summed up with a term coined by Dr. Mead, *postmenopausal zest.* These hard-core "naturalists" seemed determined to actually celebrate the end of female physiology. What we will actually really turn into they never quite delineate, but from what we've discovered in our research, we're pretty confident that it's not someone "zesty."

Gail Sheehy reported in *Silent Passages,* the "menopausal version" of her best-selling *Passages,* that Margaret Mead's daughter testified to the fact that her mother received estrogen shots once a week from midlife until she died. That's how Margaret ran the Natural History Museum, worked her way through three husbands, reported on exotic cultures, and appeared frequently on *The Tonight Show*, *The Dick Cavett Show*, and *Merv Griffin*.[4-5]

That's postmenopausal zest, *compliments of estrogen.*

Does that mean Margaret worried about "feminine freshness," as the commercials say, into her eighties? Did Margaret have a monthly period during all those years of ERT? We certainly aren't privy to that information, but if she took *enough* estrogen and any form of progesterone at all with it, she did. Progesterone, as the destroyer, in the life-giving scenario of build/destroy, build/destroy, always causes the shedding of the uterine lining if there's enough estrogen preceeding it to make progesterone receptors. Women on accurate natural hormone replacement will always have a period.

You must have a period to be *viable* in nature. Nature hates incompleteness. That's why cycles are circles and continue to be, if you're healthy. If you don't have a period, you haven't reached the peaks of hormone action that make receptors ready for the next wave of action. Without enough hormones to produce a five-day bleed, you haven't replaced enough estrogen and progesterone to protect your brain and breasts. Remember, to live in the state of grace known as youth, your body must function internally as though it's *young*. Since you're not about to go through pregnancy and lactation, the only other option is normal menstruation. That means menstrual periods *forever,* until you die, probably at a very ripe old age.

Many of us may have already lived more than a few years menses-less and find the idea of recapturing menstrual youth just a little perverse, but for your health, it's not. It *can* be messy to menstruate, but once you've accomplished accurate "replacement," it's not painful the way adolescent and perimenopausal periods can be. It can be tedious, but then so are chemotherapy, radiation, using a walker, carrying a white cane, insulin injections, a cardiac bypass, or losing your memory.

The newest clinical approach, even in natural, bio-identical hormone replacement, is that "less is more," and not for very long or very often. This pervasive fear of HRT *of any kind,* sparked by the overwhelming use and failure of synthetic hormone drugs, has colored the perception of all the available varieties of alternative hormone replacement, too.

Lingering in the background of these assumptions is the unscientific, inaccurate notion that estrogen causes cancer and that the longer you are exposed to your own estrogen in your lifetime, the greater your risk[6] of breast cancer. This assumption, unfortunately, seemed to be borne out in the epidemiological statistics of early puberty and late menopause as risk factors for cancer. We addressed that misperception in Chapter One.

Early menarche is a function of precocious puberty or high insulin, and many of those early cycles are anovulatory, as are the cycles experienced in the last ten years of reproductive life (perimenopause) before the onset of menopause. Living with all the growth factors driven by high insulin and the lack of estrogen reception from insulin resistance, coupled with no progesterone from nonovulation, cancer would seem to be inevitable, from the cellular perspective.

It was never the exposure to your own cycles that caused the increase in breast cancer seen with early menarche and late menopause, because your system stalled early on from a *lack* of estrogen reception, thanks to insulin resistance and the lack of progesterone from subsequent ovulation.

There weren't really normal cycles going on.

And even if you had a child or two, unless you breast-fed each one *naturally*, on demand for at least nine months to a year, you still truncated or missed physiologically developmental milestones that would prevent cancer.

Too Much Time on My Hands

We took the time to find out why the statistics were so gravely misinterpreted. It began with the work of anthropologist Beverly Strassmann, who teaches at the University of Michigan at Ann Arbor.[7] Strassmann spent years with the Dogon tribe in Mali, where she literally took up residence in the tribe's menstrual hut. She made a chart of the women's names and counted, over the years, their trips to the menstrual hut. Among the Dogon, she found that a woman, on average, has her first period at the age of sixteen and gives birth approximately eight times in her life. From menarche to twenty years old, she averages only seven periods overall in four years.[8] Total.

Over the next decade and a half, from twenty to thirty-five years old, she is either pregnant or breast-feeding (the Dogon breast-feed for an average of twenty months), so she averages only one period a year.[9] Then, from the age of thirty-five until menopause, around fifty, as her fertility declines, she continues to give birth and breast-feed, but she averages only four periods a year. Strassmann reasonably concluded the obvious—that normal women in the natural world had many fewer menstrual periods than their modern "civilized" counterparts.

Then Dr. Malcolm Pike, a research physician at the University of Southern California, picked up Strassmann's work, applied the "risk factor statistics" of early menarch and late menopause to it, and concluded that stopping "incessant ovulation" was the way to stop breast and ovarian cancer.[10-15] This is the kind of thinking that led to a book entitled *Is Menstrua-*

tion Obsolete?,[16] and the now-common worldview among clinicians that the least amount of hormone you can take is the best approach to replacement.

For some unfathomable reason, neither one of them ever took the obvious path of reasoning that maybe it was *what the women were doing* when they weren't visiting the menstrual hut that protected them from cancer—having and feeding babies (incessantly) for their whole lives—that, in fact, instead of the repetitious exposure to estrogen in a normal menstrual cycle being toxic, even more estrogen was needed. The escalating levels of estrogen and progesterone in pregnancy trip switches that make the breast immune to the high levels of prolactin in nursing and after menopause. But in our politically correct world, it didn't even occur to scientists looking for the *scientific* truth to venture a guess at the obvious—that perhaps to be a healthy woman, we might have to live the lives of *women* physically. Our choices to stay healthy comprise just that along with the hopeful possibility that at this late date we can try to maintain a physiological state of "potential" in nature. By becoming physiologically young, by replacing your hormones on the inside—every cell and every molecule stay prepared, waiting on "ready" to do their job, in anticipation of the big event, whether or not it ever happens.

Us and Them

How do we accomplish this miracle? More importantly, how do we accomplish this miracle against all odds, after decades of misinformation from the drug companies to the doctors whom we need to prescribe for us? Here's what we suggest your course of action be: Get your physician to order bloodwork to establish *need* and to give you a baseline so that you can adjust your own dosages, because hormone replacement is an art for which most physicians have neither the time nor the inclination. So you must learn how to be responsible for how you feel and how to prevent the health disasters of aging yourself. The art of using hormones for complete replacement has to be an individual one because everybody's different. Your response to hormone replacement will be unique to you. You are different from the woman sitting next to you, and she is not the same as her sister or daughter. Any man would tell you that that's the amazing thing about women, no two are alike, and yet we're all women.

The only way to level the playing field for your doctor is to give him the tools that clinicians work from—numbers. Normal levels of estrogen and progesterone during a twenty-eight-day menstrual ... sured in serum (bloodwork) in women of all ages fo... consensus of what the numbers should be in a "young" wo... as fact. These established peaks and valleys have numerical ra... only slightly from lab to lab.

For example, on the bloodwork requisition that a doctor will fill out th... are ranges for ages and times of the menstrual cycle. So it will say "ages 15–25, midfollicular phase." That would be the range of numbers during your *estrogen peak* on Day 11 or 12 of your cycle that you would want to reach on hormone replacement, say *350 to 500 pg (picogram)* per ml of your blood. *Progesterone* values in a young woman age 15 to 22 at the *peak* of production from the corpus luteum ("midluteal phase") is measured in double digits at values between *10 and 22 ng (nanogram).* So when you replace your progesterone from the outside, blood drawn on Day 21 of your cycle should register a number between 10 and 22, if you've got it right.[17] The key to accuracy is to always "weigh yourself on the same scale," so to speak, and always go to that same lab on the same days of your cycle at the same time of day.

These numbers will prove to your doctor that no matter how much hormone you should choose to apply, you have not exceeded *physiologic* doses. Although he may point out that the "normal" physiologic level of estrogen in a fifty-six-year-old woman is more like 40 pg per ml, remind him of the health problems in fifty-six-year-old women that you are hoping to avoid with this new approach. If he says something akin to "it just seems dangerous or unnatural," tell him that *so is living beyond reproduction for all species.* These numbers are themselves the justification for the amounts of hormones you'll need him to prescribe to reach them. Doctors have been prescribing PremPro for years at the same dose for all women, with no way to measure the effect, because there are no standards for *equilin,* horse estrogen, in the blood of a human woman.[18-19]

By charting the rising and falling hormones you are replacing for the first three months of treatment, a stable dose can be attained that can stay the same as long as you feel well. Since aging is a continuing process, checking your hormone levels every six months, after the initial dosing period of ninety days, gives you a chance to keep up increases as you need to. Fluctuating and falling hormones are no longer a concern because you returned to a "normal" rhythm as long as you continue natural hormone replacements.

e My Seesaw

should ask your doctor to order a *thyroid panel*, too, along with a C-ptide test for insulin and *prolactin* level. These measurements are the asis for evaluating aging. Dr. Uzzi Reiss, in his book *Natural Hormone Balance for Women*,[20] recommends testing for a hormone called *sex hormone binding globulin* (SHBG). SHBG binds hormones to remove them from circulation for later use. That's why some lab reports refer to *free* estrogen and *total* estrogen. The number you're looking for is the total. Although it's certainly true that only the free estrogen has effective action, SHBG occurs in inverse proportion to insulin, so the C-peptide test is a better indicator of how much "bang for the buck" you'll get from your estrogen replacement. SHBG also preferentially binds to testosterone first, before it ever gets to estrogen. We recommend Dr. Reiss's book for the marvelous job he does explaining diagnostic symptomology.

The thyroid panel, which measures thyroid stimulating hormone (TSH) from your brain and the hormones the thyroid makes, T4 and T3, will probably come back to your doctor registering "low, normal." Almost everyone's does. That doesn't mean that you don't need thyroid replacement. That's just the evidence that the test is not very accurate, because we can't possibly all have the same thyroid numbers. T4 and T3 feed back a signal to stop TSH because, when they are around, that's the signal back to the thyroid that it's made enough of them.

Thyroid hormone replacement due to the deficit in the test must be diagnosed by symptoms. Don't take no for an answer. Thyroid hormones will probably be offered to you in synthetic form. The drug Levoxyl is only T4. A more natural form is a porcine source from Armour, the makers of ham. Any woman with weight problems *must* be experiencing thyroid dysfunction as well as insulin and cortisol dysrhythmia because the thyroid is the master control on *basal metabolic rate* (BMR).

Your BMR is the rate at which you burn energy (carbohydrates), which all health professionals advise can be raised by exercising. Yes, your BMR can be raised by exercise—for about two or three hours; then you have to go do it again, and again, and again, unless you plan to ever go to sleep. Thyroid replacement of both T4 *and* T3 is the only way to truly raise your BMR reliably and permanently.

Thyroid replacement is essential to feeling well. A weak, erratic thyroid makes you fat, depressed, and bald, with dry eyes.[21-22] These sym hypothyroidism, or lack of thyroid hormone. There are two wa this condition: one is an autoimmune state called *Hashimoto's thyroiditis*, which happens when you've been without progesterone to immunosuppress for too long. The other is the end product of your thyroid's overexertion.

Your thyroid is in a rhythm with estrogen during your cycle and, of course, during pregnancy and nursing. When estrogen is up, TSH is down, because as a pregnancy ensues, estrogen escalates to depress thyroid function, so you put on weight for the upcoming lactational phase. That mechanism goes haywire in perimenopause because your estrogen just keeps declining and your thyroid starts to pour and there's no template for that. Those periods of *hypersecretion* cause racing heartbeats and sweating, usually as you're falling asleep at night or in the middle of the night when melatonin is blocking even more estrogen reception.

Before your thyroid wears out completely and you become hypothyroid, it spurts and sputters. Estrogen *replacement* can send the signal to the brain to control hyperthyroidism.[23] But if you've been without estrogen for too long, your thyroid will be spent and you'll need thyroid replacement,[24] too. Estrogen and thyroid replacement go hand in hand because thyroid hormone replacement alone, although it can stop the TSH signal and increase your BMR, will only enhance the symptoms of estrogen deprivation, because T3 creates estrogen receptors[25-27] to complete the (negative feedback) loop. So replacing estrogen and thyroid hormone at the same time can reestablish the original homeostatic balance.[28-30]

Keep Yourself Alive

The next test on the list, C-peptide, will give you an idea of where you are metabolically at midlife in terms of potential diabetes. This test is the best indicator of insulin resistance, after your weight and blood pressure. If your C-peptide is high according to the numbers provided for "normal" ranges,[31] cut out carbohydrates and alcohol and go to bed earlier. A high C-peptide level is a very accurate reading of how much insulin you are producing. You won't be overproducing insulin unless your blood sugar is up.[32]

One of the best ways to forestall Type II diabetes, especially if it runs in your family, is to utilize a device available over the counter called a blood sugar monitor. Even without the results of a C-peptide test, if you're more than twenty-five pounds overweight, you should buy a carbohydrate counter at the bookstore in the diet section and blood sugar monitor and use it before bed and again when you get up in the morning. If your blood sugar does not drop significantly to under 100 overnight, you are completely insulin resistant no matter what you weigh. In order to lose weight and normalize blood pressure, measure your blood sugar one hour after you eat and again two hours later.[33-35]

The first measurement tells you if you made the right choice of foods available—that is, how high did your blood sugar go from the amount and kind of carbohydrates you ate?[36] The second reading two hours later, or three hours after you've eaten, lets you know if your blood sugar has come down at all. That way you can choose what to have for your next meal and keep your blood sugar under one hundred. If you do that consistently for every meal all day long, until you wake up one morning with a blood sugar number that is significantly lower than when you went to bed, the weight will fall off and insulin resistance will reverse itself. You *must* reverse insulin resistance to feel young again and lose abdominal adiposity (your gut).[37-41]

Blister in the Sun

Insulin and estrogen's synergy exists because insulin in its receptor makes estrogen receptors appear because, in the grand scheme of things, the available carbohydrate in the food supply must have the control on reproduction or we'd all starve. That mechanism is why you won't receive the estrogen that you might replace unless you have estrogen receptors to do it.[42-43] If you don't control carbohydrate intake and insulin resistance, you can't get the most from your hormone replacement because you must be insulin receptive to make estrogen receptors. Insulin resistance means the insulin receptor is resistant to insulin's action, and so there are no estrogen receptors, unless your thyroid is effectively working. Thyroid hormones (T3) create estrogen receptors.[44-46]

Getting fat at menopause is a compensatory mechanism for low sex hormone levels.[47-50] The hypoglycemia and carbohydrate craving that we experience is really acute because sex hormones control your appetite for sugar, too. Estrogen all by itself is an incredible appetite suppressant.[51-52] You crave sugar to make you fat at menopause to compensate for missing estradiol with estrone production from your expanding fat base.[53-55] Cravings for specific kinds of salty and sweet foods have their own purpose, too.

For example, cravings for theobromine in chocolate[56-57] are a way to replace the GABA effects you've lost since your progesterone is missing. Alcohol consumption does the same thing, too, in relation to D-pregnelonone production. During perimenopause, as you're running out of progesterone, insulin resistance is pretty much a given because receptors cease to work as well as they once did, because progesterone, in its own receptor, affects *insulin response substrate*-2 (IRS-2),[58] which makes the insulin receptor "wake up." It's known that Type I insulin-dependent diabetics use much less insulin during pregnancy and in the luteal phase of their cycle.

Natural progesterone also immunosuppresses, and fat cells (adipocytes) are immune cells in that they put off the same immune factors—like cytokines—that T-cells and B-cells[59-60] do. So a fat cell is just another type of immune cell that "defends" you from starvation or freezing to death. The real purpose of insulin is to *insulate* you from the cold and the absence of carbohydrates when winter comes. The important cytokine for weight loss produced by fat cells is called *TNF alpha*. Fat cells produce TNF alpha in proportion to their mass.[61-62] As soon as you go past the twenty-five-pounds-overweight threshold,[63] fat cells secrete more and more TNF alpha.

TNF alpha, in turn, destroys insulin reception by fat cells.

So the fatter you get, the fatter you get, because your fat base, now that your sex hormones are gone, must make aromatase to convert what little testosterone you have into estrogen so that your brain doesn't shut down completely.

Therefore, as we said, past about twenty-five pounds overweight, the fatter you get,[64-69] the fatter you get, unless you replace you missing estrogen with natural, bio-identical estradiol to control your appetite, save what's left of your thyroid, and make progesterone receptors. Natural progesterone replacement can then step in at IRS2 and block TNF alpha activity. Natural, bio-identical, rhythmic estrogen replacement can't ever cause weight gain as long as progesterone is also replaced. Premarin causes weight gain.[70] Most important, eat some meat. Vegetarians always have lower serum estrogen levels because they're missing the cholesterol from meat that is needed to make sex hormones.[71-72]

SUMMER: Long light exposure shortens melatonin time at night

APPETITE AND METABOLISM CONTROL: Based on the timing of melatonin

M ↓ → NP ↓ → DP ↑ → L ↓ → NPY ↑ → CC ↑ → WG

WINTER: Short hours of light exposure lengthens melatonin time

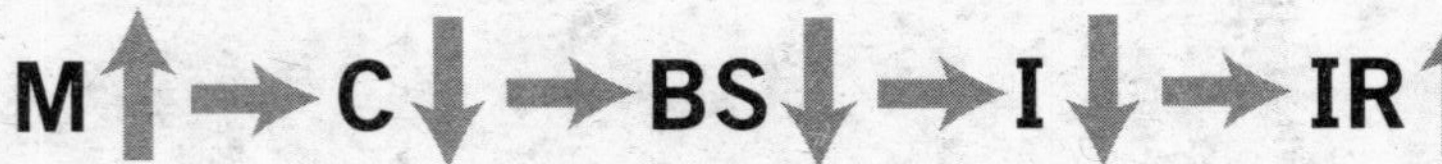

M	Melatonin	**I**	Insulin	**NP**	Nighttime Prolactin	**NPY**	NeuroPeptide Y
C	Cortisol	**IR**	Insulin Receptor	**DP**	Daytime Prolactin	**CC**	Carbo Craving
BS	Blood Sugar	**WG**	Weight Gain	**L**	Leptin	**WL**	Weight Loss

Time of the Season

If your prolactin number comes back too high, just go to bed earlier and earlier until you have a solid three and a half hours of sleep before midnight in the winter months (see chart) and talk to your doctor about a dopamine agonist (which pushes dopamine receptors into activation the way dopamine would) called *bromocriptine*.[73-74] Bromocriptine and L-dopa are widely used in Europe as anti-aging drugs because of their effects on memory enhancement, weight loss, and arthritis via prolactin. The reason bromocriptine does all this is because when dopamine is up, prolactin goes down.[75] Amphetamines like phentermine could do it, too, but most doctors won't prescribe those.

The natural way to shut down daytime production of prolactin, which is associated with breast cancer, heart disease, and autoimmunity and contributes to Alzheimer's, is to go to bed no later than three hours before midnight, and replace your hormones. Natural progesterone also blocks prolactin receptors.[76-79]

The three hours of melatonin production reset prolactin production to a "short-day," "winter" pattern, meaning less prolactin production in the daytime[80] because three hours of melatonin production before midnight is always followed by six hours of prolactin production at night to rev up the defensive arm[81] of your immune system. Any less than three hours of sleep before midnight and you are in "short night," "summer" mode. This is the norm for most Americans, who rarely get to bed before 10:00 or 11:00 P.M.

Short nights (less than three hours of melatonin production before midnight) provoke only one and a half hours of prolactin production. When that happens, prolactin is triggered by this schedule to pour again the next day in order to rev up the autoimmune arm of your immune system, because the only time in nature you would ever lose sleep in the dark is when you're nursing a baby.[82] It's devastating enough to your body to live in endless summer, aging every day in fast forward when you have sex hormones, but when you don't have them anymore, it really is the end.

Red-Eye Express

Sleeping is the key to getting your cortisol to fall, which is how you can lower your overnight blood sugar. Your blood sugar can't drop unless your because cortisol *mobilizes* blood sugar during the daytime for why when your lights are on long after normal nightfall, your cortisol stays high and so does your blood sugar. Your insulin is up as long as your blood sugar is. It's those extra hours of insulin that mimic the seasonal trigger for insulin resistance to gain weight for winter.

Since cortisol naturally begins to fall at sunset, turn the lights down wherever you are at night. You can even block some of the light by wearing sunglasses at night. Pink or red eyeglasses enhance melatonin secretion by 80 percent if you wear them after dark. In nature, the pinks and reds of sunset just before nightfall start serotonin's cascade into melatonin because red light blocks green light, and the green and blue light of daylight blocks an enzyme called *n-acetyltransferase*. This enzyme prevents serotonin from cascading into melatonin. That's actually how you stay awake all day. But the colored glasses cancel out the enzyme-blocker effect of the artificial light at night after dark and make you sleepy sooner, just like sunset does.

If you still can't sleep through the night when you first start your hormone replacement, try Tylenol PM. Acetaminophen acts directly on estrogen receptors, and diphenhydramine is an antihistamine that hits GABA receptors, so until your hormones have been back in place for a few cycles, Tylenol PM can act like estrogen and progesterone to put you to sleep.[83-87] The more you sleep through the night, the sooner your insulin resistance subsides, and the sooner your estrogen reception wakes up, too, so your hormone replacement can work.

Waking up every time you turn over or hear snoring or the cat is a low-progesterone state, but interval waking at, say, 2:00 A.M. and 4:00 A.M. or 1:00 A.M. and 3:30 A.M. is an estrogen-deprived state.[88] Knowing this will help you to adjust your replacement levels to sleep soundly *all* night.

Taking one to four 5 mg sublingual melatonin tablets from the health food store before bed (always no later than one to two hours after nightfall) can really aid in the "falling asleep" process and—if you do it early enough—staying asleep. The missing melatonin[89-90] in the sleep-wake cycle, which occurs when you lose sleep before midnight, must be replaced, too—not only to time prolactin for appetite control and cancer prevention, but to turn off estrogen and androgen receptors.[91-96] These sex hormone receptors must be blanked out for at least three hours every night to prime the rhythm of not only your immune system,[97-99] but for your hormone receptors in the brain, too. Without brain reception, estrogen's feedback to control human growth hormone's (HGH) pulsatility while you sleep[100-101] is lost, and HGH controls slow-wave sleep, the kind that keeps you asleep all night.

The most life-threatening aspect of destroying melatonin's rhythm[102] by staying up very late after sundown means that you'll be making more prolactin the next day.[103] This fact, simple alone, gives a great deal of weight to the premise that losing sleep can promote breast cancer almost as effectively as not nursing long enough.[104-111]

Breaking Us in Two

Natural hormone replacement with estrogen and progesterone can have a dramatic effect on pain management. Estrogen blocks prostaglandins like PGE2 as well as do Advil (ibuprofen) or naproxen (Aleve). Without estrogen on board, we wake up aching every morning. As estrogen falls over time as we age, every bump and knock we've ever received in our lifetimes hurts again, just as if we'd broken a bone. Progesterone, by itself, dampens the nervous system's response to pain. That's the reason pain sensitivity yoyos throughout the menstrual cycle. The huge amounts of progesterone secreted at the end of a pregnancy are, in fact, a natural analgesic provided by nature in preparation for labor. Inflammatory reactions, from arthritis to acne to Alzheimer's, are in tandem with estrogen and progesterone action, as we elucidated in Chapter Nine.

When you discuss natural hormone replacement, more likely than not your doctor will insist on ordering a bone mineral density[112-113] or bone scan test. Osteoporosis affects women eight times more than men. One in two women over age fifty will suffer at least one lifetime fracture from osteoporosis. When we run out of estrogen and progesterone, our bones start to die very quickly. Bones have their own life cycle or metabolism, a rhythm of growth and death governed by estrogen and progesterone.[114] The fall off of estrogen in perimenopause means no peak of estrogen activity to make progesterone receptors which would build bone. This is the beginning of osteoporosis. Estrogen controls *osteoclast* activity.[115] Osteoclasts are bone cells that "eat up" old bone for disposal.[116] Progesterone controls *osteoblastic* activity. Osteoblasts are bone cells that *build* fresh new bone. Progesterone, then, in this case, grows bone, and estrogen takes it away so that new bone can grow again next month. Without this balanced interplay, one of two[117] things can happen: Without estrogen, bone would overgrow into a cancer-like state, or without progesterone, unopposed estrogen would make bones thin, fragile, and porous—osteoporotic.[118]

Estrogen replacement alone, because it takes away bone, should be bad for osteoporosis and seems to be so in conventional low doses. But estrogen replacement helps for a little while because it does *prevent apoptosis* in the bone-building cells, the osteoblasts;[119] however, unless progesterone comes in to *stimulate* osteoblasts, not much bone grows[120] from estrogen replacement alone.

Drugs like Fosamax, Actonel, and Boniva stop old bone cells from being metabolized and reabsorbed, processes that must happen to assure healthy bones. When your hormones are normal in youth, the broken-down bone minerals are used to rebuild new bones again, but in menopause—without hormones—the minerals are lost, and the bones just get thinner and more brittle.

Increasing supplemental calcium is really pretty useless. No claims have ever been made by the medical establishment that increased calcium can really prevent or cure osteoporosis. Natural, transdermal, bio-identical hormone replacement prescribed in a normal cycle can do what none of those approaches[122-124] can do: revive your bones.

Don't Eat the Yellow Snow

After you've gotten the results back from your bloodwork on your estrogen and progesterone levels and your thyroid, prolactin, C-peptide, and bone scan tests, your doctor will undoubtedly tell you that with an estrogen of 40 or 70 or 140 and a progesterone of less than 2, you are within normal ranges for your age. And that's true. But remind him that it is also "normal" to see breast cancer, heart disease, diabetes, osteoporosis, fibromyalgia (pain all over), macular degeneration, autoimmunity, and the beginnings of dementia in women our age. It's really unarguable logic. If he still insists that hormones cause cancer, ask him for the studies that prove his premise in which natural, raw material hormones were used and not Premarin or progestins.

We know that he can't find any.

Replacing sex hormone action to avoid the list of possibilities in the previous paragraph will mean attaining the numbers in your bloodwork of someone not at risk for those diseases—someone twenty years old with her whole life ahead of her.[125-126] Once you have established, through a reliable testing method (bloodwork), that you are indeed in need of hormone replacement, getting a prescription for enough concentrated hormone replacement to bring you to those numbers should be your goal. Of course, you will be relentlessly offered any number of drug "hormone" products from the table in Appendix II.

Just say no.

In this book, in this chapter, you have enough information on quantity, sources, and maintenance monitoring to help your doctor help you. While finding a reliable practitioner to prescribe hormones for you in the way you want them and in the quantities you need may be very difficult, it's the only real possibility for accurate, full hormone replacement. *Our investigation of the problems and the solution indicate that any other choice will quite likely cause a serious risk to your health now and in the future.*[127] The research cited in Parts Two and Three of this book completely supports the notion that *in every case, in every way*—from breast cancer and heart attacks to Alzheimer's disease—the *raw materials* that the drug companies have adulterated to make patentable, profitable drugs do the job in your body better than anything else that is available could do, except a time machine to turn back the clock.

Natural hormone replacement can't be found over the counter, unfortunately.

While it appears, until you look more closely, that the hormones for HRT from plants are available at the health food store, it's not true. "Natural," in the case of hormone replacement, often just means that the substance can be said to have at some point come from planet Earth. But are any of the products in your health food store any more reliably scientifically grounded or effective and without side effects than the options Western medicine offers you?

Not really.

After all, every drug in Appendix II of this book started out as a *botanical derivative*, but none of them can qualify as the natural, bio-identical hormone replacement[128-131] we're supporting with the research in this book. The products at your health food or grocery store fall into the same category, but for different reasons.

Lost in the Supermarket

A growing number of postmenopausal women are trying to sidestep the decision altogether by turning to natural *supplements*.[132] In 1999, sales of progesterone containing creams, phytoestrogen extracts, and cocktails made up of vitamins, minerals, and herbs rose to $21 million in supermarkets and drugstores, more than triple 1998 sales. Sales for potentially dangerous all-in-one menopausal formulas were $36.2 million last year, which is an increase of 197 percent, according to Spins and ACNeilsen, market research firms.[133] Soy products like wild yam creams and tofu containing *phytoestrogens* and herbals like Vitex (chasteberry) and Dong Quai (Chinese)[134] containing *bioflavinoids* all promise relief from perimenopausal "symptoms," which is about all that they can do.[135-138]

Homeopathy, first practiced in the 1800s, uses increasingly diluted herbal, metallic, and gaseous formulas sprayed onto small spheres of milk sugar to affect vibrational, energetic pathways to communicate with the system to effect a cure.[139-140] Homeopathy works incredibly well on children and people with well-functioning, homeostatically intact immune systems, so although treatments for menopause like Lachesis (literally, snake oil) all guarantee alleviation of hot flashes and, sometimes, migraines, these options really can provide relief only if you have any circulating endogenous hormones left somewhere that the homeopathy can work with, like in, say, perimenopause, but not postmenopausally. Homeopathy can't affect hormones or hormone receptors that aren't there.

The hormonelike precursors in ground-up flowers and plants don't follow normal cascade patterns or create steroid receptors because they come in chronic doses that can't create "peak" levels and are for the most part oral preparations, although there are some weak creams on the market. Most natural sources of hormones without extraction and synthesis are not completely bio-available, and those that have a more potent effect are biodynamic, meaning that they have more than one hormonal effect on various receptors simultaneously.[141]

While that might seem to be an appealing idea, it's important to note that the Chinese herbal remedies available in health food stores and through alternative health practitioners have evolved, through trial and error, on *Chinese* people, which may or may not be you. It's only logical that a regimen of pseudoreplacement and symptom abatement that has been time-tested on a genetically closed group of people would work best on those people, but not necessarily on you.[142-147] Unless a licensed naturopath is making fresh extracts, tinctures, and salves from these herbs for you *personally*, designed to affect unbalanced hormones in you *personally*, you may do much more harm than good shopping for hormones at the grocery store. If you are postmenopausal, those herbs and homeopathy need receptors to work on, and you may be short on more than a few receptors depending on how long your own hormones have been gone.[148-150] At best, they are remarkably expensive compared to natural, bio-identical creams from a compounding pharmacist.

Why, then, do we keep trying to dose ourselves?

Witchy Woman

The truth is that it's probably instinct. Women throughout history have always known how to take care of themselves and each other using the materials at hand.[151] Plants containing natural hormones were the only "health food" we had before the 1960s brought us tofu and wheat sprouts. We have receptors in all of our cells for all that the Earth has to offer. We have nicotinic receptors, cannabinoid (cannabis) receptors, and even menthol receptors.[152-153]

Plants have *always* been used for medicinal purposes. Dogs eat grass when they need a laxative, and primates like chimps and gorillas may even control their own menstrual cycles by seeking out certain plants in their environment. Tried-and-true remedies like echinacea, which spikes an immune reaction or allergy, can be useful when fighting germs.[154] Many cultures use garlic as a hypoglycemic that lowers insulin by lowering blood sugar, as well as an antibacterial and an antiviral. Garlic even has an HMG-CoA blocking potential.[155] That means that garlic can act like an antibiotic, anti-diabetic, and Lipitor all at the same time.

Ginkgo biloba, from China, works at the level of prostacyclins, which are the eicosenoids that Barry Sears talks about in his book *The Zone*, for vasodilation to enhance blood flow not only in the brain but in the heart. Kava kava, used in Polynesia, actually works on brain and body receptors like benzodiazapines (Valium). Valerian root, on the other hand, doesn't work on receptors at all. Valerian decreases enzymes that cut up neurotransmitters and take them away, so in the case of valerian's soporific effects, GABA hangs around longer, much like the effect natural progesterone has when you take it orally.[156]

Song Remains the Same

Botanical sources of raw hormone material make sense pharmacologically and physiologically because plants are really just like us, on the molecular level and in terms of their response to their environment. Plants assimilate information, calculate outcomes, and respond in a complex series of molecular signaling pathways that are remarkably similar to our own. They have the power to compute, they show foresight, and they remember what's happened to them. Plants react to at least fifteen sensory signals.[157-158]

As Darwin pointed out more than a hundred years ago, "in several respects, light seems to act on plants in nearly the same manner as it does on animals by means of the nervous system."[159] Since it's only the light and food supply that our sex hormones are really responding to, plants actually mimic our own priorities.

In order to react to light, sounds, chemicals, vibrations, and touch, not to mention water, temperature, and gravity, plants have to have *hormones*, hormones just exactly like ours.[160] Botanists and ecologists have long been using terms like *foraging, competing,* and *predator evasion* when talking about plants. In order to respond proactively to their environment, plants, reacting to environmental signals, *behave* in a way to survive based on hormonal cues just as we do.

If we apply the "vase full of marbles" image from the previous chapter to the food chain, which must include plants, no matter what species sits atop another in the "great chain of being," it's always very similar molecules that are all called hormones acting "all the way down" through every species, plant and animal, to translate environmental cues into survival behaviors.

Abracadabra

Since plants are a part of the food chain and their molecules "match" ours, using their hormones to replace or bolster our health and for recreation has always been an option. The examples are endless: Beer drinking, something most of us can relate to, is really recreational sex hormone use. The cone of the hops (hops are the basis of beer) flower is full of 8-prenylnaringenine, *literally* the most estrogenic bioflavonoid on the planet.[161-162] Right now, hops are the main ingredient in those breast enhancement creams sold in TV infomercials and at the back of the grocery store tabloids.

Hormone *replacement* and manipulation for contraception from nature's bounty directly to our receptors was as natural a way to space childbirth as was nursing for fifteen months between pregnancies in the natural world.[163] Hormones in nature that fit into our receptors have been worshiped since before Christ all over the world. Universally, mistletoe may be the most celebrated of all, especially by the group of Indo-Europeans known as Aryans.[164]

When the Indo-Europeans of Asia Minor, just northwest of India, moved up into Greece and Italy and then on to Northern Europe and Scandinavia, they took with them their religion, based on the cycles of the moon, which worshiped the oak tree and its rare companion, mistletoe. Mistletoe is an evergreen semiparasitic plant that grows into a large bush on the branches of oak trees, with no roots extending to the ground. Mistletoe draws mineral salts and water from its host, the oak.[165] Mistletoe berries contain a single seed encased in a very viscous, sticky flesh. This "glue" is the way the seeds of mistletoe stick to oak branches to germinate.[166]

The Aryans found magic in the plant's ability to live without roots extending to the ground and in mistletoe's remarkable ability to stay bright green, entwining the gray dead oak even after the winter comes. Mistletoe's berries, leaves, and stems approach the bioflavanoid levels of hops.[167]

In Part Two of this book, we mentioned the story of Christmastime mistletoe. At the winter solstice, there was always, in the Celtic culture, a party. While the women prepared for the feast and orgy to come, they drank a preparation made of mead (a honey-based beer) and mistletoe berries. This potion contained the precursors of both estrogen and progesterone. After the solstice frenzy subsided, the women would experience spontaneous menstruation. This was the ancient version of the morning-after pill we know as RU-486. Any gynecologist or nurse practitioner would recognize this practice as a "progesterone challenge."

Pliny the Elder wrote in the first century B.C.E., "The Druids—and that is what the Celts call their wizards (medicine men)—hold nothing more sacred than Mistletoe and the oak on which it grows . . . it is gathered with great ceremony on the sixth day of the moon. . . . Hailing the moon in a native word that means 'universal healer of all things,' they prepare a ritual sacrifice of two white bulls. A priest in white vestments climbs the tree and with a golden sickle held in the right hand under the tunic, thrust through the left armhole cuts down the mistletoe which is caught in a white cloak."[168-169]

Pliny also goes on to say that the Druids made a potion to drink for fertility and insomnia and to rub on malignant tumors of all kinds. The writers of the time saw the results and were amazed enough to carry these "cures" back to Rome. Mistletoe was also used to "bring forth barren animals," cure epilepsy, heal ulcers, and counteract poisons of all sorts. Studies in molecular medicine bear out the truth behind these tales. Estrogen and progesterone will do all of those things. It seems that the natural hormones of mistletoe were known not just to the Druids, Gauls, and Italians as healing and regenerative, but around the world, too.[170]

The Aino of Japan and the Walos of Central Africa all held mistletoe in peculiar veneration as a medicine universally termed *all-healer*. In the Americas, Indians like the Winnebagos, Dakotas, and Sioux believed anything touched by mistletoe was brought to life again. So do we. They, like the Druids, believed that the parasite could "unlock the gates of death." These reports were based on what we would term *epidemiological science* and *experimentation* today.[171]

The ritual way in which mistletoe was harvested by the Druids was also seen among most other groups sharing the same time periods, including the Cambodians. From Sweden to Switzerland, mistletoe, to this day, figures prominently in modern European folklore. The word *mistletoe* in modern Celtic speech, in Ireland, Wales, Brittany, and Scotland, still means *all-healer.* Did these remedies made with hormones really work? The answer may lie in the fact that the number-one prescribed complementary cancer treatment in Europe is a product called *Iscador*,[172] made from mistletoe by a drug company called Weleda in Switzerland.[173]

Mixed Emotions

Iscador is administered in injections of increasing strength, almost like the progesterone peak in the menstrual cycle. A major epidemiological study published in English tracked patients who developed cancer who had and had not used Iscador. Results showed that Iscador greatly improved survival rates for a wide variety of cancers, including but not limited to breast cancer.[174] Study participants who augmented conventional therapy with mistletoe extract survived 40 percent longer compared with those who did not.

Weleda collects the saps from all parts of the mistletoe harvested twice a year, from all mistletoe found, not just that which grows on the oak. If the Druids were right about the concentration of flavonoids in the mistletoe on the sixth day of the moon, perhaps harvesting methods should be examined. Right now the efficacy of Iscador is credited to the *lectins*[175-176] in *Viscum album* (mistletoe).[177] Lectins cause an immune reaction that enhances the activity of natural killer cells.[178-179] Natural progesterone is a product of the synthesis of the phytoestrogen diosgenin, which is an isoflavone. Progesterone's ability to throw the switch for cell suicide or apoptosis is probably the effect that the concentrated phytoestrogen has. But the apoptotic merit of the flavonoids in mistletoe has all but been ignored by science until recently, when scientists reported that natural progesterone *augmented* the effects of some standard chemotherapy.[180-181]

Where Have All the Flowers Gone?

Besides hops and mistletoe, many plants contain phytoestrogens. The parent sources of phytoestrogens, *isoflavones,* contain flavonoids, of which there are at least 3,000 that have been identified.[182-183] Ginseng flowers exert a luteotrophic effect, meaning that they act like luteinizing hormone (LH) in your body. LH causes ovulation if you have any eggs left. So does the berry of *Vitex agnus-castus*, or chasteberry plant.[184-185] Across the board in nature, the flowers or berries of a plant have "female" or ovarian and pituitary hormone effects, and the stems and leaves have androgenic effects.[186] The flowers of blue cohosh, for example, have a very weak estrogenic effect on receptors similar to estriol, the third-down-the-line metabolite (the end product of enzyme reactions on steroid hormones) of 17-beta estradiol. That's why blue cohosh doesn't do much for hot flashes.

Natural estrogen replacement ameliorates hot flashes by raising the core body temperature's sweating threshold.[187-189] Black cohosh, on the other hand, has a vasodilatory effect that works better on vasomotor symptoms,[190] which are the *flushing* part of hot flashes. Some isoflavones, like licorice root, which works on cortisol receptors, and poke root, which works on thyroid receptors, act like steroid and peptide hormones,[191] not sex hormones. The *phytoestrogens*[192] that the media and over-the-counter drug marketers push so hard as solutions for menopause are all flavonoids. Red clover, burdock root, horny goat weed, red raspberry leaf, and peppermint are all filled with *phytoestrogens*.[193] These plant hormones are 1,000 times weaker than the hormones found in your body or in bio-identical natural hormone replacement.

Lignans, found in fiber, are not really phytoestrogens. They turn into biologically active estrogenic compounds in your gut through enzyme activity. Phytoestrogens taken in from plants can compete with your own endogenous estrogen for binding sites on genes and receptors. So taking these over-the-counter supplements once you have hormone replacement can confuse your receptors and diminish the effects of replacement.[194] Seeds are full of phytoestrogens, too.[195-197] Linseed, evening primrose oil, and pomegranates are all full of phytoestrogenic compounds. But, again, since they have one-thousandth of the potency of natural hormones by prescription, you'd need to rub on or ingest a thousand times more every day. That's why synthesis in the lab in prescription-strength natural hormones increases potency enough to make hormone replacement convenient and cheap without the side effects of drugs.

Genistein and diosgenin are the phytoestrogens most often synthesized out of plants to make the natural bio-identical hormones that were used in all the studies we've presented in this book that were not done with the hormone drugs[198] (see Appendix II).

It's easier to extract phytoestrogens from legumes (beans like soy) and tubers like wild Mexican yams than to use hops flowers or mistletoe. While phytoestrogens from plant matter like crushed flowers or berries can have a weak estrogenic action on estrogen receptors, progestagenic activity from any phytoestrogen in a plant substance can only happen in *premenopausal* women. Progestagenic plants can *encourage* (through LH action) an actual luteal or progesterone-driven phase by causing ovulation of the eggs you have left. Postmenopausal women can experience no progestagenic action from phytoestrogens, because there's no potential for a corpus luteum, unless they're synthesized and concentrated into a bio-identical molecule in the lab.

The way the lab does it is much like it's done in our own body's cells.

Groovin' Is Easy

Remember that in your body, choles*terol* that you eat from fats or make from carbohydrates through HMG CoA, coupled with the action of other various enzymes, becomes steroid sex hormones, first pregnelonone, then progesterone, to DHEA or testosterone, which can eventually become 17-beta estradiol. This process can be reenacted in the lab. The precursor to steroid hormones in plants—like sex steroids or cortisol (hydrocortisone itch cream is made this way)—is ubiquitous in plants as diverse as mistletoe to sarsaparilla to wild Mexican yams and even soybeans. The lab technicians do the same thing with the plant hormones genistein or diosgenin and enzymes in a petri dish that your body does with cholesterol.[199]

The botanical "progesterone" from plant sources in the lab can easily become testosterone and then estradiol. It is somewhere in between, during the creation of these three bio-identical hormone molecules that your body's receptors would recognize, that contains all of the potential hormonelike chimeras that are patentable as unique drugs for companies like Wyeth-Ayerst.

These molecules that can be synthesized in between the two bio-identical hormone molecules progesterone and testosterone are called *progestin drugs*, which often have estrogenic or androgenic effects (testosteronelike) versus progestagenic effects on receptors,[200] even though they started out as natural progesterone. Progestins can confuse your receptors and immune system,[201-204] because they aren't bio-identical to the hormone molecules in humans.

Progestins and some 17-beta estradiol in various combinations are what's in any version of the Pill.[205] Seventeen-beta estradiol is the strongest form of estrogen occurring in your body, which just means that it is the most "active" form. Seventeen-beta estradiol fits in both alpha and beta estrogen receptors. As 17-beta estradiol is metabolized or used up, the products created along the way are *different* forms of estrogen with different names. They are called E3-*estriol* and E1-*estrone*. Until very recently, the first and most infamous synthesized estrogen was diethylstilbesterol (DES), which was used to prevent miscarriage, in cancer treatments, and to dry up a mother's milk supply.

It's a Mistake

Estriol is really never produced in any quantity in your body except in the third trimester of pregnancy, and it's produced by the adrenal glands of the baby, not mom.[206] Estriol is found as the major waste product in the urine of young women because as the third or end product it's the bulk of estrogen in waste. As hormone replacement, it will act on vaginal tissues for dryness, but estriol is the third metabolite down the line in the process of metabolizing estradiol and as such has very weak effects all over your body.[207]

Uninformed doctors, who are afraid of prescribing the most active form of estrogen, real bio-identical 17-beta estradiol, often think that estriol is better than nothing; worse yet, some think that estriol can act as a "natural" SERM (in replacement for tamoxifen and its derivatives) to keep estradiol from reaching receptors, as if that's a good thing.[208-209]

It also looks as if the trend toward prescribing testosterone, with other hormones or alone, to relatively perimenopausal women may be *very* dangerous. In 1999, the journal *Carcinogenesis* published a report from the University of Hong Kong on the role of androgens (testosterone) in breast cancer.[210] It was a rat study using 17-beta estradiol and testosterone to induce cancer. They found that low levels of 17-beta estradiol initiated the cancer growth, but in combination with testosterone, the incidence of cancer skyrocketed.

They said that "our data showed that after treatment with testosterone, either alone or in combination with 17-beta estradiol, there was overexpression of the androgen receptor in ductal epithelial cells." Testosterone not only makes its own receptor occur, it downregulates the function of any estrogen receptor next to it.[211] That means that if you've stopped ovulating, because of low chronic estrogen levels, or a practitioner prescribes both estrogen and testosterone, it may increase your chances of breast cancer significantly.

The trendy alternative to PremPro offered by "open-minded" providers is called *Tri-Est*.[212] It's an illogical, unscientific, very-low-dose combination of bio-identical clones of the three estrogens naturally occurring in your body—estradiol, estriol, and estrone. Since 17-beta estradiol will always metabolize into the other two by the action of enzymes also naturally occurring in your body, taking all three is not only redundant, it's physiologically just odd and probably confuses receptors. It seems to be more of a marketing ploy to the "natural" movement because, theoretically at least, in its tenets, it's closer to health food than to genuine endocrinology.

On the subject of marketing ploys, this year the pharmaceutical company Duramed got the FDA to approve the first new conjugated estrogen since Premarin in the 1970s. It's called Cenestin.[213-214] It's still Premarin,[215] at least the same molecular structure as Premarin, but with the horse urine hormone derivative removed. Even though they've replaced animal estrogen with soy-derived 17-beta estradiol and some other synthetics, it's still a formula and a chronic dose that your body can't use. This is just a marketing ploy by a drug company to make Premarin and to make the animal rights people (PETA) leave them alone.

They're having enough trouble with the American Heart Association right now.[216]

Bang on the Drum All Day

The hormones that we share with plants work best when absorbed through the skin.[217-219] The raw materials of natural progesterone and 17-beta estradiol can be suspended in creams or an alcohol gel.[220-222] Hormones have very different effects when taken by mouth. Solvay Pharmaceuticals makes the most widely marketed natural progesterone pill, Prometrium, which is made from the raw material progesterone in an oil base, in doses of 100 and 200 mg. It has the potential—just as progesterone does—to be a neurosteroid and act like a neurotransmitter when it crosses the blood-brain barrier. Natural progesterone, from your ovaries or transdermally applied, hits GABA receptors all over to calm the brain. Prometrium[223-224] taken orally must go through the liver instead of directly into the bloodstream. Prometrium, after being metabolized in the liver, becomes a molecule with more druglike, intoxicating side effects on GABA.[225-227]

Anything ingested orally must face the first-pass liver detox. That fact alone means that any drug or hormone that comes in a pill must be overdosed to have any effect at all. By the time a pill makes it through your system, you've only absorbed about 10 percent, so you've ingested 90 percent more of any drug taken by mouth than you needed to than if you had just taken it transdermally. Molecules that pass through your skin are rated at 60 to 70 percent absorption and potency. On the skin of your arm, what you don't absorb ends up on your sleeve; once you've swallowed it, God knows where the excess might land or what it might be turned into.

But the best reason to use hormones through the skin is *timing*.[228]

And We Danced

Any endocrinologist worth his salt knows that hormones are not chronically pouring into your system. Hormones, all hormones, have *pulsatility* and *amplitude*. That means that hormones have a "beat" like music or your heart. Think of a single drumbeat—*boom, boom, boom*—or your pulse. That's pulsatility.[229] Now hear it go faster and louder—*boom, boom, boom, boom*. That's amplitude. In the same way your heart races if you open the closet and find a monster, your hormones can "race" depending on the needs of your system and the environmental cues to which it's responding.

Transdermal hormones can deposit through your skin[230-234] into your fat base below, where it will sit, waiting to seep into your bloodstream. With every pulse of your heartbeat, your resting baseline of estrogen or progesterone seeps through capillaries into the blood rushing by. When you are under stress and your heart beats faster, the amplitude of hormone release is faster, too. This system of delivery of hormone to your bloodstream will bring you internally as close to being twenty years old as you'll ever get when putting in hormones from the outside.[235-236] The potential that the newly available insulin pump created for Type II diabetics, which pulses insulin automatically and more normally when you eat, will ever be modified for sex hormone replacement anytime soon is, sadly, just a dream.

The transdermal mode of delivery is physiologically more identical to the pulse and amplification of the beat of your own orchestrated hormones than any pill or patch can possibly, with their chronically low application of hormone, ever approach. But from *where* your doctor orders your hormone cream matters a lot.[237] Your doctor can't just order your hormone replacement cream from just any "drug" store. He must order it from a drugstore that has a *compounding* pharmacist. Most drugstores, certainly not the large chains—like Walgreen's, Duane Reade, CVS, or Rite Aid—do not compound hormones from scratch. This fact, however, is no reason to think it's difficult to get bio-identical hormone creams.

Potion #9

Some smaller drugstores have pharmacists who compound. But more than likely, your physician will order your hormones from a compounding pharmacy that does nothing but compounding. That means no pills supplied by large drug companies like Pfizer or Eli Lilly or Wyeth-Ayerst. Pharmacists now are dispensers of drug company–supplied pills. Occasionally they mix a powder with distilled water to make a syrup or liquid medicine, mostly for children. That's what has happened to the science of pharmacy in the last sixty years, since World War II and the rise of the giant pharmaceutical companies. Before World War II, there were only compounding pharmacy.

In the last 30,000 years,[238] generations of pharmacists have been mixing medicines. Preparing and dispensing compounds of herbs was what the original shaman did for his tribe. Fertility and resurrection magic from herbal sources was, from time immemorial, a healing specialty, along with intoxicants. Treating wounds with pastes made from plants and minerals, or moxabustion in Chinese medicine—the practitioner places gently burning, smoking plants under overturned glass cups on sore joints or muscles—is a testament to the effectiveness and origins of transdermal compounded preparations.

In Europe today, the drug companies not only provide estrogen, testosterone, and progesterone gels and creams, but more standard fare, like analgesics such as ibuprofen, are made into transdermal gels. Prior to 1960, the art and skill of compounding pharmacy was an integral part of pharmacy school. However, as compounding took a back seat to dispensing pills sent in giant boxes from large pharmaceutical companies, the pharmacist's need for compounding skills decreased, too. Eventually, the belief that manufactured drugs could replace the need for individualized medications became more prevalent. It is often assumed that an individual with a pharmacy degree possesses all of the training necessary to compound.[239]

That's not true.

The majority of pharmacists can "mix" medicines, but have very little training in the true art of compounding from raw ingredients like pure micronized hormone powders such as USP progesterone and 17-beta estradiol. Most pharmacists will have had only a semester of basic compounding after four years of pharmacy school. In defense of pharmacy programs everywhere, it's pretty difficult to fund and support advanced compounding classes when, in fact, these classes would put the pharmacist in direct competition with the manufacturers of *commercial* pharmaceutical preparations like Androgel, a transdermal gel preparation of raw testosterone from Solvay, a large pharmaceutical company.[240]

Elected

In order for your doctor to order from a compounder, he'll need your help. Doctors often form relationships with pharmacists who are particularly helpful or efficient. Most likely your doctor would turn to his preferred pharmacist to order your hormones. Since you don't want to run into a brick wall if his pharmacist is not a compounder, you will want to have options ready to share with your doctor, like the phone numbers of some compounding pharmacies that you have already interviewed.

We have included in Appendix I the phone number for the Professional Compounding Centers of America (PCCA) and the number for the International Association of Compounding Pharmacists (IACP). These agencies will fax you a list of recommended compounding pharmacists in your area. Pick a couple and call them. The questions to ask are:

- Have you taken continuing education courses on compounding?
- How many years experience do you have compounding?
- Do you possess a database or hard copy of formulations?
- Do you possess, on the premises, the equipment necessary to compound and package the formula as prescribed?

- Where do you purchase your raw pharmaceuticals?
- How many compounded prescriptions do you dispense in a week?
- Will you mail my prescription promptly? How much notice do you need for a refill?
- Do you regularly have your formulas evaluated by a third-party outside authority for potency, accuracy, and contamination?

If the pharmacists you reach have no time to speak to you or return your call, move on to the next name on the list. If the pharmacists you finally speak to are defensive or indignant about your list of questions, move on to the next name on the list. Once you've found one or two pharmacies that satisfy you, make sure that the pharmacy will package your hormone creams in 3cc syringes with capped ends.

This is very important.

The packaging for compounded preparations varies widely from pharmacy to pharmacy. The difference between receiving your hormones in a tub or tube with a measuring spoon or via a small (3cc) syringe with lines marked off to guide your application is the difference between an accurate dose for accurate replacement and the over-the-counter phytoestrogen creams available at the health food store. Take two copies of your list of preferred compounders with you to your doctor's appointment—one for the doctor and one for his nurse/receptionist, who will actually call in or fax your prescription.

Change Partners

You will, by your second visit, have bloodwork proving need. At this second visit, you can discuss your preferences. While it's most likely that your doctor will prescribe transdermal natural hormones, it's very *unlikely* that he will provide a prescription for the quantity of hormone that it will take to reach the blood levels we outlined earlier of a twenty-year-old woman.

You may face an incredulous professional who will, at best, look confused by your plan (to use the hormones in increasing amounts and check your blood levels twice a month on Days 11 and 21 of your cycle until full replacement is attained) or, at worst, laugh at you and flat-out refuse. If this doctor is an old, trusted family friend or a young, open-minded, hungry-to-build-a-practice novice physician, hand him this book.

Offer to sign a waiver saying you've been informed, but still want to plan your own treatment. Always try to use simple logic: remind him that *young women rarely have osteoporosis, macular degeneration, or osteoarthritis, and they rarely die of cancer, heart disease, Type II diabetes, or Alzheimer's disease. Young women, too, on the whole, are not incontinent, too cold, too hot, or plagued by unrelenting insomnia. They have regular periods when they aren't pregnant or breast-feeding.*[241] So it makes good sense that you would want to replace *all* of your hormones *accurately* to the levels of optimum health.

That small piece of logic means that in order to ensure reliable good health, your endocrine physiology *must mimic youth.*[242-244] If he's smart, he'll get it. If not, move on. Find a doctor or nurse practitioner who's interested in a new approach to real evidence-based medicine, not the standard of care.

You are a consumer, you have the right to shop.

You may be constrained by what your HMO or insurance will pay for; that's why you picked at least two pharmacists to choose from. Now pick the cheapest. Ask about pricing: "How much is a prescription for 40 mg of E2 (estrogen)?" Ask this same question of all of the pharmacists you interview, then compare prices. These hormones may be handmade; but the raw materials are inexpensive and the pricing is uncontrolled. That combination means that some compounders can get greedy. The pharmacist should offer to help you file your insurance claim. Argue for reimbursement with your insurance company; they pay for birth control pills, Viagra, and Premarin—don't let them off the hook for the hormones or the bloodwork.

Day by Day

Because hormone creams are purported to be available over the counter, at your local health food store or pharmacy, there're great misconceptions about their efficacy. The truth is that they are only available by prescription, and since most doctors are often unaware of their existence or of how effective they are, not only is their effect on cancer only a whisper among molecular biologists, but their reliability as HRT is somewhat scoffed at by the clinicians who *have* heard of them.[245] Be firm. You've done your homework; it's at the back of this book. Offer the research to your doctor. Ask for four bloodwork requisitions with the same tests ordered in advance—one each for Day 11 and Day 21 to check hormone levels on peak days for the next two months. Your doctor just needs to call one of the Wiley Registered Pharmacies™ on the list at www.thewileyprotocol.com and say to the pharmacist there "The Wiley Protocol®" and your name. You will receive two packages stamped "^{28}WP" in the upper-left-hand corner: a purple one for progesterone and a green one for estrogen. The right amount of hormones and a patient instruction sheet with both a personal and a lunar calendar will be included. If you have any questions the Wiley Registered Pharmacy™ pharmacist can't answer, go back to the website. The Registered Pharmacies™ on the website have agreed to make the hormones exactly the same, with the same materials, packaging and pricing every time; so someday we can run a national study using the standardized compunded hormone regimen, *something that's never been done before.*

You will apply your hormones in "lines" to any hairless part of your body with a fat pad (inner thigh, upper arm). Transdermal hormones are dosed BID (morning and night).

The numbers under the wave pattern chart (see Appendix I) reflect this twice-a-day dosing.

Don't forget the blood draws on Days 11 or 12 and 21, or you can't adjust the dose for accuracy. Day 12's estrogen and progesterone readings should be inverse to Day 21's, for example, Day 12, E-425, P-1.7 versus Day 21, E-150, P-21. Lab values vary, but remember that the "age range and phase of cycle" is always printed somewhere on the lab report. When you have your lab work done, ask them to carbon copy the patient and give them your fax number.

Natural Woman

ESTROGEN: The first five days of your cycle are a low twice-a-day dose of 4 lines BID during the course of your period. If you haven't had a period in a while, use the lunar calendar provided with your hormones and go with the phases of the moon as we described in Chapter Two. Any period after your first cycle that is less than four days long means you still don't have enough estrogen to build an adequate lining in the uterus. On Days 6, 7, and 8, the dose builds to six lines twice a day. On Days 9, 10, and 11, the dose increases

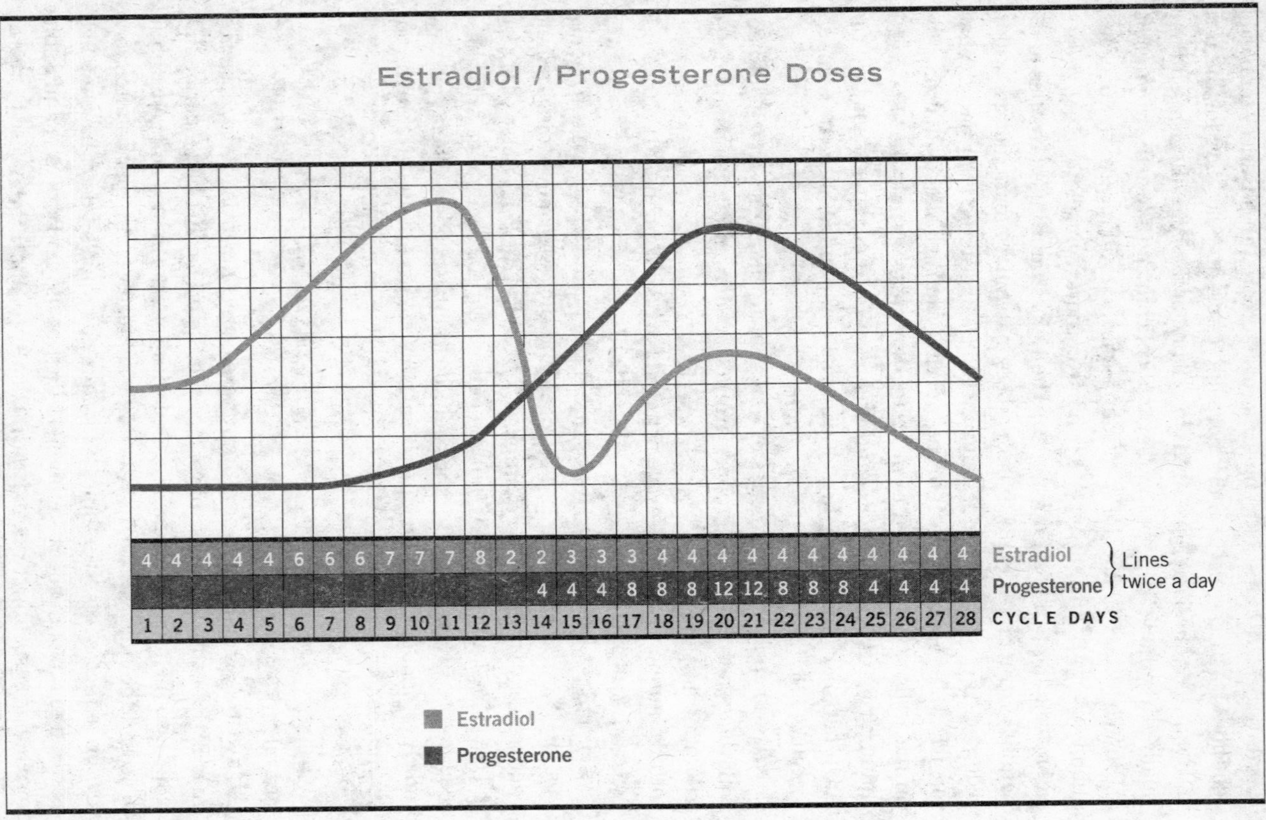
Estradiol / Progesterone Doses
Estradiol 4 4 4 4 4 6 6 6 7 7 7 8 2 2 3 3 3 4 4 4 4 4 4 4 4 4 4 4
Progesterone 4 4 4 8 8 8 12 12 8 8 8 4 4 4 4
Lines twice a day
CYCLE DAYS 1 2 3 4 5 6 7 8 9 10 11 12 13 14 15 16 17 18 19 20 21 22 23 24 25 26 27 28
Estradiol
Progesterone

to seven lines BID, and on Day 12, at the peak of the estrogen cycle, it's eight lines BID.

The standard-of-care-standard-issue Vivelle or Climara estrogen patches usually supplied for HRT contain a continuous static dose of .5 or one-half of 1 mg transdermally. So the idea that you are asking for twelve times that much twice a day, even just for two days out of twenty-eight, may have your doctor near hysterics. Good luck. Remind him of "all young women"—that is, if high episodic doses of estrogen caused cancer, all young women would be dead. Moreover, all pregnant women would be dead, because the *physiologic* dose of estrogen a pregnant woman is exposed to in the third trimester can reach blood levels above 1,600, or over three times as high as you are aiming for.[246]

On Days 13 and 14, go back to two lines BID. On Days 15, 16, and 17, three lines BID. Days 18 through 28 are four lines BID again, where we started. Check the chart[247-248] (see Appendix I).

PROGESTERONE: *Your progesterone is not dosed like the estrogen.* Progesterone is much stronger. Progesterone is added to your schedule on the morning of Day 14. Start with 4 lines BID on Days 14 and 15. That's four lines each dose morning and night. Increase the dose to eight lines BID Days 16 and 17. On Days 18 and 19, increase it to ten lines. Day 20 is twelve lines, and at the peak, Day 21, the dose is fourteen lines on the syringe, which is just about half of a syringe.

This amount and concentration will completely block your estrogen reception. It could give you a headache,[249] but during the first cycle, it's unlikely. If so, next month take one line less BID on Days 18 through 21. The first few cycles of progesterone can also act like a diuretic, increasing urinary frequency.[250] You should be sleeping better by now. If you're not, on Day 1 of your next cycle, use one to two lines of progesterone at night just to sleep, along with your regular estrogen.

On Day 22, go back down to twelve lines BID. On Days 23 and 24, drop the dose to ten lines BID. On Days 25 and 26, you're at eight lines BID, and Days 27 and 28 are back to four lines BID.

THEN STOP THE PROGESTERONE FOR FOURTEEN DAYS, but *never stop the estrogen again*. Just keep cycling over and over and over and over, just like when you were young and took birth control pills for years without stopping, only this time the rhythm's right[251-252] (see Appendix I).

Ruby Tuesday

The first five days of the twenty-eight-day cycle prescribed must be your menstrual period. *Even if you do not menstruate now, you will in the next one or two cycles.*[253-254] It doesn't matter how long ago your period stopped. It will return.[255]

Your replacement hormone levels must be high enough to build a uterine lining and then shed it once a month. As we've seen in the research, this hormone action of build and shed extends all the way to the myelin sheath encasing the neurons in your brain. If there is no evidence of this happening in your uterus, then it's not happening in your breasts and brain, either. This "virtual fertility" will fool Mother Nature into believing you have your whole life ahead of you, when in fact you've already lived what you were allowed in nature.

And here's a maybe-you-can-save-your-fertility heads-up: If you are in your twenties or very early thirties and *can't* have a baby yet, there is very strong evidence, *theoretically,* that 17-beta estradiol mimicking the levels found in twenty-year-olds will keep oocytes (your eggs) from aging along with you.[256-262] In other words, ablating your own *aging* rhythm with a new bio-identical, natural hormone rhythm created with transdermal creams *might* make your eggs more viable as soon as you can have a child. Or, as the scientists say, "It can't be excluded from the research that this method should show significant success."

When you are able to have a baby, you'd just stop the progesterone half of the cycle until you conceive—then you'd be making your own estrogen and progesterone. However, every year that you wait, you increase your chances of breast cancer from delaying pregnancy and lactational rhythms.[263-264]

If you don't have a uterus, this prescription is still the same. Many women all over the country, with and without cancer, have volunteered to use this protocol of treatment. *The concentrations of hormones in the cream and the doses have been arrived at by trial and error in human subjects over the last seven years.*[265]

Any doctor or health care practitioner who offers you "hormone" replacement that does *not* result in a four- to five-day period of bleeding at the end of twenty-eight days has not provided you with a natural hormone replacement cycle. The birth control pill, offered to menopausal women to ablate fluctuating cycles by imposing their own rhythm, does not qualify as hormone *replacement*, even though you may bleed at the end of a cycle, because the cycle birth control pills create what looks more like a zigzag line than two peaks of hormonal activity.

Replacing only *some* of your endocrine function, or replacing the pattern of endocrine function that you have now with the wrong pattern, does nothing but create *different* disease or, in the case of chronic, low-dose, unopposed estrogen without progesterone, sometimes even cancer.

We must respect the music.

Conclusion

An estimated 203,500 women in the United States are expected to develop invasive breast cancer in the year 2002. Breast cancer increased about 4.5 percent a year during the 1980s, and continued to increase, but at a slower pace, through 2000, which is the most recent year that has been reported.[1] In addition to *invasive* breast cancer, 54,300 new cases of in situ breast cancer, which is not metastatic, are expected to occur in 2002. Approximately 88 percent of those will be ductal carcinoma in situ (DCIS), undetectable to physical exam.

The increase in the detection of DCIS cases is a direct result of mammography.

Although the curve of past and presently occurring breast cancers, as depicted on a graph, matches exactly the cresting wave of aging in the baby boomer generation[2] of women passing through perimenopause and menopause, medical authorities examining the problem never even entertain the possibility that falling hormone levels may be the cause of this "epidemic." Unfortunately for us as women, simply replacing the falling endogenous hormones with the synthetic ones marketed by the drug companies not only exacerbates breast cancer *and heart disease*, but the hormone-like drugs create a whole host of new iatrogenic diseases.

Dancing in the Dark

We are told instead by our physicians to lower the fat in our diets,[3-5] exercise,[6-7] practice breast self-exams,[8] and rely on mammography for early detection[9] of a disease that to date medicine can only measure "cure" for in five-year increments.[10] Mammography has recently been deemed no better as a means of early detection than breast self-exam.[11] And after a carefully conducted eleven-year study following 266,064 factory workers in Shanghai, China, breast self-exam has been exposed as ineffective, too. Doctors in the *Journal of the National Cancer Institute* have now concluded that it makes no difference whether or not women learn to examine their own breasts or not.[12] After eleven years there was no difference between the group of women who were taught and supervised on how to do their own breast self-exams and those who were given no information at all.

Our doctors are consistently being misled by drug companies that cite independent research to endorse their products. The pharmaceutical industry increasingly uses references to clinical trials to back up claims that are bogus. Pilar Villaneuva and Salvador Peiro at the Valencia School of Health Studies in Spain published in the *Lancet* that of the 102 ads they investigated, 45 of the claims for greater effectiveness, safety, or convenience were not supported by the corresponding references.[13] Robert Fletcher, an epidemiologist at Harvard Medical School, agrees that this problem is universal.

The *New York Times* reported on December 4, 2002, that promotional spending by drug companies in 2001 approached $19.1 billion. Some drug companies have repeatedly disseminated misleading ads for prescription drugs even after being cited for violations. Millions of people see the deceptive commercials before the government can try to halt them. Pfizer, for example, has received several letters[14] over the last four years from the FDA requesting them to stop making misleading claims about Lipitor, as has Proctor and Gamble, for its osteoporosis drug, Actonel. Approximately 8.5 million viewers, us, request and receive prescriptions for specific drugs after seeing ads for those products. Consumer advertising for drugs has shot up 150 percent since 1997.[15]

Money for Nothing

The *New York Times* reported on Sunday, January 26, 2003, that cancer specialists, oncologists, in private practice are pocketing hundreds of millions of dollars each year by selling drugs to patients that they buy directly from drug companies and mark up for profit. Typically, doctors give patients prescriptions for drugs that are then filled at pharmacies. But oncologists buy chemotherapy drugs themselves, often at prices discounted by drug companies trying to sell more of their products, and then administer them intravenously to patients in their offices.[16]

Oncologists began selling drugs directly more than a decade ago, after they persuaded insurers that it would be less expensive to administer the drugs in their offices than in the hospitals. This was part of a trend of doctors, specialists, being paid much more to perform services and treatments in their offices than in hospitals. (Other specialists, like urologists, also profit from chemotherapy drugs, but administer them to only some of their patients.)[17]

Drug companies, on average, give oncologists discounts as high as 86 percent on some chemotherapy drugs. Oncologists can make huge sums—often the majority of their practice revenue—from the difference between what they pay for the drugs and what they charge insurance companies and government programs. While compensation for most specialists has increased 19 percent on average since 1997, private-practice oncologists' compensation has risen slightly more than 40 percent.[18]

Among cancer doctors, this practice is referred to as a "cancer *concession*." This practice creates an obvious conflict of interest. The current system creates a perverse incentive. This "concession" may lead some doctors to recommend chemotherapy when patients may not benefit.[19]

In a 2001 study of cancer patients in Massachusetts conducted by a team of researchers from the NIH, the authors found that a third of those patients received chemo in the last six months of their lives after their cancers were deemed "unresponsive" to chemotherapy. The NIH said that "those findings strongly suggested *overuse* of chemotherapy at the end of life." While oncologists contend that they are just trying to respond to their patients' wishes for a chance, no matter how slim, of living longer, the reality is that the patients are really enduring more suffering.[20] The only group interested in stopping this practice is the insurance industry, which finds it untenable that another group might actually make money at their expense.

Mama Weer All Crazee Now

In the meantime, schools debate whether or not to give school nurses the option to hand out birth control pills at high schools in rural areas[21] where it's difficult to get to a pharmacy, even though teen pregnancies are way down thanks to rising infertility in younger and younger women.[22] Researchers are now promising women a *new* birth control pill that will prevent pregnancy and *delay* menopause, just to keep the option open to older women to have babies they won't live to raise.

They're calling it the "career" pill.[23]

It's very important to remember here that it is one of the remarkable "truths of the ages" that if something seems too good to be true, it probably is. There may, in fact, be a career pill coming, but it will be at a price none of us can afford, because mammograms, self-exams, our doctors, and all of the drug companies and their "cooked" numbers on the research can't save us.

There is no science fiction, future-shock medical miracle coming to save us from being women in a world driven by the rules that apply only to the needs of men's physiology. The fact that we can play as hard, run as fast, and outthink them on any given day does not, in any given way, exempt us from the laws of nature and our own biology.

An estimated 40,000 deaths are anticipated from breast cancer in 2002.[24] The National Institutes of Health estimate the overall costs for cancer in the year 2002 at $156.7 *billion* for direct medical costs (total of all health expenditures); $15.4 billion for indirect morbidity costs (total of lost productivity due to illness); and $84.7 billion for indirect mortality costs[25] (cost of lost productivity due to premature death). And yet they report breast cancer deaths declining, ever so slightly, due to the false bias of early detection not actually deferring date of death, because medicine can't bear the idea that they can't save us from being, in the end, *women*.

American Woman

The "collaborative reanalysis of individual data," published in July 2002 in the *Lancet*,[26] from 47 studies in 30 countries, including 50,302 women with breast cancer and 96,973 woman without the disease, researchers concluded that if women in developed nations like the United States breast-fed nine months longer than the norm, which is three months, breast cancer deaths would be reduced by 25,000 lives. Furthermore, and most importantly, if women breast-fed twelve months longer, or fifteen months in total, as is the norm in developing nations, lives saved from breast cancer each year would approach 50,000. Since only 40,000 of us are expected to die from breast cancer this year, that's all of us who would be saved.[27]

If that statistic sounds too good to be true, British author Mel Greaves reports in his book *Cancer: The Evolutionary Legacy*[28] "that the Chinese

Tanka or boat people in Southern China and Hong Kong traditionally breast-feed their infants unilaterally (with the right breast only) because they row the boats with their other arm. In these women, the risk of breast cancer postmenopausally has been reported to be significantly more likely to occur, if it occurs at all, in the unsuckled breast. There is similar suggestion that among Canadian Inuit women, who practice the same technique, the outcome is the same."[29]

All of the inability "to see the forest for the trees" in medicine and science in the twenty-first century has led a proposal for the *final solution*, a drastic "cure" offered up as a hope by desperate leaders with no answers, prophylactic mastectomy to any woman over thirty years old. Published on September 27, 2002, from Queen's University in Ulster, a major new study by top scientists in Ireland suggests that "women will have a better chance of avoiding the disease of breast cancer if they have their ovaries and breasts removed."[30]

Rock and Roll Part II

In this book we are proposing a *drastic* final solution of our own to breast cancer that is far more logical, given the scientific evidence. We propose that instead of incrementally shedding, by dissection, the physiological evidence of our gender, we instead actually become full-fledged healthy women again through the magic of natural hormone replacement, young and old.

We propose using the raw materials that the drug companies have altered to make money, in rhythmic replacement across a cycle of twenty-eight days. These plant-derived hormones, correctly prescribed, will make you sleep, stop hot flashes, erase mind noise, alleviate heel and joint pain, bring back your memory and libido, give you strong bones twelve ways along with an unstoppable heart, and—because you can mimic the physiology of a twenty-year-old on real bio-identical hormones—and maybe *no cancer*, thick hair,[31] a thin waist,[32-34] a great sex life,[35-36] clear skin,[37-38] and pheromones.[39]

The proof, of course, that this premise will work is epidemiological—the cohort is *all young women*. If high rhythmic levels cyclically of hormones occuring naturally didn't protect all young women from the diseases and tribulations of old age such as cancer, heart disease, and Alzheimer's, we wouldn't call them young—we'd call them sick.

If that proposal sounds too good to be true, we offer a study from the *Journal of the National Cancer Institute*, published May 16, 2001, entitled "Hormone Replacement Therapy After a Diagnosis of Breast Cancer in Relation to Recurrence and Mortality."[40] The title is pretty straightforward.

So are the results reported. What is important to note here is that these results were gleaned from a study using predominantly Premarin. In this case, it's particularly obvious that *any*, even minor, estrogenic effect is better than none.

Results: "The rate of breast cancer recurrence was 17 per 1000 person-years in women who used HRT (the bad stuff) after diagnosis and 30 per 1000 person-years in non-users. Breast cancer mortality rates were 5 per 1000 person-years in HRT users and 15 per 1000 person-years in non-users." Translation: HRT users had half the rate of recurrence of nonusers and one-third the rate of death, or put another way, women not on hormone replacement were twice as likely to have a recurrence of their cancer and three times as likely to die from it as users of HRT. Only 3 percent of these women had access to topical estradiol and none of them got any natural progesterone at all, and they were still better off than the women with breast cancer who received no replacement of any kind.[41]

Fakin' It

In fact, when it comes to the real effects of toxic synthetic hormones, another study from the *Journal of the National Cancer Institute*, "Effects of Long-Term Estrogen Deprivation on Apoptotic Responses of Breast Cancer Cells to 17-beta Estradiol,"[42] makes our point quite nicely. In it, *high* concentrations of natural estradiol in vitro resulted in a 60 percent reduction in the growth of breast cancer cells and a *sevenfold increase* in cell death. This study was done to figure out what *unnatural* synthetic hormone would do the same job because they *need* a patentable drug to make money.[43]

This study was done at the NIH and paid for with a grant from the Public Health Service. The authors admitted that the supersynthetic DES[44] was replaced by tamoxifen's chronic effect (remember, tamoxifen sits on and occupies the estrogen receptor until the blaring signal burns out the feedback from your pituitary and you are eventually estrogenless) in the treatment of breast cancer in the late 1970s for marketing reasons. Back then it was known that women on DES survived twice as long as women on tamoxifen, but DES had become politically incorrect because of its generational effects on cervical-uterine cancer.[45] The greed jumps from the paper.

At the bottom of all of it, it's still the old shell game. They seem to know what really works with no side effects and they keep trying to find a way to make money, instead of just curing cancer. Rose Kushner knew that big surgeries with long recoveries made more money than a lumpectomy or simple biopsy. In fact, it's such a bargain that in order for the doctors to make ends meet, you're now treated to the standard of care—lumpectomy, radiation, chemotherapy, and tamoxifen for your DCIS, which wouldn't have been found at all without a mammogram and would have become invasive cancer in 25 percent of cases if left alone. (It's interesting to note here that between the years 1979 and 1986 the incidence of DCIS in women fifty years and older increased by 235 percent compared with a 50 percent increase in the incidence of regular localized breast cancer. For women under age fifty, a 138 percent increase during the period occurred, thanks to mammography.)[46]

But this slight percentage of cancers that will metastasize has grown because once you're diagnosed with DCIS, the standard of care treatment is injury to the site (lumpectomy), more ionizing radiation, and, more often today, chemoprotection in the guise of tamoxifen. According to molecular biology studies, as well as epidemiology and anecdotal evidence–based medicine *natural hormone replacement in high concentrations is actually the answer*.[47] On the other hand, the treatment that is now de rigueur should most certainly push a DCIS lying undiscovered nearby in the same breast over the edge into invasive metastatic cancer. That means *logically* that the treatment prescribed for localized, nonmetastatic breast cancers (DCIS), often found in women at midlife, through injury, radiation, and hormone ablation, should create, over time, a much worse cancer upon recurrence.

Just say "No, thank you."

All She Wants to Do Is Dance

In conclusion, do what Rose Kushner did: Be responsible for your own life and health. Don't relinquish the care of your body and mind to anyone else.

Realize that your doctor is just as human and fallible as you are and under just as much stress financially and at work. His opinion is just an *opinion*, hopefully based on evidence-based medical research, but maybe not.

Don't believe what you see and hear on television, especially if it's a drug ad or a news flash. Take magazine articles with a grain of salt and be careful on the Internet—stay with PubMed and away from WebMD. Find some chat rooms and talk to other women about what their experiences have been and what they know. Tell each other.

And tell your daughters the truth wherever you find it.

Babies and long-term breast-feeding are the natural answer to stopping the epidemic of breast cancer in American women today.[48] There are options for being healthy that women around the world have that we don't. In Scandinavia, mothers and fathers are granted ninety-six weeks of "parental" leave, fifty-two weeks of that at 80 percent of their salary, the rest of the time on a sliding pay scale,[49] versus our option of *seven weeks unpaid* maternity leave, only at companies of fifty employees or more.[50] Mothers and fathers there have sixty days of paid sick leave, too, when caring for their older children. Now that's what we call addressing women's rights.

Take the initiative to lobby Congress for longer maternity leaves for *both* parents by writing letters to your representative. Any woman who's ever really breast-fed on demand, night and day, for more than a year knows it's an impossible task alone. Dad deserves the right to be a caregiver, too. Women by nature take care of each other, men, and their children; if you can do that, everything else will be okay.

Remembering to be a woman in *this* world, that's the hard part.

Appendix I

For lists of Certified Doctors and Registered Pharmacies providing the authentic Wiley Protocol™ to women everywhere or if you are a pharmacy willing to join us in standardizing the Protocol™ or a doctor seeking certification, please go to www.thewileyprotocol.com for links and information.

What the Wiley Protocol™ is not:

- It is not synthetic drugs with hormone-like effects.
- It is not over-the-counter.
- It is not called anything but "The Wiley Protocol™."
- It is not done with pills or patches or olive oil.
- It is not a chronic static daily dosing schedule with radical peaks on days 12 and 21.
- It is not accomplished with half doses or quarter doses.
- It is not prescribed in gels or lotions or ketchup packets of soy oil.
- It does not come in a pump bottle or jar with a spoon or tube.
- It is not dispensed in anything but capped "3cc" syringes and mylar ziplock bags with the ²⁸WP logo on the bag.
- It is not like any other HRT regimen that will be offered to you anytime soon.

IMPORTANT:
It is not the Wiley Protocol™ if it is not compounded for you by a Wiley Registered Pharmacy.

Appendix II

HORMONE-LIKE DRUGS TO AVOID

All of these *drugs* are originally derived from botanical sources, but that does not make them "natural," rhythmic, cyclical HRT. Very few of these products are just the "raw" materials or can be dosed in a natural escalating and descending pattern transdermally.

ORAL ESTROGENS			
Name	**Drug Company**	**Type**	**Dosage**
Bi-Est	Compounding pharmacy	Estradiol and estriol (usually in a 20–80% ratio) (capsule, cream, or gel)	1.25, 2.5, 5 mg
Cenestin	Duramed	Conjugated estrogens (from plant sources)	.625, .0 mg
Estrace	Bristol-Myers Squibb	Micronized estradiol (from plant sources)	.5, 1, 2 mg
Estratab	Solvay	Esterified estrogens (from plant sources)	.3, .625, 1.25, 2.5 mg
Estriol	Compounding pharmacy	Estriol	2 to 8 mg
Gynodiol	Fielding	Micronized estradiol (from plant sources)	.5, 1.5, 2 mg
Menest	Monarch	Esterified estrogens (from plant sources)	.3, .625, 1.25, 2.5 mg
Ogen	Pharmacia/Upjohn	Estropipate (piperazine estrone sulfate)	.625, 1.25, 2.5, 5 mg
Ortho-est	WomanFirst	Estropipate	.625, 1.25 mg
Premarin	Wyeth-Ayerst	Conjugated estrogens (equine)—45% estrone sulfate, 55% equine estrogens	.3, .625 (standard), .9, 1.25, 2.5 mg
Tri-Est	Compounding pharmacy	Estradiol, estrone, and estriol (usually in a 10-10-80% ratio) (capsule, cream, or gel)	1.25, 2.5, 5 mg

ESTROGEN PATCHES			
Name	**Drug Company**	**Type**	**Dosage**
Alora	Proctor & Gamble	Matrix patch—estradiol	.05, .075, .1 mg
Climara	Berlex	Matrix patch—estradiol	.025, .05, .0075, .1 mg

ESTROGEN PATCHES			
Name	**Drug Company**	**Type**	**Dosage**
Esclim	Women First HealthCare	Matrix patch—estradiol	.025, .0375, .050, .075, .1 mg
Estraderm	Novartis	Transdermal patch—estradiol	.05, 1 mg
Fempatch	Parke-Davis	Matrix patch—estradiol	.05 mg
Vivelle and Vivelle Dot	Novogyne Pharmaceuticals	Matrix patch—estradiol	.0375, .05, .075, .1 mg

PROGESTERONES AND PROGESTINS			
Name	**Drug Company**	**Type**	**Dosage**
Aygestin	ESI Lederle	Norethindrone acetate	2.5, 5 mg
Cycrin	ESI Lederle	Medroxyprogesterone acetate	2.5, 5, 10 mg
Generic	MPA Varies	Medroxyprogesterone acetate	2.5, 5, 10 mg
Generic progesterone	Compounding pharmacy	Natural micronized progesterone	100, 200 mg
Micronor	Ortho	Norethindrone	.35 mg
Mirena	Schering	Levonorgestral IUD	20 mcg daily (lasts for 5 years)
Norlutate	Parke-Davis	Norethindrone acetate	2.5, 5, 10 mg
Prochieve (formerly Crinone)	Columbia Labs	Natural progesterone vaginal gel	4% gel (delivering 45 mg of progesterone)
Prometrium	Solvay Pharmaceuticals	Natural micronized progesterone	100, 200 mg
Provera	Pharmacia and Upjohn	Medroxyprogesterone acetate	2.5, 5, 10 mg

COMBINATION ESTROGEN/PROGESTIN			
Name	**Drug Company**	**Type**	**Dosage**
Activella	Pharmacia and Upjohn	Continuous, oral: estradiol, norethindrone acetate	1 mg estradiol, .5 mg norethindrone acetate
CombiPatch	Novartis	Continuous, patch: estradiol, norethindrone acetate	.05 mg estradiol; .04 mg NDA
FemHRT	Duramed (distributed by Parke-Davis)	Continuous, oral: ethinyl estradiol, norethindrone acetate	5 mcg ethinyl estradiol; 1 mg NDA
Ortho-Prefest	Ortho-McNeil	Continuous, oral: estradiol, norgestimate	1 mg estradiol; .09 mg norgestimate sequential (progestin delivered every 3 days for 3 days)

COMBINATION ESTROGEN/PROGESTIN

Name	Drug Company	Type	Dosage
Premphase	Wyeth-Ayerst	Cyclial, oral: conjugated estrogens (Premarin) medroxyprogesterone acetate (Cycrin)	.625 mg estrogen; 2.5 mg progestin (progestin included in last 2 weeks only)
Prempro	Wyeth-Ayerst	Continuous, oral: conjugated estrogens (Premarin); medroxyprogesterone acetate (Cycrin)	.625 mg estrogen; 2.5 mg progestin

TESTOSTERONE AND COMBINATION ESTROGEN/TESTOSTERONE

Name	Drug Company	Type	Dosage
Android-10	ICN	Methyltestosterone	10 mg
Estratest	Solvay	Esterified estrogens, methyltestosterone	1.25 mg estrogen; 2.5 mg testosterone
Estratest H.S.	Solvay	Esterified estrogens, methyltestosterone	.625 mg estrogen; 1.25 mg testosterone
Methyl-testosterone	Generic	Methyltestosterone	10 mg
Premarin with methyltestosterone	Wyeth-Ayerst	Conjugated estrogens; methyltestosterone	.0625 mg estrogen; 5 or 10 mg testosterone

ORAL CONTRACEPTIVES

Name	Company	Type	Dosage
Alesse	Wyeth-Ayerst	Ethinyl estradiol; levonorgestrel	20 mcg estrogen; .10 mg progestin
Desogen	Organon	Ethinyl estradiol; desogestrel	30 mcg estrogen; 0.15 mg progestin
Estrostep Fe	Parke-Davis	Ethinyl estradiol; norethindrone acetate	Phasic estrogen (20 mcg first week; 30 mcg second week; 35 mcg third week); 1 mg progestin
Levlen	Berlex	Ethinyl estradiol; levonorgestrel	30 mcg estrogen; 0.15 mg progestin
Levlite	Berlex	Ethinyl estradiol; levonorgestrel	20 mcg estrogen; .10 mg progestin
Lo/Ovral	Wyeth-Ayerst	Ethinyl estradiol; norgestrel	30 mcg estrogen; 0.30 mg progestin

ORAL CONTRACEPTIVES			
Name	**Company**	**Type**	**Dosage**
Loestrin	Parke-Davis	Ethinyl estradiol; norethindrone acetate	30 mcg estrogen; 1.50 mg progestin
Loestrin 1/20	Parke-Davis	Ethinyl estradiol; norethindrone acetate	20 mcg estrogen; 1 mg progestin
Mircette	Organon	Ethinyl estradiol; desogestrel	20 mcg estrogen; .15 mg progestin
Nordette	Wyeth-Ayerst	Ethinyl estradiol; levonorgestrel	30 mcg estrogen; 0.15 mg progestin
NuvaRing	Organon	Ethinyl estradiol; etonogestrel	Releases 15 mcg estradiol and 120 mcg etonogestrel daily
Ortho Evra (patch)	Ortho-McNeil	Ethinyl estradiol; norelgestromin	Releases 20 mcg estradiol; 150 mcg progestin daily
Ortho-Cept	Ortho	Ethinyl estradiol; desogestrel	30 mcg estrogen; 0.15 mg progestin
Ortho-Cyclen	Ortho ethinyl	Ethinyl estradiol; norgestimate	35 mcg estrogen; 0.25 mg progestin
Tri-Levlen	Berlex	Ethinyl estradiol; levonorgestrel	Phasic estrogen (30, 40, 30 mcg); phasic progestin (0.05, 0.075, 0.125 mg)
Triphasil	Wyeth-Ayerst	Ethinyl estradiol; levonorgestrel	Phasic estrogen (30, 40, 30 mcg); phasic progestin (0.05, 0.075, 0.125 mg)
Yasmin	Berlex	Ethinyl estradiol; drospirenone	30 mcg estrogen; 3 mg progestin

TRANSDERMAL ESTROGENS			
Name	**Company**	**Type**	**Dosage**
Estrasorb	Novavax, Inc.	oil	4.3 mg BID estradiol In soy oil
Estrogel	Solvay	alcohol based gel	1.25 g daily
Femring	Warner Chilcott	vaginal ring	.05 mg – .1 mg doses of Estradiol acetate

Notes

CHAPTER ONE

1. Buus, D. Desires in human mating. *Ann N Y Acad Sci* 2000; 907: 3949.
2. Cheng, M, Peng, J, Johnson, P. Hypothalamic neurons preferentially respond to female nest coo stimulation: demonstration of direct acoustic stimulation of leuteinizing hormone release. *J Neurosci* 1998; 18: 5477–89.
3. Steidl, S, Li, L, Yeomans, J. Conditioned brain-stimulation reward attenuates the acoustic startle reflex in rats. *Behav Neurosci* 2001; 115: 710–7.
4. Suzuki, A, Kozloski, J, Crawford, J. Temporal encoding for auditory computation: physiology of primary afferent neurons in sound-producing fish. *J Neurosci* 2002; 22: 6290–301.
5. Naganuma, H, Tokumasu, K, Okamoto, M, et al. Three-dimensional analysis of morphological aspects of the human saccular macula. *Ann Oto Rhinol Laryngol* 2001; 110: 1017–21.
6. Russolo, M. Sound-evoked postural responses in normal subjects. *Acta Otolaryngol* 2001; 122: 21–7.
7. Motluk, A. Just gotta dance. *New Scientist Magazine* 1996; 151: 10.
8. Ochi, K, Ohashi, T. Sound-evoked myogenic potentials and responses with 3-ms latency in auditory brainstem response. *Laryngoscope* 2001; 111: 1818–21.
9. McIntosh, A, Gonzalez-Lima, F. Large-scale functional connectivity in associative learning: interrelations of the rat auditory, visual, and limbic systems. *J Neurophysiol* 1998; 80: 3148–62.
10. Wilczynski, W, Allison, J. Acoustic modulation of neural activity in the hypothalamus of the leopard frog. *Brain Behav Evol* 1989; 33: 317–24.
11. Nakamura, H. Neurobiology of physical environmental stress. *Nippon Eiseiwigaku Zasshi* 1992; 47: 785–97.
12. Backous, D, Minor, L, Aboujaoude, E, et al. Relationship of the utriculus and the sacculus to the stapes footplates: anatomic implications for sound and/or pressure acoustic activation. *Ann Otol Rhinol Laryngol* 1999; 108: 548–53.
13. Watson, S, Halmagyi, G, Colebatch, J. Vestibular hypersensitivity to sound. *Neurology* 2000; 54: 722–8.
14. U.S. Census Bureau, 2000 Census.
15. Saegusa, M, et al. Down-regulation of bc1-2 expression is closely related to squamous differentiation and progesterone therapy in endometrial carcinomas. *J Pathol* 1997 Aug; 182(4): 429–36.
16. Ishiwata, I, et al. Effects of progesterone on human endometrial carcinoma cells in vivo and in vitro. *J Natl Cancer Inst* 1978 May; 60(5): 947–54.
17. Dai, D, Wolf, D, Litman, E, et al. Progesterone inhibits human endometrial cancer growth and invasiveness: down-regulation of cellular adhesion molecules through progesterone B receptors. *Cancer Res* 2002; 62: 881–6.

18. Lu, LJ, et al. Decreased ovarian hormones during a soya diet: implications for breast cancer prevention. *Cancer Res* 2000 Aug 1; 60(15): 4112–21.
19. Rossouw, JE, et al. Risks and benefits of estrogen plus progestin in healthy postmenopausal women: principal results from the women's health initiative randomized controlled trial. *JAMA* 2002 Jul 17; 288(3): 321–33.
20. World health organization study of neoplasia and steroid contraceptives. Breast cancer and depot medroxyprogesterone acetate: A multinational study. *Lancet* 1991; 338: 833.
21. Paul, C, et al. Depot medroxyprogesterone (Depo-Provera) and risk of breast cancer. *Br Med J* 1989; 299: 759.
22. Skegg, DC, et al. Depot medroxyprogesterone acetate and breast cancer: a pooled analysis of the WHO and New Zealand studies. *JAMA* 1995; 273: 799.
23. *Physician's Desk Reference*, 55th ed. Medical Economics Co., Inc., Montvale, NJ, 2001. Pages 3434–3439.
24. Majumdar, SR, et al. Promotion and prescribing of hormone therapy after report of harm by the Women's Health Initiative. *JAMA*. 2004 Oct 27; 292(16): 1983–8.
25. Paul, C, et al. Depot medroxyprogesterone (Depo-Provera) and risk of breast cancer. *Br Med J* 1989; 299: 759.
26. Skegg, DC, et al. Depot medroxyprogesterone acetate and breast cancer: a pooled analysis of the WHO and New Zealand studies 1995; *JAMA* 273: 799.
27. Schwallie, PC, et al. Contraceptive use—efficacy study utilizing medroxyprogesterone acetate administered as an intramuscular injection once every 90 days. *Fertil Steril* 1973; 24: 331.
28. *Physician's Desk Reference,* 55th ed. Medical Economics Co., Inc., Montvale, NJ, 2001. Pages 3429–3432.
29. Ibid. 55th ed. Pages 3434–3439.
30. World Health Organization Study of Neoplasia and Steroid Contraceptives. Breast Cancer and depot medroxyprogesterone acetate: a multinational study. *Lancet* 1991; 338: 833.
31. Paul, C, et al. Depot medroxyprogesterone (Depo-Provera) and risk of breast cancer. *Br Med J* 1989; 299: 759.
32. Skegg, DC, et al. Depot medroxyprogesterone acetate and breast cancer: a pooled analysis of the WHO and New Zealand studies. *JAMA* 1995; 273: 799.
33. Schwallie, PC, et al. Contraceptive use—efficacy study utilizing medroxyprogesterone acetate administered as an intramuscular injection once every 90 days. *Fertil Steril* 1973; 24: 331.
34. Neergaard, L. Health agency says type of hormone therapy hurts instead of helping women's hearts and causes breast cancer. *AP World Politics*, 2002 Jul 9.
35. Majumdar, SR, et al. Promotion and prescribing of hormone therapy after report of harm by the Women's Health Initiative. *JAMA*. 2004 Oct 27; 292(16): 1983–8.
36. Ball, G, Rites, I, Balthazart, J. Neuroendocrinology of song behavior and avian brain plasticity: multiple sites of action of sex steroid hormones. *Front Neuroendocrinol* 2002; 23: 137–78.

37. Dyer, F. The biology of the dance language. *Annu Rev Entomol* 2002; 47: 917–49.
38. Law, S. The regulation of menstrual cycle and its relationship to the moon. *Acta Obstet Gynecol Scand* 1986; 65: 45–8.
39. Moon, C, Fifer, W. Evidence of transnatal auditory learning. *J Perinatol* 2000; 20: S37–44.
40. Law, S. The regulation of menstrual cycle and its relationship to the moon. *Acta Obstet Gynecol Scand* 1986; 65: 45–8.
41. Law, S. The regulation of menstrual cycle and its relationship to the moon. *Acta Obstet Gynecol Scand* 1986; 65: 45–8.
42. Whitmore, D. Light acts directly on organs and cells in culture to set the vertebrate circadian clock. *Nature* 2000; 404: 87–91.
43. Ceriani, M, Darlington, T, Staknis, D, et al. Light-dependent sequestration of timeless by cryptochrome. *Science* 1999; 285: 553–56.
44. Goldman, B. The circadian timing system and reproduction in mammals. *Steroids* 1999; 64: 679–85.
45. Copinschi, G, Van Reeth, O, Van Cauter, E. Biologic rhythms. *Presse Med* 1999; 28: 942–6.
46. Morris, K. New day dawns for research on circadian rhythms. *The Lancet* 1999; 353: 990.
47. Copinschi, G, et al. Biologic rhythms. Effect of aging on the desynchronization of endogenous rhythmicity and environmental conditions. *Presse Med.* 1999 May 1–8; 28 (17): 942–6. Review.
48. Akari, N. Lighting up the nucleus. *Science* 2000; 288: 821–22.
49. Leproult, R, Colecchia, E, Van Cauter, E. Transition from dim to bright light in the morning induces an immediate elevation of cortisol levels. *J Clin Endocrinol Metab* 2001; 86: 151–57.
50. Duncan, W. Circadian rhythms and the pharmacology of effective illness. *Pharmacol Ther* 1996; 71: 253–312.
51. Korth, C. A co-evolutionary theory of sleep. *Med Hypotheses* 1995; 45: 304–10.
52. Spiegel, K, Leproult, van Carter, E. Impact of sleep debt on metabolic and endocrine function. *The Lancet* 1999; 354: 1435–39.
53. van Cauter, E, Blackman, J, Roland, D. Modulation of glucose regulation and insulin secretion by circadian rhythmicity and sleep. *J Clin Invest* 1991; 88: 934–42.
54. Kornhauser, J, Mayo, K, Takahashi, J. Light, immediate-early genes, and circadian rhythms. *Behav Genet* 1996; 26: 221–40.
55. Arendt, J. Biological rhythms: the science of chronobiology. *JR Coll Physicians Lond* 1998; 32: 27–35.
56. Morell, V. A 24-hour circadian clock is found in the mammalian retina. *Science* 1995; 272: 349.
57. Roush, W. Can "resetting" hormonal rhythms treat illness? *Science* 269: 1220–21.
58. Boden, G, Ruiz, J, Urbain, J, et al. Evidence for a circadian rhythm of insulin secretion. *Am J Physiol* 1996; 271: E246–52.
59. Wehr, T, Moul, D, Barbato, G, et al. Conservation of photoperiod-responsive mechanism in humans. *Am J Physiol* 1993; 265: R846–57.
60. Shweiki, D. Earth-moon evolution: implications for the mechanism of the biological clock? *Med Hypotheses* 2001; 56: 647–51.

61. Selye, H. Forty years of stress research: principal remaining problems and misconceptions. *Can Med Assoc J* 1976 Jul 3; 115 (1): 53–6.
62. Perdrizet, GA. Hans Selye and beyond: responses and stress. *Cell Stress Chaperones.* 1997 Dec; 2(4): 214–9.
63. Hahn, R. Profound bilateral blindness and the incidence of breast cancer. *Epidemiology* 1991; 2: 208–10.
64. Joseph, V, Marriet, J, Lee, F, et al. Prenatal hypoxia impairs circadian synchronisation and response of the biological clock to light in adult rats. *J Physiol* 2002; 543: 387–95.
65. Braam, J, Davis, R. Rain-, wind-, and touch-induced expression of calmodulin and calmodulin-related genes in Arabidopsis. *Cell* 1990; 60: 357–64.
66. Schernhammer, E, Laden, F, Speizer, E, et al. Rotating night shifts and risk of breast cancer in women participating in the nurses' health study. *J Natl Cancer Inst* 2001; 93:1563–68.
67. Stumpf, W, Privette, T. The steroid hormone of sunlight soltriol (vitamin D) as a seasonal regulator of biological activities and photoperiodic rhythms. *J Steroid Biochem Mol Biol* 1991; 39: 283–9.
68. McFerran, D, Stirland, J, Norris, A, et al. Persistent synchronized oscillations in prolactin gene promotor activity in living pituitary cells. *Endocrinology* 2001; 142: 3255–60.
69. Nishihara, K, Horiuchin, S, Eto, H, et al. The development of infants' circadian rest-activity rhythm and mothers' rhythm. *Physiol Behav* 2001; 77: 91.
70. Nishihara, K, Horiuchi, S, Eto, H, et al. Mother's wakefulness at night in the post-partum period is related to their infants' circadian sleep-wake rhythm. *Psychiatry Clin Neurosci* 2000; 54: 805–6.
71. Rensing, L, Ruoff, P. Temperature effect on entrainment, phase shifting, and amplitude of circadian clocks and its molecular basis. *Chronobiol Int* 2002; 19: 807–64.
72. Nielsen, H, Georg, B, Hannibal, J, et al. Homer-1 mRNA in the rat suprachiasmatic nucleus is regulated differentially by the retinohypothalamic tract transmitters pituitary adenylate cyclase activating polypeptide and glutamate at time points where light phase-shifts the endogenous rhythm. *Brain Res Mol Brain Res* 2002; 105: 79–85.
73. Redwine, L, Hauger, R, Gillin, J, et al. Effects of sleep and sleep deprivation on interleukin-6, growth hormone, cortisol, and melatonin levels in humans. *J Clin Endocrinol Metab* 2000; 85: 3597–3603.
74. Mercer, J, Moar, K, Hoggaard, A. Photoperiod regulates arcuate nucleus POMC, AGRP, and leptin receptor mRNA in the hypothalamus. *Am J Physiol Regul Integr Comp Physiol* 2000; 278: R271–81.
75. *http://www.nih.gov/health/chip/nia/aging/biochem.html.*
76. Toussaint, O, Remacle, J, Dierick, J, et al. Approach of evolutionary theories of aging, stress, senescence-like phenotypes, calorie restriction and hormesis from the viewpoint of far-from-equilibrium thermodynamics. *Mech Ageing Dev* 2002; 123: 937–46.
77. Hauptman, S. A thermodynamic interpretation of malignancy: do the genes come later? *Med Hypotheses* 2002; 58: 44–7.
78. Toussaint, O, Raes, M, Remacle, J. Aging as a multi-step process characterized by a low-

ering of entropy production leading the cell to a sequence of defined stages. *Mech Aging Dev* 1991; 61: 45–64.

79. Demetrius, L. Thermodynamics and evolution. *T Theor Biol* 2000; 206: 1–16.
80. Skulachev, V. Aging is a specific biological function rather than the results of a disorder in complex living systems: biochemical evidence in support of Weismann's hypothesis. *Biochemistry (Moscow)* 1997; 62: 1191–95.
81. Carey, JR, et al. Slowing of mortality rates at older ages in large medfly cohorts. *Science* 1992 Oct 16; 258 (5081): 457–61.
82. Sgro, C, Partridge, L. A delayed wave of death from reproduction in drosophila. *Science* 1999; 286: 2521–3.
83. Matsui, D, Sakari, M, Sato, T, et al. Transcriptional regulation of mouse steroid 5alpha-reductase type 2 gene by progesterone in brain. *Nucleic Acids Res* 2002; 30: 1387–93.
84. Tang, M, et al. Progesterone receptor activates its promoter activity in human endometrial stromal cells. *Mol Cell Endocrinol*. 2002 Jun 28; 192 (1–2): 45–53.
85. Formby, B, et al. Progesterone inhibits growth and induces apoptosis in breast cancer cells: inverse effects on Bc1-2 and p53. *Ann Clin Lab Sci*. 1998 Nov–Dec; 28 (6): 360–9.
86. Formby, B, Wiley, T. Bc1-2, survivin and variant CD44 v7-v10 are downregulated and p53 is upregulated in breast cancer cells by progesterone: inhibition of cell growth and induction of apoptosis. *Mol Cell Biochem* 1999; 202: 53–61.
87. Hovey, R, Trott, J, Ginsburg, E, et al. Transcriptional and spatiotemporal regulation of prolactin receptor mRNA and cooperativity with progesterone receptor function during ductal branch growth in the mammary gland. *Dev Dyn* 2001; 222: 192–205.
88. Talukder, A, Wang, R, Kuman, R. Expression and transactivating functions of the bZIP transcription factor GADD153 in mammary epithelial cells. *Oncogene* 2002; 21: 4289–300.
89. Lantinga-Van Leweuwen, I, Timmermans-Sprang, E, Mol, J. Cloning and characterization of the 5'-flanking region of the canine growth hormone gene. *Mol Cell Endocrinol* 2002; 197: 133–41.
90. Yu, S, Lee, M, Shin, S, et al. Apoptosis induced by progesterone in human ovarian cancer cell line SNU-840. *J Cell Biochem* 2001; 82: 445–51.
91. Malet, C, Spritzer, P, Guillaumin, D, et al. Progesterone effect on cell growth, ultrastructural aspect and estradiol receptors of normal human breast epithelial cells in culture. *J Steroid Biochem Mol Biol* 2000; 73: 171–81.
92. Formby, B, et al. *Tolerance to the fetal-placental allograft: molecular mechanism of progesterone immunosuppression*. Plenum Pub corp., 2003, in press.
93. Bu, S, Yin, D, Ren, X et al. Progesterone induces apoptosis and up-regulation of p53 expression in ovarian carcinoma cell lines. *Cancer* 1997; 79: 1944–50.
94. Ahgmed-Sorour, H, Bailey, C. Role of ovarian hormones in the long-term control of glucose homeostasis, glycogen formation and glyconeogenesis. *Ann Nutr Metab* 1981; 25: 208–12.
95. McKenna, N, O'Malley, B. Nuclear receptor coactivators. *Endocrinology* 2002; 143: 2461–5.

96. Wolkow, C. Life span: getting the signal from the nervous system. *Trends Neurosci* 2001; 25: 212–6.
97. DeMayo, F, Zhao, B, Takamoto, N, et al. Mechanisms of action of estrogen and progesterone. *Ann N Y Acad Sci* 2001; 955: 48–59.
98. Groner, B. Transcription factor regulation in mammary epithelial cells. *Domest Anim Endocrinol* 2002; 23: 25–32.
99. Formby, B, Wiley, T. Bc1-2, survivin and variant CD44 v7-v10 are downregulated and p53 is upregulated in breast cancer cells by progesterone: inhibition of cell growth and induction of apoptosis. *Mol Cell Biochem* 1999; 202: 53–61.
100. Fitzpatrick, J, Mize, A, Wade, C, et al. Estrogen-mediated neuroprotection against beta-amyloid-amyloid toxicity requires expression of estrogen receptor alpha or beta and activation of the MAPK pathway. *J Neurochem* 2002; 82: 674–82.
101. Nilsen, J, Briton, R. Impact of progestins on estrogen-induced neuroprotection: synergy by progesterone and 19-norprogesterone and antagonism by medroxyprogesterone acetate. *Endocrinology* 2002; 143: 205–12.
102. Dai, D, Wolf, D, Litman, E, et al. Progesterone inhibits human endometrial cancer growth and invasiveness: down-regulation of cellular adhesion molecules through progesterone B receptors. *Cancer Res* 2002; 62: 881–6.
103. Mendelsohn, M. Genomic and nongenomic effects of estrogen in the vasculature. *Am J Cardiol* 2002; 90: 3F–6F.
104. Castagnetta, L, Granata, O, Traina, A, et al. A role for sex steroids in autoimmune diseases: a working hypothesis and supporting data. *Ann N Y Acad Sci* 2002; 966: 193–203.
105. Vassen, L, Wegrzyn, W, Klein-Hitpass, L. Human insulin receptor substrate-2 (IRS-2) is a primary progesterone response gene. *Mol Endocrinol* 1999; 13: 485–94.
106. Saad, Z, Bramwell, V, Wilson, S. Expression of genes that contribute to proliferative and metastatic ability in breast cancer resected during various menstrual phases. *Lancet* 1998; 351: 1170–73.
107. Strassman, R, Qualls, C, Lisansky, E, et al. Elevated rectal temperature produced by all-night bright light is reversed by melatonin infusion in men. *J Appl Physiol* 1991; 71: 2178–82.
108. Krauchi, K, et al. Thermoregulatory effects of melatonin in relation to sleepiness. *Chronobiol Int*. 2006; 23(1–2): 475–84.
109. Jackson, JG, et al. Insulin receptor substrate-1 is the predominant signaling molecule activated by insulin-like growth factor-I, insulin, and interleukin-4 in estrogen receptor-positive human breast cancer cells. *J Biol Chem*. 1998 Apr 17; 273 (16): 9994–10003.
110. Turkington, Carol A. Precocious puberty. *Gale Encyclopedia of Medicine,* 1995 January 01.
111. Rosenfield, Robert L, et al. Current age of onset of puberty. *Pediatrics* 2000 September 1.
112. Gale Group. Girls reaching puberty earlier. 2000 January. www.findarticles.com.
113. Pathomvanich, A, et al. Early puberty: a cautionary tale. *The American Academy of Pediatrics*. 2000 March; 105: 115–116.

114. Bennett, Maryann. Beyond their years: precocious puberty steals years of growth from kids at an early age. ABCNEWS.com.
115. Giddens, Herman, ME, et al. Secondary sexual characteristics and menses in young girls seen in office practice: a study from the Pediatric Research and Office Settings Network. *Pediatrics* 1997; 99: 505–512.
116. Hillier, SG, et al. Control of preovulatory follicular estrogen biosynthesis in the human ovary. *J Clin Endocrinol Metab* 1996; 81: 1401.
117. Judd, HL, et al. Serum androstenedione and testosterone levels during the menstrual cycle. *J Clin Endocrinol Metab* 1973; 36:475.
118. McLachlan, RI, et al. Serum inhibin levels during the periovulatory interval in normal women: Relationships with sex steroid and gonadotrophin levels. *Clin Endocrinol (Oxf)* 1990; 32:39.
119. Groome, NP, et al. Measurement of dimeric inhibin B throughout the human menstrual cycle. *J Clin Endocrinol Metab* 1996; 81: 1401.
120. Sano, Y, et al. Changes in enzyme activities related to steroidogenesis in human ovaries during the menstrual cycle. *J Clin Endocrinol Metab* 1981; 52: 994.
121. Erickson, GF. Follicular maturation and atresia. In Lamigni, C, Givens, JR, *The Gonadotropins: Basic Science and Clinical Aspects in Females*. Academic Press, New York, 1982. Page 171.
122. Hsueh, AJ, et al. Intraovarian mechanisms in the hormonal control of granulosa cell differentiation in rats. *J Reprod Fertil* 1983; 69: 325.
123. Yen, SS, et al. Modulation of pituitary responsiveness to LRF by estrogen. *J Clin Endocrinol Metab* 1974; 39: 170.
124. Marshall, JC, et al. Selective inhibition of follicle-stimulating hormone secretion by estradiol. Mechanism for modulation of gonadotropin responses to low dose pulses of gonadotropin-releasing hormone. *J Clin Invest* 1983; 71: 248.
125. Yen, SS, Samuel, SC, et al. *Reproductive Endocrinology*. W.B. Saunders Co., Philadelphia, PA, 1999. Page 682.
126. Scott, JA, et al. Factors affecting pituitary gonadotropin function in users of oral contraceptive steroids. *Am J Obstet Gynecol* 1978; 130: 8817.
127. Bracken, MB, et al. Conception delay after oral contraceptive use: The effect of estrogen dose. *Fertil Steril* 1990; 53:21.
128. Kitzinger, S, et al. *Being born*. Grosset & Dunlap, New York, NY, 1986.
129. Meyer, A. Hox gene variation and evolution. *Nature* 1998; 391: 225–6.
130. Raman, V, Tamori, A, Vali, M, et al. HOXA5 regulates expression of the progesterone receptor. *J Biol Chem* 2000; 275: 26551–55.
131. Srebrow, Anabella, et al. Expression of Hoxa-1 and Hoxb-7 is regulated by extracellular matrix-dependent signals in mammary epithelial cells. *Journal of Cellular Biochemistry* 1998; 69: 377–391.
132. Cillo, C, Cantile, M, Failla, A. Homeobox genes in normal and malignant cells. *J Cell Physiol* 2001; 188: 161–69.
133. Castronovo, V, Kusaka, M, Chariot, A, et al. Homeobox genes: potential candidates for the

transcriptional control of the transformed and invasive phenotype. *Biochem Pharmacol* 1994; 47: 137–43.

134. Williams, RW. Plant homeobox genes: many functions stem from a common motif. *Bioessays* 1998 Apr; 20 (4): 280–2.
135. Cermik, Dilek, et al. HOXA10 expression is repressed by progesterone in the myometrium: differential tissue-specific regulation of HOX gene expression in the reproductive tract. *The Journal of Clinical Endocrinology & Metabolism* 2001; 86 (7) 3387–3392.
136. *http://www.celldeath-apoptosis.org/HistOfApoptosis.html.*
137. Corn, P, Wafik, S. Derangement of growth and differentiation control in oncogenesis. *Bioessays* 2002; 24: 83–90.
138. Lehner, R, et al. Localization of telomerase hTERT protein and survivin in placenta: relation to placental development and hydatidiform mole. *Obstet Gynecol* 2001 Jun; 97 (6): 965–70.
139. Cillo, C, Faiella, A, Cantile, M, et al. Homeobox genes and cancer. *Exp Cell Res* 1999; 248: 1–9.
140. Kirchner, T, Muller, S, Hattori, T, et al. Metaplasia, intraepithelial neoplasia and early cancer of the stomach are related to dedifferentiated epithelial cells defined by cytokeratin-7 expression in gastritis. *Wirchows Arch* 2001; 439: 512–22.
141. Moss, Ralph W. *Questioning chemotherapy.* Equinox Press, Brooklyn, NY, 1995. Pages 95–96.
142. Taylor, SG, et al. Combination chemotherapy vs. tamoxifen as initial therapy for stage IV breast cancer in elderly women. *Ann Int Med* 1986; 104: 455–461.
143. Physician's Desk Reference. *www.pdr.net.*
144. Song, R, Mor, G, Naftolin, F, et al. Effect of long-term estrogen deprivation on apoptotic responses of breast cancer cells to 17beta-estradiol. *J Natl Cancer Inst* 2001; 93: 1714–23.
145. Natrajan, P, Gambrell, R. Estrogen replacement therapy in patients with early breast cancer. *Am J Obstet Gynecol* 2002; 187: 289–94.
146. Vassilopoulou-Sellin, R, Asmar, L, Hortobagyi, G, et al. Estrogen replacement therapy after localized cancer: clinical outcome of 319 women followed prospectively. *J Clin Oncol* 1999; 17: 1482–7.
147. O'Meara, E, Rossing, M, Daling, J, et al. Hormone replacement therapy after diagnosis of breast cancer in relation to recurrence and mortality. *J Natl Cancer Inst* 2001; 93: 754–5.
148. Natrajan, P, Gambrell, R. Estrogen replacement therapy in patients with early breast cancer. *Am J Obstet Gynecol* 2002; 187: 289–94.
149. O'Meara, E, et al. Hormone replacement therapy after diagnosis of breast cancer in relation to recurrence and mortality. *J Natl Cancer Inst* 2001; 93: 754–5.
150. Gliozzo, B, Sung, C, Scalia, P, et al. Insulin-stimulated cell growth in insulin receptor substrate-1-deficient ZR-75-1 cells is mediated by phosphatidylinositol-3-kinase-independent pathway. *J Cell Biochem* 1998; 70: 268–80.
151. Weiderpass, E, Gridley, G, Persson, L, et al. Risk of endometrial and breast cancer in patients with diabetes mellitus. *Int J Cancer* 1997; 71: 360–63.

152. Formby, B, Wiley, T. Insulin modulates expression of the estrogen-induced genes bc1-2, c-fos and luca-2 in MCF-7 breast tumor cells: an association with breast cancer risk in type 2 diabetic patients? *Diabetes* 1998; 47(suppl1): 952.
153. Wiley, TS, et al. Bc1-2, survivin and variant CD44 v7-v10 are downregulated and p53 is upregulated in breast cancer cells by progesterone: inhibition of cell growth and induction of apoptosis. *Mol Cell Biochem* 1999; 202: 53–61.
154. Bu, S, Yin, D, Ren, X, et al. Progesterone induces apoptosis and up-regulation of p53 expression in ovarian carcinoma cell lines. *Cancer* 1997; 79: 1944–50.
155. Saegusa, M, et al. Down-regulation of bc1-2 expression is closely related to squamous differentiation and progesterone therapy in endometrial carcinomas. *J Pathol* 1997 Aug; 182 (4): 429–36.
156. Groshong, S, et al. Biphasic regulation of breast cancer cell growth by progesterone: role of the cyclin-dependent kinase inhibitors, p21 and p27. *Mol Endocrinol* 1997; 11: 1593–1607.
157. Sivaraman, L, Conneely, O, Medina, D, et al. p53 is a potential mediator of pregnancy and hormone-induced resistance to mammary carcinogenesis. *Proc Natl Acad Sci (USA)* 2001; 98: 12379–84.
158. Yang, J, Yoshizawa, K, Nandi, S, et al. Protective effects of pregnancy and lactation against N-methyl-N-nitrosourea-induced mammary carcinomas in female Lewis rats. *Carcinogenesis* 1999; 20: 623–28.
159. DiMartino-Nardi, J. Pre-and postpubertal findings in premature adrenarche. *J Pediatr Endocrinol Metab* 2000; 13 (Suppl5): 1265–9.
160. Ibanez, L, Potau, N, Dunger, D, et al. Precocious puberty in girls and the development of androgen excess. *J Pediatr Endocrinol Metab* 2000; 13 (suppl 5): 1261–3.
161. Wathen, P, Henderson, M, Witz, C. Abnormal uterine bleeding. *Med Clin North Am* 1995; 79: 329–44.
162. Jasen, P. Breast cancer and the language of risk, 1750–1950. *Social History of Medicine* 2002; 15: 17–43.
163. Data source: National Cancer Institute, Epidemiology, and end results program. 2001.
164. Moradi, T, Adami, H, Ekbom, A, et al. Physical activity and risk of breast cancer: a prospective cohort study among Swedish twins. *Int J Cancer* 2002; 100: 76–81.
165. Terry, P, Suzuki, R, Hu, E, et al. A prospective study of major dietary patterns and the risk of breast cancer. *Cancer Epidemiol Biomarkers Prev* 2001; 10: 1281–5.
166. Hgorn-Ross, P, Hoggatt, K, West, D, et al. Recent diet and breast cancer risk: the California teachers study (USA). *Cancer Causes Control* 2002; 13: 407–15.
167. Chen, H, Xiao, J, Hu, G, et al. Estrogenicity of organophosphorous and pyrethroid pesticides. *J Toxicol Environ Health* 2002; 65: 1419–35.
168. Gammon, M, Wolff, M, Neugut, A, et al. Environmental toxins and breast cancer on Long Island. II organochlorine compound levels in blood. *Cancer Epidemiol Biomarkers Prev* 2002; 11: 686–97.
169. Jeffy, B, Chirrnomas, R, Romagnolo, D. Epigenetics of breast cancer: polycyclic aromatic hydrocarbons as risk factors. *Environ Mol Mutagen* 2002; 39: 235–44.
170. Speroff, L. The effect of again on fertility. *Curr Opin Obstet Gynecol* 1994; 6:115–20.

CHAPTER TWO

1. Carr, B, Blackwell, R. *Textbook of reproductive medicine*, 2d ed. Appleton & Lange, Stamford, Conn. 1988. Page 271.
2. Musey, V, Collins, D, Musey, P, et al. Long-term effect of a first pregnancy on the secretion of prolactin. *N Engl J Med* 1987; 316: 229–34.
3. Musey, V, Collins, C, Brogan, D, et al. Long term effect of the first pregnancy on the hormonal environment: estrogens and androgens. *J Clin Endocrinol Metab* 1987; 64: 111–8.
4. Musey, V, Collins, D, Musey, P. Age-related changes in the female hormonal environment during reproductive life. *Am J Obstet Gynecol* 1987; 157: 321–7.
5. Tryggvadottir, L, Tulinius, H, Byfjord, J, et al. Breast cancer risk factors and age at diagnosis: An icelandic cohort study. *Int J Cancer* 2002; 98: 604–8.
6. Shah, M, Maibach, H. Estrogen and skin. An overview. *Am J Clin Dermatol* 2001; 2: 143–50.
7. Chambliss, K, Shaul, P. Estrogen modulation of endothelial nitric oxide synthase. *Endocr Res* 2001; 23: 665–86.
8. Simoncini, T, Fornari, L, Mannella, P, et al. Novel non-transcriptional mechanisms for estrogen receptor signaling in the vascular system. Interaction of estrogen receptor alpha with phosphatidylinositol 3-OH kinase. *Steroids* 2002; 67: 935–9.
9. Inoue, A, Yoshida, N, Omoto, Y, et al. Development of cDNA microarray for expression profiling of estrogen-responsive genes. *J Mol Endocrinol* 2002; 29: 175–92.
10. Burger, D, Dayer, J. Cytokines, acute-phase proteins and hormones: IL-1 and TNF-alpha production in contact-mediated activation of monocytes by T lymphocytes. *Ann N Y Acad Sci* 2002; 966: 464–73.
11. McEwen, B. Estrogen actions throughout the brain. *Recent Prog Horm Res* 2002; 57: 357–84.
12. Schwartz, D, Mayaux, M. Female fecundity as a function of age. *N Engl J Med* 1982; 306: 404–11.
13. Gindoff, P. Reproductive potential in the older women. *Fertil Steril* 1986; 46: 989–92.
14. Rowe-Finkbeiner, Kristin. Oops, I forgot to have kids. *Bust Magazine*. 2002 Summer; 44–49.
15. *http://www.ppsinc.org/men/men01.htm.*
16. Breast cancer and breastfeeding: collaborative reanalysis of individual data from 47 epidemiological studies in 30 countries including 50,302 women with breast cancer and 96,973 women without the disease. *The Lancet* 2002; 360: 187–206.
17. Rensing, L, Meyer-Grahle, U, Ruoff, P. Biological timing and the clock metaphor: oscillatory and hourglass mechanisms. *Chronobiol Int* 2001; 18: 329–69.
18. Palmert, M, Boepple, P. Variation in the timing of puberty: clinical spectrum and genetic investigation. *J Clin Endocrinol Metab* 2001; 86: 2364–68.
19. Apter, D, Sipila, I. Development of children and adolescents: physiological, pathophysiological, and therapeutic aspects. *Curr Opin Obstet Gynecol* 1993; 5: 764–73.
20. Apter, D, Butzow, T, Laughlin, G, et al. Gonadotropin-releasing hormone pulse generator

activity during pubertal transition in girls: pulsative and diurnal patterns of circulating gonadotropins. *J Clin Endocrinol Metab* 1993; 76: 940–9.

21. Palmert, M, Hayden, D, Mansfield, M, et al. The longitudinal study of adrenal maturation during gonadal suppression: evidence that adrenarche is a gradual process. *J Clin Endocrinol Metab* 2001; 86: 1536–42.
22. Meerlo, P, Koehl, M, van der Borght, F, et al. Sleep restriction alters the hypothalamic-pituitary-adrenal response to stress. *J Neuroendocrinol* 2002; 14: 397–402.
23. Matthews, S. Early programming of the hypothalamo-pituitary-adrenal axis. *Trends Endocrinol Metab* 2002; 13: 373–5.
24. Leal, A, Moreira, A. Food and the circadian activity of the hypothalamic-pituitary-adrenal axis. *Braz J Med Biol Res* 1997; 30: 1391–405.
25. Karlsbeek, A, van Heerikhuize, J, Wortel, J, et al. A diurnal rhythm of stimulatory input to the hypothalamo-pituitary-adrenal system as revealed by timed intrahypothalamic administration of the vasopressin VI antagonist. *J Neurosci* 1996; 16: 5555–65.
26. *http://www.pbs.org/healthweek.*
27. Veldhuis, J, Metzger, D, Martha, P, et al. Estrogen and testosterone, but not a nonaromatizable androgen, direct network integration of the hypothalamo-somatotrope (growth hormone)-insulin-like growth factor I axis in the human: evidence from pubertal pathophysiology and sex-steroid hormone replacement. *J Clin Endocrinol Metab* 1997; 82: 3414–20.
28. Silva, J, Price, C. Insulin and IGF-1 are necessary for FSH-induced cytochrome P450 aromatase but not cytochrome P450 side-chain cleavage gene expression in oestrogenic bovine granulosa cells in vitro. *J Endocrinol* 2002; 174: 499–507.
29. McTernan, P, Anderson, L, Anwar, A. Glucocorticoid regulation of P450 aromatase activity in human adipose tissue: gender and site differences. *J Clin Endocrinol Metab* 2001; 87: 327–35.
30. Apter, D, Hermanson, E. Update on female pubertal development. *Curr Opin Obstet Gynecol* 2001; 14: 475–81.
31. Moschos, S, Chan, J, Mantzopros, C. Leptin and reproduction. *Fertil Steril* 2001; 77: 433–44.
32. Mann, D, Plant, T. Leptin and pubertal development. *Semi Reprod Med* 2002; 20: 93–102.
33. Laberge, L, Petit, D, Simard, C, et al. Development of sleep patterns in early adolescence. *J Sleep Res* 2001; 10: 59–67.
34. van Cauter, E, Blackman, J, Roland, D, et al. Modulation of glucose regulation and insulin secretion by circadian rhythmicity and sleep. *J Clin Invest* 1991; 88: 934–42.
35. MacGillivray, M, Morishima, A, Conte, F, et al. Pediatric endocrinology update: an overview. The essential roles of estrogens in pubertal growth, epiphyseal fusion and bone turnover: lessons from mutations in the genes for aromatase and the estrogen receptor. *Horm Res* 1998; 49 (Suppl): 2–8.
36. Hillier, S. Current concepts of the roles of follicle stimulating hormone and luteinizing hormone in folliculogenesis. *Hum Reprod* 1994; 9: 188–91.
37. Law, S. The regulation of menstrual cycle and its relationship to the moon. *Acta Obstet Gynecol Scand* 1986; 65: 45–8.

38. Tsuboi, S, Kotani, Y, Ogawa, K, et al. An intramolecular disulfide bridge as a catalytic switch for serotonin N-acetyltransferase. *J Biol Chem* 2002; 288: 4323–32.
39. Blask, D, Sauer, L, Dauchy, R. Melatonin as a chronobiotic/anticancer agent: cellular, biochemical, and molecular mechanisms of action and their implications for circadian-based cancer therapy. *Curr Top Med Chem* 2002; 2: 1130–32.
40. Kiefer, T, Ram, P, Yuan, L, et al. Melatonin inhibits estrogen receptor transactivation and cAMP levels in breast cancer cells. *Breast Cancer Res Treat* 2002; 71: 37–45.
41. Ram, P, Kiefer, T, Silverman, M, et al. Estrogen receptor transactivation in MCF-7 breast cancer cells by melatonin and growth factors. *Mol Cell Endocrinol* 1998; 141: 53–64.
42. Rato, A, Pedrero, J, Martinez, M, et al. Melatonin blocks the activation of estrogen receptor for DNA binding. *FASEB J* 1999; 13: 857–68.
43. Kiefer, T, et al. Melatonin inhibits estrogen receptor transactivation and cAMP levels in breast cancer cells. *Breast Cancer Res Treat* 2002; 71: 37–45.
44. Yuan, L, et al. MT(1) melatonin receptor overexpression enhances the growth suppressive effect of melatonin in human breast cancer cells. *Mol Cell Endocrinol* 2002; 192: 147–5.
45. Cahill, D, et al. Expected contribution to serum estradiol from individual ovarian follicles in unstimulated cycles. *Hum Reprod* 2000; 15: 1909–12.
46. Shoham, Z. The clinical therapeutic window for luteinizing hormone in controlled ovarian stimulation. *Fertil Steril* 2002; 77: 1170–7.
47. Cutler, W, Friedmann, E, McCoy, N. Pheromonal influences on sociosexual behavior in men. *Arch Sex Behav* 1998; 27: 1–13.
48. Cohn, B. In search of human skin pheromones. *Arch Dermatol* 1994; 130: 1048–51.
49. Singer, A. A chemistry of mammalian pheromones. *J Steroid Biochem Mol Biol* 1991; 39: 627–32.
50. Sorensewn, P. Biological responsiveness to pheromones provides fundamental and unique insight into olfactory function. *Chem Senses* 1996; 21: 245–56.
51. Mustaparta, H. Central mechanisms of pheromone information processing. *Chem Senses* 1996; 21: 269–75.
52. Cowley, J, Brooksbank, B. Human exposure to putative pheromones and changes in aspects of social behaviour. *J Steroid Biochem Mol Biol* 1991; 39: 647–59.
53. McKlintock, M. On the nature of mammalian and human pheromones. *Ann N Y Acad Sci* 1998; 855: 390–2.
54. Janssen, F, Zavazava, N. How does the major histocompatibility complex influence behavior? *Arch Immunol Ther Exp* 1999; 47: 139–42.
55. Porter, R, Cernoch, J, Balogh, R. Odor signatures and kin recognition. *Physiol Behav* 1985; 34: 445–8.
56. Eklund, A, Belshak, M, Lapidos, K, et al. Polymorphisms in the HLA-linked olfactory receptor genes in the Hutterites. *Hum Immunol* 2000; 61: 711–7.
57. Rikowski, A, Grammer, K. Human odour, symmetry and attractiveness. *Proc R Soc Lond B* 1999; 266: 869–71.
58. Schiestl, F, Ayasse, M, Paulus, H, et al. Sex pheromones mimicry in the early spider orchid: patterns of hydrocarbons as the key mechanism for pollination by sexual deception. *J Comp Physiol [A]* 2000; 186: 567–74.

59. Wong, B, Schiestl, F. How an orchid harms its pollinator. *Proc R Soc Lond B Biol Sci* 2002; 269: 1529–32.
60. Farmer, E. Surface-to-air signals. *Nature* 2001; 411: 854–6.
61. Fraser, Robert, et al. *Golden bough*. Palgrave Macmillan Publishing, New York, NY, 2002. Page 681.
62. Wedekind, C, Seebek, T, Bettens, F, et al. MHC-dependent mate preferences in humans. *Proc R Soc Lond B Biol Sci* 1995; 260: 245–9.
63. Jocob, S, McKlintock, M, Zelano, B, et al. Paternally inherited HLA alleles are associated with women's choice of male odor. *Nat Genet* 2002; 30: 175–9.
64. Janssen, E, Zavazava, N. How does the major histocompatibility complex influence behavior? *Arch Immunol Ther Exp* 1999; 47: 139–42.
65. Porter, R, Cernoch, J, Balogh, R. Odor signatures and kin recognition. *Physiol Behav* 1985; 34: 445–8.
66. Eklund, A, Belshak, M, Lapidos, K, et al. Polymorphisms in the HLA-linked olfactory receptor genes in the Hutterites. *Hum Immunol* 2000; 61: 711–7.
67. Davis, J, Rueda, B. The corpus luteum: an ovarian structure with maternal instincts and suicidal tendencies. *Front Biosci* 2001; 7: 11949–78.
68. Collaer, M, et al. Human behavioral sex differences: a role for gonadal hormones during early development. *Psychological Bull* 1995; 118: 55–107.
69. Lehner, R, Bobak, J, Kim, N, et al. Localization of telomerase hTERT protein and survivin in placenta. *Am Obstet Gynecol* 2001; 97: 965–70.
70. Formby, B, Wiley, TS. Breast cancer cell growth and programmed death by progesterone. In *Breast Cancer* ed. Pasqualini, A. Marcel Dekker, New York, NY, 2002.
71. Formby, B, Wiley, TS. Bc1-2, survivin and variant CD44 v7-v10 are downregulated and p53 is upregulated in breast cancer cells by progesterone: inhibition of cell growth and induction of apoptosis. *Mol Cell Biol* 1999; 202: 53–61.
72. Bu, S, Yin, D, Ren, X, et al. Progesterone induces apoptosis and up-regulation of p53 expression in human ovarian carcinoma cell lines. *Cancer* 1997; 79: 1944–50.
73. Yu, S, Lee, M, Shin, S. Apoptosis induced by progesterone in human ovarian cell line SNU-840. *J Cell Biochem* 2001; 82: 445–51.
74. Lewin, J, Cooper, A, Birch, B. Progesterone: a novel adjunct to intravesical chemotherapy. *BJU Int* 2002; 90: 736–41.
75. Garcia-Gasca, A, Spyropoulos, D. Differential mammary morphogenesis along the antero-posterior axis in Hoxc6 gene targeted mice. *Dev Dyn* 2000; 219: 261–76.
76. Raman, V, Tamori, A, Vali, M, et al. HOXA5 regulates expression of the progesterone receptor. *J Biol Chem* 2000; 275: 26551–5.
77. Taylor, H, Igarashi, P, Olive, D. Sex steroids mediate HOXA11 expression in the human peri-implantation endometrium. *J Clin Endocrinol Metab* 1999; 84: 1129–35.
78. Quenby, S, Gazvani, M, Brazeau, C, et al. Oncogenes and tumor suppressor genes in the first trimester human fetal gonadal development. *Mol Hum Reprod* 1999; 5: 737–41.
79. Snell, E, Scemama, J, Stellwag, E. Genomic organization of the HoxA4-Hoxa10 region from Morone saxatilis; implications for hox gene evolution among vertebrates. *J Exp Zool* 1999; 285: 41–49.

80. Hodgkin, J. The remarkable ubiquity of DM domain factors as regulators of sexual phenotype: ancestry or aptitude? *Genes Dev* 2002; 16: 2322–6.
81. Humphreys, R, Lydon, J, O'Malley, B, et al. Mammary gland development is mediated by both stromal and epithelial progesterone receptors. *Mol Endocrinol* 1997; 11: 801–11.
82. Schepers, G, Teasdale, R, Koopman, P. Twenty pairs of sox: extent, homology, and nomenclature of the mouse and human sox transcription factor gene families. *Dev Cell* 2002; 3: 167–70.
83. Carpenter, E. Hox genes and spinal cord development. *Dev Neurosci* 2002; 24: 24–34.
84. Taylor, H, Arici, A, Olive D, et al. HOXA10 is expressed in response to sex steroids at the time of implantation in the human endometrium. *J Clin Invest* 1998; 101: 1379–84.
85. Sivaraman, L, Conneely, O, Medina, D, et al. P53 is a potential mediator of pregnancy and hormone-induced resistance to mammary carcinogenesis. *Proc Natl Acad Sci (USA)* 2001; 98: 12379–84.
86. Rajkumar, L, Guzman, R, Yang, J, et al. Short-term exposure to pregnancy levels of estrogen prevents mammary carcinogenesis. *Proc Natl Acad Sci (USA)* 2001; 98: 11755–59.
87. Medina, D, Sivaraman, L, Hilsenbeck, S, et al. Mechanisms of hormonal prevention of breast cancer. *Ann NY Acad Sci* 2001; 952: 23–35.
88. Rosner, B, Colditz, G, Willett, W. Reproductive risk factors in a prospective study of breast cancer: the Nurses' Health Study. *Am J Epidemiol* 1994; 139: 819–35.
89. Breast cancer and breastfeeding: collaborative reanalysis of individual data from 47 epidemiological studies in 30 countries including 50,302 women with breast cancer and 96,973 women without the disease. *Lancet* 2002; 360: 187–206.
90. Kelsey, I. Breast cancer epidemiology summary and future directions. *Epidemiol Rev* 1993; 15: 256–63.
91. Vitzthum, V. Nursing behaviour and its relation to duration of post-partum amenorrhoea in an Andean community. *J Biosoc Sci* 1989; 21: 145–60.
92. Heinig, M, Mommsen-Rivers, L, Peerson, J, et al. Factors related to duration of postpartum amenorrhoea among USA women with prolonged lactation. *J Biosoc Sci* 1994; 26: 517–27.
93. Diaz, S, Seron-Ferre, M, Cardenas, H, et al. Circadian variation of basal plasma prolactin, prolactin response to suckling, and length of amenorrhea in nursing women. *J Clin Endocrinol Metab* 1989; 68: 946–55.
94. Hrdy, SB. *Mother nature: a history of mothers, infants, and natural selection.* Pantheon Books, New York, 1999. Page 194.
95. Breast cancer and breastfeeding: collaborative reanalysis of individual data from 47 epidemiological studies in 30 countries, including 50,302 women with breast cancer and 96,973 women without the disease. *Lancet* 2002; 360: 187–95.
96. U.S. Census Bureau Statistics, 2002.
97. Hrdy, SB. *Mother nature: a history of mothers, infants, and natural selection.* Pantheon Books, New York, 1999. Page 175.
98. Datha, C. *Social forces, feminism, and breastfeeding.* Pages 556–61.

99. American Cancer Society. *Surveillance Research*. 2001.
100. Yalom, Marilyn. *A history of the breast*. Alfred A. Knopf, New York, NY, 1997. Page 141.
101. Datha, BC. *Social forces, feminism, and breastfeeding*. Pages 556–61.
102. Yalom, Marilyn. *history of the breast*. Alfred A. Knopf, New York, NY, 1997. Page 142.
103. Ibid. Page 141.
104. *NY Times* April 7, 1988.
105. Robins, Gay. Illustration of a Vessel in the Form of a Lactating Woman. *Women in ancient egypt*. Harvard Univ. Press, Harvard, MA, 1993. Pages 90–91.
106. Yalom, Marilyn. *History of the breast*. Alfred A. Knopf, New York, NY, 1997. Page 206.
107. Svensson, M, Sabharwal, H, Hakansson, A, et al. Molecular characterization of alpha-lactalalbumin folding variants that induce apoptosis in tumor cells. *J Biol Chem* 1999; 274: 6388–96.
108. Svensson, M, Duringer, C, Hallgren O, et al. Hamlet—a complex from human milk that induces apoptosis in tumor cells but spares healthy cells. *Adv Exp Med Biol* 2002; 503: 125–32.
109. Svensson, M, Sabharwal, H, Hakansson, A, et al. Molecular characterization of alpha-lactalalbumin folding variants that induce apoptosis in tumor cells. *J Biol Chem* 1999; 274: 6388–96.
110. Svensson, M, Duringer, C, Hallgren, O, et al. Hamlet—a complex from human milk that induces apoptosis in tumor cells but spares healthy cells. *Adv Exp Med Biol* 2002; 503: 125–32.
111. Yalom, Marilyn. *A history of the breast*. Alfred A. Knopf, New York, NY, 1997. Page 207.
112. De Moulin, D. *A short history of breast cancer.* The Hague, 1983. Page 2.
113. Sabbaj, S, Edwards, B, Ghosh, M, et al. Human immunodeficiency virus-specific CD8+ T cells in human breast milk. *J Virology* 2002; 76: 7365–73.
114. HIV transmission via breast milk in Ugandan women limited. *AIDS Weekly Plus* 1996 Sep 23; 17.
115. Guay, LA, et al. Detection of human immunodeficiency virus type 1 (HIV-1) DNA and p24 antigen in breast milk of HIV-1-infected Ugandan women and vertical transmission. *Pediatrics* 1996 Sep; 98 (3 Pt 1): 438–44.
116. Towers, CV, et al. A "bloodless cesarean section" and perinatal transmission of the human immunodeficiency virus. *Am J Obstet Gynecol* 1998 Sep; 179 (3 Pt 1): 708–14.
117. Weiss, P, et al. Long-term follow-up of infants of mothers with type 1 diabetes: evidence for hereditary and nonhereditary transmission of diabetes and precursors. *Diabetes Care* 2000; 23: 905–11.
118. Lemke, H, et al. Is there a maternally induced immunological imprinting phase? *Scand Immunol* 1999; 50: 348–54.
119. Creatsas, George, et al. The young woman at the rise of the 21st century. *Annals of the New York Academy of Sciences* Volume 900; 2000. Page xiii.
120. Shah, I. Fertility and contraception in Europe. *Eur. J. Contracept. Rep. Health Care* 1997; 2: 53–61.
121. Fleming, Sir Alexander; In 1928, while working on influenza virus, he observed that mould secreted an active substance he named *penicillin*. *See* Nobel lecture, 1945.

122. Greaves, Mel. *Cancer: the evolutionary legacy.* Oxford University Press Inc., New York, NY, 2000. Pages 144–145.
123. Harris, Jay R. et al. *Diseases of the Breast.* Lippincott-Raven Publishers, New York, 1996. Page 162.
124. MacMahon, B, et al. Age at first birth and breast cancer risk. *Bull WHO* 1970; 43: 209.

CHAPTER THREE

1. Pearce, Fred. Mamma Mia. *New Scientist* 2002 July 20 38–41.
2. Rinzler, Carol Ann, et al. *Estrogen and breast cancer: a warning to women.* Macmillan Publishing Co., New York, NY, 1993. Page xvii.
3. Jasen, P. Breast cancer and the language of risk, 1750–1950. *Social History of Medicine* 2002; 15: 17–43.
4. ABC News. *The century: america's time: vol. 3.* Buena Vista Home Entertainment, Inc., Burbank, CA, 2000.
5. U.S. Census Bureau, 2000 Census.
6. Wiley, TS, et al. *Lights Out: Sleep, Sugar and Survival.* Pocket Books, New York, NY, 2000.
7. Cross, Jason. Velocitized. *www.over-your-head.com.* May 1, 2001.
8. Musey, V, Collins, D, Musey, P, et al. Age-related changes in the female hormonal environment during reproductive life. *Am J Obstet Gynecol* 1987; 157: 312–7.
9. Timiras, Paola S, et al. *Hormones and aging.* CRC Press, New York, NY, 1995. Page 124.
10. Canivenc, R, et al. Histophysiologie de l'ovaire a la peri- et la postmenopause. *Proc. Journées d'Endocrinologie Clinique* 1979 November 16–17; Foundation de Recherche en Hormonologie, SEPE Publ., France, 1980; 43.
11. Robertson, D, Burger, H. Reproductive hormones: aging and the perimenopause. *Acta Obstet Gynecol Scand* 2002; 81: 612–6.
12. Creatsas, George, et al. The young woman at the rise of the 21st century. *Annals of the New York Academy of Sciences.* Volume 900 2000. Page 6.
13. Attanasio, A, et al. Circadian rhythms in serum melatonin from infancy to adolescence. *J Clin Endocrin. Metabolism* 1985; 61: 388.
14. Cavallo, A, et al. Relation between nocturnal melatonin profile and hormonal markers of puberty in humans. *Horm Res* 1992; 37: 185.
15. Messinis, IE, et al. Effect of varying concentrations of follicle stimulating hormone on the production of gonadotropin surge attenuating factor (GnSAF) in women. *Clin Endocrin* 1993; 39: 45–50.
16. Messinis, IE, et al. Effect of follicle stimulating hormone or human chorionic gonadotrophin treatment on the production of gonadotrophin surge attenuating factor (GnSAF) during the luteal phase of the human menstrual cycle. *Clin Endocrinol (Oxf)* 1996 Feb; 44 (2): 169–75.
17. Messinis, IE, et al. Effect of an increase in FSH on the production of gonadotrophin-surge-attenuating factor in women. *J Reprod Fertil* 1994 Aug; 101 (3): 689–95.
18. Collett, ME, et al. The effect of age upon the pattern of the menstrual cycle. *Fertil Steril* 1954; 5: 437.
19. Sherman, BM, et al. The menopausal transition: analysis of LH, FSH, estradiol, and

progesterone concentrations during menstrual cycles of older women. *J Clin Endocrinol Metab* 1976 Apr; 42 (4): 629–36.

20. Richardson, SJ, et al. Follicular depletion during the menopausal transition: evidence for accelerated loss and ultimate exhaustion. *J Clin Endocrinol Metab* 1987 Dec; 65 (6): 1231–7.
21. Faddy, MJ, et al. Accelerated disappearance of ovarian follicles in mid-life: implications for forecasting menopause. *Hum Reprod* 1992 Nov; 7 (10): 1342–6.
22. Quenby, S, Gazvani, M, Brazeau, C, et al. Oncogenes and tumor suppressor genes in the first trimester human fetal gonadal development. *Mol Hum Reprod* 1999; 5: 737–741.
23. Windham, G, Elkin, E, Fenster, L, et al. Ovarian hormones in premenopausal women: variation by demographic, reproductive and menstrual characteristics. *Epidemiology* 2002; 13: 675–84.
24. Bernstein, J. Epidemiology of endocrine-related risk factors for breast cancer. *J Mammary Gland Biol Neoplasia* 2002; 7: 65–76.
25. Hovey, R, Trott, J, Vonderhaar, B. Establishing a framework for the functional mammary gland: from endocrinology to morphology. *J Mammary Gland Biol Neoplasia* 2002; 7: 17–38.
26. Sivaraman, L, Medina, D. Hormone-induced protection against breast cancer. *J Mammary Gland Biol Neoplasia* 2002; 7: 77–92.
27. Wysowski, D, Comstock, G, Helsing, H, et al. Sex hormones in serum in relation to the development of breast cancer. *Am J Epidemiol* 1987; 125: 791–9.
28. Hankinson, S, Willett, W, Manson, J, et al. Plasma sex steroids hormone levels and risk of breast cancer in postmenopausal women. *J Natl Cancer Inst* 1998; 90: 1292–9.
29. Kwa, H, Cleton, F, Wang, D, et al. A prospective study of plasma prolactin levels and subsequent risk of breast cancer. *Int J Cancer* 1981; 28: 673–6.
30. Hankinson, S, Willett, W, Michaud, D, et al. Plasma prolactin levels and subsequent risk of breast cancer in postmenopausal women. *J Natl Inst Cancer* 1999; 91: 629–34.
31. Wennbo, H, Gebre-Medhin, M, Linde, A, et al. Activation of the prolactin receptor is important for induction of mammary tumors in transgenic mice. *J Clin Invest* 1997; 100: 2744–51.
32. Vonderhaar, B. Prolactin involvement in breast cancer. *Endocrine-Related Cancer* 1999; 6: 389–404.
33. Clevenger, C, Chang, W, Ngo, W, et al. Expression of prolactin and prolactin receptor in human breast carcinoma. Evidence for an autocrine/paracrine loop. *Am J Pathol* 1995; 146: 695–705.
34. Touraine, P, Martini, J, Zafrani, B, et al. Increased expression of prolactin receptor gene assessed by quantitative polymerase chain reaction in human breast tumors versus normal breast tissues. *J Clin Endocrinol Metab* 1998; 83: 667–74.
35. Ingram, D, Nottage, E, Roberts, A. Prolactin and breast cancer risk. *Med J Aust* 1990; 153: 469–73.
36. Ewans, K, Shyamala, G, Ravani, S, et al. Latent transforming growth factor-beta activation in mammary gland: regulation by ovarian hormones affects ductal and alveolar proliferation. *Am J Pathol* 2002; 160: 2081–93.
37. Boyd, N, Stone, J, Martin, L, et al. The association of breasts mitogens with mammographic densities. *Br J Cancer* 2001; 87: 876–82.

38. Clevenger, C, Plank, T. Prolactin as an autocrine/paracrine factor in breast tissue. *J Mammary Gland Biol Neoplasia* 1997; 2: 59–68.
39. Dickson, RB, et al. Growth regulation of normal and malignant breast epithelium. In Bland, KI, et al., *The Breast*, W.B. Saunders, Philadelphia, PA, 1991. Page 363.
40. Fenton, SE, et al. Prolactin inhibits epidermal growth factor (EGF)-stimulated signaling events in mouse mammary epithelial cells by altering EGF receptor function. *Mol Biol Cell* 1993 Aug; 4 (8): 773–80.
41. Bezault, J, et al. Human lactoferrin inhibits growth of solid tumors and development of experimental metastases in mice. *Cancer Res* 1994 May 1; 54 (9) 2310–2.
42. Snedeker, SM, et al. Expression and functional properties of transforming growth factor alpha and epidermal growth factor during mouse mammary gland ductal morphogenesis. *Proc Natl Acad Sci* (USA) 1991 Jan 1; 88 (1): 276–80.
43. Coleman-Kmacik, S, et al. Differential temporal and spatial gene expression of fibroblast growth factor family members during mouse mammary gland development. *Mol Endocrinol* 1994 Feb; 8 (2): 218–29.
44. Collins, MK, et al. Growth factors as survival factors: regulation of apoptosis. *Bioessays* 1994 Feb; 16 (2): 133–8.
45. Russo, J, et al. Development of the human mammary gland. In Neville, MC, et al. *The Mammary Gland*. Plenum, New York, NY, 1987. Page 67.
46. Daniel, C, et al. Local effects of growth factors. In Lippman, ME, et al., *Regulatory Mechanisms in Breast Cancer*. Kluwer, Boston, MA, 1990. Page 79.
47. Yen, Samuel, SC, et al. *Reproductive endocrinology.* W.B. Saunders Co., Philadelphia, PA, 1999. Pages 286–287.
48. Neville, MC, et al. Endocrine regulation of nutrient flux in the lactating woman. Do the mechanisms differ from pregnancy? *Adv Exp Med Biol* 1994;352:85–98.
49. Schmitt-Ney, M, et al. Mammary gland-specific nuclear factor activity is positively regulated by lactogenic hormones and negatively by milk stasis. *Mol Endocrinol* 1992 Dec; 6 (12): 1988–97.
50. Tourkine, N, et al. Activation of STAT factors by prolactin, interferon-gamma, growth hormones, and a tyrosine phosphatase inhibitor in rabbit primary mammary epithelial cells. *J Biol Chem* 1995 Sep 8; 270 (36): 20952–61.
51. Nishikawa, S, et al. Progesterone and EGF inhibit mouse mammary gland prolactin receptor and beta-casein gene expression. *Am J Physiol* 1994 Nov; 267 (5 Pt 1): C1467–72.
52. London, SJ, et al. Lactation and risk of breast cancer in a cohort of US women. *Am J Epidemiol* 1990 Jul; 132 (1): 17–26.
53. De Bortoli, M, et al. Hormonal regulation of c-erbB-2 oncogene expression in breast cancer cells. *J Steroid Biochem Mol Bio* 1992 Sep; 43 (1–3): 21–5.
54. Bates, N, Hurst, H. An intron 1 enhancer element mediates oestrogen-induced suppression of ERBB2 expression. *Oncogene* 1997; 15: 473–81.
55. Yarden, R, Wilson, M, Chrysogelos, S. Estrogen suppression of EGFR expression in breast cancer cells. A possible mechanism to modulate growth. *J Cell Biochem* 2001; 81: 232–46.
56. Gotzsche, P, Olsen, O. Is screening for breast cancer with mammography justifiable? *Lancet* 2000; 355:129–34.

57. Olsen, O, Goetsche, P. Cochrane review on screening for breast cancer with mammography. *Lancet* 2001; 358: 1340–42.
58. Moradi, T, Adami, H, Ekbom, A, et al. Physical activity and risk for breast cancer: a prospective cohort study among Swedish twins. *Int J Cancer* 2002; 100: 76–81.
59. De Waard, F, Trichopoulos, D. A unifying concept of the aetiology of breast cancer. *Int J Cancer* 1988; 41: 666–669.
60. Horn-Ross, P, Hoggatt, K, West, D, et al. Recent diet and breast cancer risk: the California teachers study (USA). *Cancer Causes Control* 2002; 13: 407–15.
61. Nechushtan, H, Peretz, T. Tamoxifen and breast cancer. *Harefuah* 2002; 141: 718–20.
62. Hendrix, S, McNeeley, S. Effect of selective estrogen receptor modulators on reproductive tissues other than endometrium. *Ann N Y Acad Sci* 2001; 949: 243–50.
63. Grann, V, Jacobson, J. Population screening for cancer-related germline gene mutations. *Lancet Oncol* 2002; 3: 3412–8.
64. Foulkes, W, Rosenblatt, J, Chappuis, P. The contribution of inherited factors to the clinicopathological features and behavior of breast cancer. *J Mammary Gland Biol Neoplasia* 2001; 6: 453–65.
65. Ginger, M, Gonzalez-Rimbau, M, Gay, J, et al. Persistent changes in gene expression induced by estrogen and progesterone in the rat mammary gland. *Mol Endocrinol* 2001; 15: 1993–2009.
66. Gudas, J, Nguyen, H, Li, T, et al. Hormone-dependent regulation of BRCA1 in human breast cancer cells. *Cancer Res* 1995; 55: 4561–5.
67. Medina, D, Sivaraman, L, Hilsenbeck, S, et al. Mechanisms of hormonal prevention of breast cancer. *Ann N Y Acad Sci* 2001; 952: 23–35.
68. Sivaraman, L, Medina, D. Hormone-induced protection against breast cancer. *J Mammary Gland Biol Neoplasia* 2002; 1: 77–92.
69. Guzman, R, Yang, J, Rajkumar, L, et al. Hormonal prevention of breast cancer: mimicking the protective effect of pregnancy. *Proc Natl Acad Sci* (USA) 1999; 96: 2520–5.
70. Fossati, R, et al. Cytotoxic and hormonal treatment for metastatic breast cancer: a systematic review of published randomized trials involving 31,510 women. *J Clin Oncol* 1998; 16: 3439–60.
71. Vinyals, A, Peinado, M, Gonzalez-Garrigues, M, et al. Failure of wild-type p53 gene therapy in human cancer cells expressing a mutant p53 protein. *Gene Ther* 1999; 6: 22–33.
72. Sacco, M, Soldati, S, Mira, C, et al. Combined effects on tumor growth and metastasis by antiestrogenic and antiangiogenic therapies in MMTV-neu mice. *Gene Ther* 2002; 9: 1338–41.
73. Klein, C, Blankenstein, T, Schmidt-Kittler, O, et al. Genetic heterogeneity of single disseminated tumour cells in minimal residual cancer. *Lancet* 2002; 360: 683–9.
74. Fossati, R, Confalonieri, C, Torri, V, et al. Cytotoxic and hormonal treatment for metastatic breast cancer: a systematic review of published randomized trials involving 31,510 women. *J Clin Oncol* 1998; 16: 8439–60.
75. Jasen, P. Breast cancer and the language of risk 1750–1950. *Social History of Medicine* 2002; 15: 17–43.
76. Moss, Ralph W. *Questioning chemotherapy.* Equinox Press, Brooklyn, NY, 1995. Pages 84–85.
77. Early breast cancer trialists' collaborative group. Favorable and unfavorable effects of

long-term survival of radiotherapy for early breast cancer: an overview of the randomised trials. *Lancet* 2000; 355: 1757–70.

78. Starr, Paul. *The social transformation of american medicine*. Basic Books, Inc., Publishers, New York, NY, 1982. Page 135.
79. Sivaraman, L, Hilsenbeck, SG, Zhong, L, et al. Early exposure of the rat mammary gland to estrogen and progesterone blocks co-localization of estrogen receptor expression of proliferation. *J Endocrinol* 2001; 171: 75–83.
80. Kirchner, T, Muller, S, Hattori, T, et al. Metaplasia, intraepithelial neoplasia and early cancer of the stomach are related to dedifferentiated epithelial cells defined by cytokeratin-7 expression in gastritis. *Wirchows Arch* 2001; 439: 512–22.
81. Cillo, C, Faiella, A, Cantile, M, et al. Homeobox genes and cancer. *Exp Cell Res* 1999; 248: 21–9.
82. Smalley, M, Dale, T. Wut signalling in mammalian development and cancer. *Cancer Metastasis Rev* 1999; 18: 215–30.
83. Introna, M, Golay, J. How can oncogenic transcription factors cause cancer: a critical review of the myb story. *Leukemia* 1999; 13: 1301–6.
84. Adida, C, Crotty, P, McGrath, J, et al. Developmentally regulated expression of the novel cancer anti-apoptosis gene survivin in human and mouse differentiation. *Am J Pathol* 1998; 152: 43–9.
85. Breast cancer and breastfeeding. Collaborative reanalysis of individual data from 47 epidemiological studies in 30 countries, including 50,302 women with breast cancer and 96,973 women without the disease. *Lancet* 2002; 360: 187–95.

CHAPTER FOUR

1. Melrow, D, et al. The link between female infertility and cancer: epidemiology and possible aetiologies. *Hum Reprod Update* 1996; 2: 63–75.
2. Venn, A, et al. Risk of cancer after use of fertility drugs with in-vitro fertilization. *Lancet* 1999; 354: 1586–90.
3. Franco, C, et al. Ovulation induction and the risk of ovarian tumors. *Minerva Ginecol* 2000; 52: 103–9.
4. Wakeley, K. Reproductive technologies and risk of ovarian cancer. *Curr Opin Obstet Gynecol* 2000; 12: 43–7.
5. Venn, A, et al. Characteristics of ovarian and uterine cancers in a cohort of in vitro fertilization patients. *Gynecol Oncol* 2001; 82: 64–8.
6. Glud, E, et al. Fertility drugs and ovarian cancer. *Epidemiol Rev* 1998; 20: 237–57.
7. Rossing, M, et al. Ovarian tumors in a cohort of infertile women. *N Engl J Med* 1994; 331: 771–6.
8. Whittemore, A, et al. Characteristics relating to ovarian cancer risk: collaborative analysis of 12 US case-control studies II Invasive epithelial ovarian cancers in white women. Collaborative ovarian cancer group. *Am J Epidemiol* 1992; 136: 1184–203.
9. Lee, John. *Natural progesterone: the multiple roles of remarkable hormone*. Jon Carpenter Publishing, Charlbury, Oxon, Wales, 1999.
10. Traina, A, et al. Oral contraceptive use and breast cancer risk in areas with different incidence. A case-control study among young women. *Ann N Y Acad Sci* 1996; 784: 564–9.

11. Pinkerton, G, et al. Post-pill anovolution. *Med J Aust* 1976; 1: 220–8.
12. Marchbanks, P, et al. Oral contraceptives and the risk of breast cancer. *N Engl J Med* 2002; 346: 2025–32.
13. Robb-Nicholson, C. By the way doctor. I'm 47 and my menstrual periods are quite irregular, so my doctor started me on birth control pills. How will I know when I enter menopause and when to switch to HRT? *Harv Womens Health Watch* 1999; 7: 8.
14. Somkuti, S, et al. The effect of oral contraceptive pills on markers of endometrial receptivity. *Fertil Steril* 1996; 65: 484–8.
15. Kay, C, et al. Breast cancer and the pill—a further report from the Royal College of General Practitioners' oral contraception study. *Br J Cancer* 1988; 58: 675–80.
16. Rookus, M, et al. Oral contraceptives and risk of breast cancer in women aged 20–54 years. *Lancet* 1994; 344: 844–51.
17. Terry, M, et al. Oral contraceptive use and Cyclin D1 overexpression in breast cancer among young women. *Cancer Epidemiol Biomarkers Prev* 2002; 11:1100–3.
18. Prehn, A, et al. Increase in breast cancer incidence in middle-aged women during the 1990s. *Ann Epidemiol* 2002; 12: 476.
19. Chilvers, C, et al. The effect of patterns of oral contraceptive use on breast cancer risk in young women. The UK national case-control study group. *Br J Cancer* 1994; 69: 922–3.
20. *www.playboy.com.*
21. Fraser, JG, et al. *Golden bough*. Simon and Schuster, New York, NY. 2002. Page 577.
22. Ventura, S, et al. Trends in pregnancy rates for the United States, 1976–97: an update. *Natl Vital Stat Rep* 2001; 49: 1–9.
23. Armitage, B, Babb, P. Population review: (4). Trends in fertility. *Popul Trends* 1996; 84: 7–13.
24. Francis, D. New global forecast: population decline in sight. *The Christian Science Monitor* 03/02. 2002 March 11.
25. Becker, Jill B, et al. *Behavioral endocrinology.* A Bradford Book, MIT Press, Cambridge, MA, 1992. Page 3.
26. Henry, J. Biological basis of the stress response. *Integr Physiol Behav Sci* 1992; 27: 66–83.
27. Caufriez, A, et al. Immediate effects of an 8-h advance shift of the rest-activity cycle on 24-h profiles of cortisol. *Am J Physiol Endocrinol Metab* 2002 May; 282 (5): E1147–53.
28. Sandman, CA, et al. Maternal stress, HPA activity, and fetal/infant outcome. *Ann NY Acad Sci* 1997 Apr 24; 814: 266–75.
29. Glover, V. Maternal stress or anxiety during pregnancy and the development of the baby. *Pract Midwife* 1999 May; 2 (5): 20–2.
30. Herrenkohl, LR. Prenatal stress disrupts reproductive behavior and physiology in offspring. *Ann NY Acad Sci* 1986; 474: 120–8.
31. Essex, M, et al. Maternal stress beginning in infancy may sensitize children to later stress exposure: effect on cortisol and behavior. *Biol Psychiatry* 2002; 52: 776–79.
32. Seckl, J. Physiologic programming of the fetus. *Clin Perinatol* 1998; 25: 939–62.
33. Jirtle, R, et al. Genomic imprinting and environment disease susceptibility. *Environ Health Perspect* 2000; 108: 271–8.
34. Jacobovits, A, et al. Interactions of stress and reproduction. *Zentralbl Gynekol* 2002; 124: 189–93.

35. Herrenkohl, L. Prenatal stress disrupts reproductive behavior and physiology in offspring. *Ann NY Acad Sci* 1986; 474: 20–8.
36. Glover, V. Maternal stress or anxiety during pregnancy and the development of the baby. *Pract Midwife* 1999; 2: 20–2.
37. Herrenkohl, L. Prenatal stress reduces fertility and fecundity in female offspring. *Science* 1979; 206: 1097–9.
38. Caufriez, A, et al. Immediate effects of an 8-h advance shift of the rest-activity cycle on 24-h profiles of cortisol. *Am J Physiol Endocrinol Metab* 2002; 282: E1147–53.
39. Wiley, TS, et al. *Lights out: sleep, sugar and survival.* Pocket Books, New York, NY, 2000.
40. Van Cauter, E, et al. Metabolic effects of short-term elevations of plasma cortisol are more pronounced in the evening than in the morning. *J Clin Endocrinol Metab* 1999; 84: 3082–92.
41. Campbell, Scott, et al. Extraocular circadian phototransduction in humans. *Science* 1998 Jan 16; 279 (5349): 396–399.
42. Regulation of endocrine pancreas secretions (insulin and glucagon) during the periodic lethargy-walking cycle of the hibernating mammal. *Diabete et Metabolisme* 1987 June; 13 (3): 176–181.
43. Diamond, Michael, et al. Suppression of counterregulatory hormone response to hypoglycemia by insulin. *Journal of Clin Endo Metab* 1990; 72 (6): 1388–1390.
44. Spiegel, K, et al. Impact of sleep dept on metabolic and endocrine function. *Lancet* 1999; 354: 1435–9.
45. Henry, JP. Biological basis of the stress response. *Integrated Physiological Behavioral Sciences* 1992 Jan; 27 (1): 66–83.
46. Roennenberg, T, et al. Annual rhythm of human reproduction: biology, sociology, or both? *J Biol Rhythms* 1990; 5: 195–216.
47. Ashley, M. Season of birth: stability of the pattern in Canada. *Can J Public Health* 1988; 79: 101–3.
48. Stryer, L. *Biochemistry*, 3d ed. W. Freedman and Company, New York, NY, 1988. Page 315.
49. Nebert, D, et al. Clinical importance of the cytochromes P450. *Lancet* 2002; 360: 1155–62.
50. Endoh, A, et al. CYP21 pseudogene transcripts are much less abundant than those from the active gene in normal human adrenocortical cells under various conditions in culture. *Mol Cell Endocrinol* 1998; 137: 13–9.
51. Kristiansen, S, et al. Induction of steroidogenic enzyme genes by insulin and IGF-1 in cultured adult human adrenocortical cells. *Steroids* 1997; 62: 258–65.
52. Chang, C, et al. The response of 21-hydroxylase messenger ribonucleic acid levels to adenosine 3',5'-monophosphate and 12-O-tetradecanoylphorbol-13-acetate in bovine adrenalcortical cells is dependent on culture conditions. *Endocrinology* 1991; 128: 604–10.
53. Sudha, S, et al. Influence of streptozotocin-induced diabetes and insulin treatment on the pituitary-testicular axis during sexual maturation in rats. *Exp Clin Endocrinol Diabetes* 2000; 108: 14–20.

54. McGee, E, et al. The effect of insulin and insulin-like growth factors on the expression of steroidogenic enzymes in a human ovarian thecal-like tumor cell model. *Fertil Steril* 1996; 65: 87–93.
55. Luboschitzky, R, et al. Decreased melatonin secretion in a phenotypically male 46, XX patient with classic 21-hydroxylase deficiency. *Exp Clin Endocrinol Diabetes* 2000; 108: 237–40.
56. Collaer, M, et al. Human behavioral sex differences: a role for gonadal hormones during early development: *Psychological Bull* 1995; 118: 55–107.
57. Arnold, A, et al. Gonadal steroid induction of structural sex differences in the central nervous system *Annu Rev Neurosci* 1984; 7: 413–42.
58. Migeon, C, Wisniewski, A. Sexual differentiation: from gender to gender. *Horm Res* 1998; 50: 245–51.
59. Okada, A, et al. Effect of estrogens on ontogenetic expression of progesterone receptor in the fetal female reproductive tract. *Mol Cell Endocrinol* 2002; 195: 55–64.
60. Lemmen, J, et al. Detection of oestrogenic activity of steroids present during mammalian gestation using oestrogen receptor alpha- and oestrogen receptor beta-specific in vitro assays. *J Endocrinol* 2002; 174: 435–46.
61. Miller, Kenneth R, et al. *Biology*; new ed. Prentice Hall, Needham, MA, 1993. Pages 204–225.
62. Collaer, M, et al. Human behavioral sex differences. A role for gonadal hormones during early development. *Psychological Bull* 1995; 118: 55–107.
63. Domer, G, et al. Stressful events in prenatal life of bi- and homosexual men. *Exp Clin Endocrinol* 1983; 81: 83–7.
64. Luboschitzky, R, et al. Decreased melatonin secretion in a phenotypically male 46, XX patient with classic 21-hydroxylase deficiency. *Exp Clin Endocrinol Diabetes* 2000; 108: 237–40.
65. Dorner, G, et al. Gene- and environment-dependent neuroendocrine etiogenesis of homosexuality and transsexualism. *Exp Clin Endocrinol* 1991; 98: 141–50.
66. Goodman, R. Understanding human sexuality in terms of chaos theory and fetal development. *Med Hypotheses* 1997; 48: 237–43.
67. Bailey, J, et al. A test of the maternal stress theory of human male homosexuality. *Arch Sex Behav* 1991; 20: 277–93.
68. U.S. Census, 2000. *Reported Same Sex Couples*.
69. Kirby, David. The next generation: open-minded and well-adjusted, children with gay parents say their families are a gift. *The Advocate* 1999 June 22.
70. Lorde, Audre. How gay was the Harlem Renaissance? *www.women in the life.com*, 2000.
71. Committee makes recommendations for California schools. *San Francisco Chronicle* 2001 April 13.
72. Vilaine, E. Genetics of sexual development. *Annv Rev Sup Res Review*. 2000; 11: 1–25.
73. Becker, Jill B, et al. *Behavioral endocrinology*. A Bradford Book, MIT Press, Cambridge, MA, 1992.
74. Katz, Esther. Margaret Sanger papers project: boi of Margaret Sanger. 2001 October 1. *www.nyu.edu/projects/sanger/ms-bio.htm*.

75. Seaman, Barbara, et al. *Women and the crisis in sex hormones*. Bantam Books, Inc., New York, 1977.
76. Ibid. Page 79.
77. Ibid.
78. Rock, John, M.D. *The time has come: a Catholic doctor's proposals to end the battle over birth control.* Alfred A. Knopf, New York, NY, 1963.
79. Seaman, Barbara, et al. *Women and the crisis in sex hormones*. Rawson Associates Publishers, Inc., New York, NY, 1977. Pages 82–83.
80. Ibid. Page 83.
81. Rowe-Finkbeiner, Kristin. Oops, I forgot to have kids. *Bust Magazine* 2002 Summer. Pages 44–49.
82. Abdel-Sayed, W, et al. Some metabolic and hormonal changes in women using long acting injectable contraception. *Alex J Pharm Soc* 1989; 3: 29–32.
83. Harlow, B, Signotello, L. Factors associated with early menopause. *Maturitas* 2000; 35: 3–9.
84. Murphy, L, et al. Mechanisms involved in the evolution of progestin resistance in human breast cancer cells. *Cancer Res* 1991; 51: 2051–7.
85. Rachon, D., et al. Effects of estrogen depletion on IL-6 production by peripheral blood cells in postmenopausal women. *J Endocrinol* 2002; 172: 387–95.
86. Oyelola, O, et al. Steroidal contraceptives and changes in individual plasma phospholipids: possible role in thrombosis. *Adv Contracept* 1990; 6: 93–206.
87. Vasilakis-Scaramozza, C, et al. Risk of venous thromboembolism with cyproterone or levonorgestrel contraceptives. *Lancet* 2001; 358: 1427–9.
88. Kemmeren, J, et al. Third generation oral contraceptives and risk of venous thrombosdisease: meta-analysis. *BJM* 2001; 323: 1–9.
89. Seaman, Barbara, et al. *Women and the crisis in sex hormones*. Rawson Associates Publishers, Inc., New York, 1977. Page 83.
90. Ibid. Pages 87–88.
91. Petersen, K, et al. Metabolic and fibrinolytic response to changes insulin sensitivity in users of oral contraceptives. *Contraception* 1999; 60: 337–44.
92. Kumle, M, et al. Use of oral contraceptives and breast cancer risk. The Norwegian-Swedish women's lifestyle and health cohort study. *Cancer Epidemiol Biomarkers Prev* 2002; 11: 1375–81.
93. *www.yasmin.com.*
94. *http://www.orthotri-cyclen.comanswer/birth=_answers/quickfacts.html.*
95. Rossouw, JE, et al. Risks and benefits of estrogen plus progestin in healthy postmenopausal women: Principal results from the women's health initiative randomized controlled trial. *JAMA* 2002 Jul 17; 288(3): 321–33.
96. Gibaldi, Milo. Drug evaluation: media celebrates the pill's 40th birthday. *Milo Gibaldi Pharmaceutical Report* 2000 June 15; www.aaps.org/news/articles/2000.
97. Diethylstilbestrol and media coverage of the "morning after" pill. *http://www.iusb.edu/;sljournal/1999/Paper10.html.*
98. Baumslag, Naomi, et al. *Milk, money and madness: the culture and politics of breastfeeding.* Bergin and Garvey, Westport, CT, 1995.

99. Diethylstilbestrol and media coverage of the "morning after" pill. *http://www.iusb.edu/;sljournal/1999/Paper10.html.*
100. Yalom, Marilyn. *A history of the breast.* Alfred A. Knopf, New York, NY 1997. Page 128.
101. Ibid. Page 141.
102. Baumslag, Naomi, et al. *Milk, money and madness: the culture and politics of breastfeeding.* Bergin and Garvey, Westport, CT, 1995.
103. Palmer, Gabrielle. *The politics of breast-feeding.* Pandora, London, 1988.
104. Starr, Paul. *The social transformation of american medicine.* Basic Books, Inc., Publishers, New York, NY, 1982. Pages 139–140.
105. Baby Milk Action. Briefing paper. History of the campaign. *www.babymilkaction.org.*
106. Fomon, S. Infant feeding in the 20th century: formula and breast. *J Nutr* 2001 Feb; 31 (2): 409S–20S.
107. Palmer, Gabrielle. *The politics of breast-feeding.* Pandora, London, 1988.
108. Baumslag, Naomi, et al. *Milk, money and madness: the culture and politics of breastfeeding.* Bergin and Garvey, Westport, CT, 1995.
109. Leslynotes.com. Childbirth information for women & men. Brief history.
110. *Nutrition During Lactation.* National Academy Press. 1991. Page 29.
111. Weiss, H, et al. Prenatal and perinatal risk factors for breast cancer in young women. *Epidemiology* 1997; 8: 181–7.
112. Becker, Jill B, et al. *Behavioral Endocrinology.* A Bradford Book, Cambridge, MA, 1992. Pages 58–59.
113. Breast cancer and breastfeeding. Collaborative reanalysis of individual data from 47 epidemiological studies in 30 countries, including 50,302 women with breast cancer and 96,973 women without the disease. *Lancet* 2002; 360: 187–95.
114. Ibid.
115. Brind, J, et al. Induced abortion as an independent risk factor for breast cancer: a comprehensive review and meta-analysis. *J Epidemiol Community Health* 1996; 50: 481–96.
116. Daling, J, et al. Risk of breast cancer in young women: relationship to induced abortion. *J Natl Cancer Inst* 1994; 86: 1584–92.
117. Hadjimichael, OC, et al. Abortion before first livebirth and risk of breast cancer. *Br J Cancer* 1986; 53: 281–4.
118. Russo, J, et al. Susceptibility of mammary gland to carcinogenesis. Pregnancy interruption as a risk factor in tumor incidence. *Am J Pathol* 1980; 100: 497–512.
119. Vatten, L, et al. Pregnancy related protection against breast cancer depends on length of gestation. *Br J Cancer* 2002; 87: 289–90.
120. Kalb, Claudia. Should you have your baby now? *Newsweek* 2001 August 13.
121. Ibid.
122. Kalb, Claudia. Should you have your baby now? *Newsweek*, 2001 August 13.
123. Rowe-Finkbeiner, Kristin. Oops, I forgot to have kids. *Bust Magazine* 2002 Summer; 44–49.
124. Hart, Betsy. Science and the "sisterhood": why is mixing feminism and facts not kosher? *Jewish World Review* 2001 August 14. *www.jewishworldreview.com.*

125. Thompson, WD, et al. Maternal age at birth and risk of breast cancer in daughters. *Epidemiology* 1990 Mar; 1(2): 101–6.
126. Newcomb, P, et al. Lactation and a reduced risk of premenopausal breast cancer. *N Engl J Med* 1994; 330: 81–7.
127. Ibid.
128. Rowe-Finkbeiner, Kristin. Oops, I forgot to have kids: *Bust Magazine* 2002 Summer; 44–49.
129. Key, T, et al. Epidemiology of breast cancer. *Lancer Oncol* 2001; 2: 33–40.
130. Sivaraman, L, et al. Early exposure of the rat mammary gland to estrogen and progesterone blocks co-localization of estrogen receptor expression and profileration. *J Endocrinol* 2001; 171: 75–83.
131. Medina, D, et al. Mechanisms of hormonal prevention of breast cancer. *Ann N Y Acad Sci* 2001; 978: 23–35.
132. Sivaraman, L, et al. p53 is a potential mediator of pregnancy and hormone-induced resistance to mammary carcinogenesis. *Proc Natl Acad Sci* (USA) 2001; 98: 12379–84.

CHAPTER FIVE

1. National Library of Medicine, fact sheet. *http://www.nlm.nih.gov/pubs/factsheets/nlm.html.*
2. *http://www.ncbi.nlm.nib.gov/entrez/query.fogi.*
3. Cicinelli, E, et al. Twice-weekly transdermal estradiol and vaginal progesterone as continuous combined hormone replacement therapy in postmenopausal women: a 1-year prospective study. *Am J Obstet Gynecol*, 2002 Sep; 187 (3): 556–60.
4. Levine, H, et al. Comparision of the pharmacokinetics of crinone 8% administered vaginally versus prometrium administered orally in postmenopausal women (3). *Fertil Steril* 2000 Mar; 73 (3): 516–21.
5. Shantha, S, et al. Natural vaginal progesterone is associated with minimal psychological side effects: a preliminary study. *J Womens Health Gend Based Med* 2001 Dec; 10(10): 991–7.
6. *Physicians' desk reference*, 55th ed. Medical Economics Co., Inc., Montvale, NJ, 2001. Page 1418.
7. *su1http://www.tmc.edu/thi/diagimeds.html.*
8. Sains, A. Health care in Europe. The rules are changing. *Europe* 2002; 420: 6–9.
9. Samuels, N. Acupuncture for cancer patients. Why not? *Harefuah* 2002; 141: 608–610.
10. Kubo, T, et al. Targeted systemic chemotherapy using magnetic liposomes with incorporated adriamycin for osteosarcoma in hamsters. *Int J Oncol* 2001 Jan; 18 (1): 121–5.
11. *www.lectlaw.com/files/exp24.htm.*
12. Morrow, M, et al. Standard for the management of ductal carcinoma in situ of the breast (DCIS). *CA Cancer J Clin* 2002; 52:256–76.
13. Levine, R, et al. Ethical considerations in translating epidemiologic evidence into medical practice. *Ann Epidemiol* 2002; 12: 532–4.
14. Moss, RA. *Questioning chemotherapy*. Equinox Press, Brooklyn, NY, 1995. Page 114.
15. Patterson, K. What doctors don't know (almost everything). *The New York Times Magazine* 2002 May 5: 74–80.
16. Rossouw, JE, et al. Risks and benefits of estrogen plus progestin in healthy post-

menopausal women: principal results from the women's health initiative randomized controlled trial. *JAMA* 2002 Jul 17; 288 (3): 321–33.

17. Fujimoto, J, et al. Progestins suppress estrogen-induced expression of vascular endothelial growth factor (VEGF) subtypes in uterine endometrial cancer cells. *Cancer Lett* 1999 Jul 1; 141 (1–2): 63–71.
18. Nilsen, J, Briton, R. Impact of progestins on estrogen-induced neuroprotection: synergy by progesterone and 19-norprogesterone and antagonism by medroxyprogesterone acetate. *Endocrinology* 2002; 143: 205–12.
19. Yao, D, et al. Synthesis and reactivity of potential toxic metabolites of tamoxifen analogues: droloxifene and toremifene 0-quinones. *Chem Res Toxicol* 2001; 14: 1643–53.
20. Stiborova, M, et al. New selective inhibitors of cytochromes P450 2B and their application to antimutagenesis of tamoxifen. *Arch Biochem Biophys* 2002; 403: 41–9.
21. McLuckie, K, et al. DNA adducts formed from 4-hydroxytamoxifen are more mutagenic than those formed by alpha-acetyitamoxifen in a shuttle vector target gene replicated in human Ad293 cells. *Biochemistry* 2002; 41: 8899–906.
22. Goldstein, S, et al. Adverse events that are associated with the selective estrogen receptor modulator levormeloxifene in an aborted phase III osteoporosis treatment study. *Am J Obstet Gynecol* 2002; 187: 521–7.
23. Nechushtan, H, et al. Tamoxifen and breast cancer. *Harefuah* 2002; 141: 718–20.
24. Groshong, S, et al. Biphasic regulation of breast cancer cell growth by progesterone: Role of the cyclin-dependent kinase inhibitors, p21 and p27. *Mol Endocrinol* 1997; 11: 1593–1607.
25. Formby, B, Wiley, TS. Bcl-2, survivin and variant CD44 v7-v10 are downregulated and p53 is upregulated in breast cancer cells by progesterone: inhibition of cell growth and induction of apoptosis. *Mol Cell Biochem* 1999; 202: 53–61.
26. Hilakivi-Clarke, L, et al. Does estrogen always increase breast cancer risk? *J Steroid Biochem Mol Biol* 2002; 80: 163–74.
27. Pardee, AB. GI events and regulation of cell proliferation. *Science* 1989 Nov 3; 246 (4930): 603–8.
28. Fujimoto, J, et al. Progestins suppress estrogen-induced expression of vascular endothelial growth factor (VEGF) subtypes in uterine endometrial cancer cells. *Cancer Lett* 1999 Jul 1; 141 (1–2): 63–71.
29. Decensi, A, et al. Effect of transdermal estradiol and oral conjugated estrogen on C-reactive protein in retinoid-placebo trial in healthy women. *Circulation* 2002; 106: 1224–8.
30. Lacreuse, A, et al. Estradiol, but not raloxifene, improves aspects of spatial working memory in aged ovariectomized rhesus monkeys. *Neurobiol Aging* 2002; 23: 589–600.
31. Chuang, T, et al. Principles of evidence-based medicine using stage I-II melanoma as a model. *Int J Dermatol*, 2002; 41: 721–8.
32. Goodman, N. Evidence-based medicine needs proper critical reviews. *Anest Analg* 2002; 95: 1817–8.
33. Kichener, H. Evidence-based medicine applied to cervical cancer. *Virus Res* 2002; 89: 175–81.

34. Gerson, L. Screening for esophageal adenocarcinoma: an evidence-based approach. *Am J Med* 2002; 113: 499–505.
35. Wallach, P, et al. The profession of medicine: an integrated approach to basic principles. *Acad Med* 2002; 77: 1168–9.
36. Wilson, K, et al. Teaching evidence-based complimentary and alternative medicine. Appraising the evidence for papers on therapy. *J Altern Compliment Med* 2002; 8: 673–9.
37. Thornton, Hazel. Breast screening seems driven by belief rather than evidence. *BMJ* 2002 March 16; 324: 677.
38. Susan, Mayor. Row over breast cancer screening shows that scientists bring "some subjectivity into their work." *BMJ* 2001 Oct 27; 323: 956.
39. Clegg, Li F, et al. Cancer survival among US whites and minorities: a SEER (Surveillance, Epidemiology, and End Results) program population based study. *Arch Intern Med* 2002; 162: 1985–93.
40. Fossati, R, et al. Cytotoxic and hormonal treatment for metastatic breast cancer: a synthetic review of published randomized trials involving 31,510 women. *J Clin Oncol* 1998; 10: 3489–99.
41. Rigby, JE, et al. Can physical trauma cause breast cancer? *Eur J Cancer Prev* 2002 Jun; 11 (3): 307–11.
42. Kopans, DB. Physical trauma and breast cancer. *Lancet* 1994 May 28; 343 (8909): 1364–5.
43. Van Netten, JP, et al. Physical trauma and breast cancer. *Lancet* 1994 Apr 16; 343 (8903): 978–9.
44. Cooper, LF, et al. Estrogen-induced resistance to osteoblast apoptosis is associated w/increased hsp27 expression. *J Cell Physiol* 2000 Dec; 185 (3): 401–7.
45. Formby, B, Wiley, TS. Bcl-2, survivin and variant CD44 v7-v10 are downregulated and p53 is upregulated in breast cancer cells by progesterone: inhibition of cell growth and induction of apoptosis. *Mol Cell Biochem* 1999; 202: 53–62.
46. Bu, S, et al. Progesterone induces apoptosis and up-regulation of p53 expression in human ovarian carcinoma cell lines. *Cancer* 1997; 79: 1944–50.
47. http://www.health.org/nongovpvbs/alcocancer/. The National Toxicology Program.
48. Norberg, T, et al. Increased p53 mutation frequency during tumor progression—results from a breast cancer cohort. *Cancer Res* 2001; 61: 8317–21.
49. Simpson, A. The natural somatic mutation frequency and human carcinogenesis. *Adv Cancer Res* 1997; 71: 209–40.
50. Rainey, P. Evolutionary genetics: the economics of mutation. *Curr Biol* 1999; 9: R371–3.
51. Tomlinson, J, et al. The mutation rate and cancer. *Proc Natl Acad Sci* (USA) 1996; 93: 14800–3.
52. Tycko, Benjamin. Epigenetic gene silencing in cancer. *The Journal of Clinical Investigation* 2000 Feb; 105 (4).
53. Mattick, John S, et al. The evolution of controlled multitasked gene networks: the role of introns and other noncoding RNAs in the development of complex organisms. *Mol Biol Evol* 2001; 18 (9): 1611–1630.
54. Liu, M, et al. P53 gene mutations: case study of a clinical marker for solid tumors. *Semin Oncol* 2002 Jun; 29(3): 246–57. Review.

55. Hill, KA, et al. p53 as a mutagen test in breast cancer. *Environmental Molecular Mutagen* 2002; 39: 216–227.
56. Gasso, P, et al. The p53 pathway in breast cancer. *Breast Cancer Research* 2002; 4: 70–76.
57. Prince, V. The hox paradox: More complex(es) than imagined. *Dev Biol* 2002 Sep 1; 249 (1): 1–15. Review.
58. Samson, SL, et al. Role of Sp 1 in insulin regulation of gene expression. *J Mol Endocrinol* 2002 Dec; 29 (3): 265–79.
59. Hernandez-Boussard, T, et al. Sources of bias in the detection and reporting of p53 mutations in human cancer: analysis of the IARC p53 mutation database. *Genet Anal* 1999; 14: 229–33.
60. Strauss, B. Role in tumorigenesis of silent mutations in the TP53 gene. *Mutat Res* 2000; 457: 93–104.
61. Farid, N. P53 mutations in thyroid carcinoma: tidings from an old foe. *J Endocrinol Invest* 2001; 24: 536–45.
62. Strauss, B. Silent and multiple mutations in p53 and the question of the hypermutability of tumors. *Carcinogenesis* 1997; 18: 1445–52.
63. Offner, S, et al. p53 gene mutations are not required for early dissemination of cancer cells. *Proc Natl Acad Sci* (USA) 1999; 96: 6942–46.
64. Tomlinson, I, et al. Selection, the mutation rate and cancer: ensuring that the tail does not wag the dog. *Nature Med* 1999; 5: 11–12.
65. Strauss, Bernard S. Silent and multiple mutation in p53 and the question of the hypermutability of tumors. *Carcinogenesis* 1997; 18(8): 1445–1452.
66. Tomlinson, Ian, et al. Selection, the mutation rate and cancer: ensuring that the tail does not wag the dog. *Nature Medicine* January 1999; 5 (1).
67. Luecke, RH, et al. Mathematical modeling of human embryonic and fetal growth rates. *Growth Dev Aging* 1999 Spring-Summer; 63 (1–2): 49–59.
68. Edwards, BK, et al. Annual report to the nation on the status of cancer, 1973–1999, featuring implications of age and aging on U.S. cancer burden. *Cancer* 2002 May 15; 94 (10): 2766–92.
69. Cicinelli, E, et al. Twice-weekly transdermal estradiol and vaginal progesterone as continous combined hormone replacement therapy in postmenopausal women: A 1-year prospective study. *Am J Obstet Gynecol* 2002; 187: 556–60.
70. Formby, B, Wiley, T. Progesterone inhibits growth and induces apoptosis in breast cancer cells. *Ann Clin Lab Sci* 1998; 28: 360–9.
71. Formby, B, Wiley, T. Bcl-2, survivin and variant CD44 v7-v10 are downregulated and p53 is upregulated in breast cancer cells by progesterone: inhibition of cell growth and induction of apoptosis. *Mol Cell Biochem* 1999; 202: 53–61.
72. Yu, S, Lee, M, Shin, S, et al. Apoptosis induced by progesterone in human ovarian cancer cell line SNU-840. *J Cell Biochem* 2001; 82: 445–51.
73. Pardee, AB. G1 events and regulation of cell proliferation. *Science* 1989 Nov 3; 246 (4930): 603–8. Review.
74. Hunter, T. Cooperation between oncogenes. *Cell* 1991 Jan 25; 64 (2): 249–70. Review.

75. Goustin, A, et al. Growth factors and cancer. *Cancer Res* 1986 Mar; 46(3): 1015–29. Review.
76. Huggins, C, et al. *Cancer Res* 1941; 1: 293.
77. Huggins, C. Endocrine-induced regression of cancers. Nobel Lecture, 1966 Dec. 13.
78. Huggins, C, et al. Extinction of experimental mammary cancer. I estradiol-17beta and progesterone. *Proc Natl Acad Sci* (USA) 1962; 48: 379–86.
79. Huggins, C, et al. Estradiol benzoate and progesterone in advanced human-breast cancer. *JAMA* 1962; 182: 136–40.
80. Huggins, C, et al. Studies on prostatic cancer: I. the effect of castration, of estrogen and of androgen injection on serum phosphatases in metastatic carcinoma of the prostate. 1941. *J Urol* 2002 Jul; 168 (1): 9–12.
81. Huggins, C, et al. *Cancer Res* 1941; 1: 293.
82. Partin, AW, et al. Prostate-specific antigen as a marker of disease activity in prostate cancer. *Oncology (Huntigt)* 2002 Sep; 16 (9): 1218–24; discussion 1224, 1227–8.
83. Cherry, C, et al. Ovarian cancer screening and prevention. *Semin Oncol Nurs* 2002 Aug; 18 (3): 167–73.
84. Moss, DW. Diagnostic aspects of alkaline phosphatase and its isoenzymes. *Clin Biochem* 1987 Aug; 20 (4): 225–30.
85. Fishman, WH. Alkaline phosphatase isozymes: recent progress. *Clin Biochem* 1990 Apr; 23 (2): 99–104.
86. Huggins, C, et al. Studies on prostatic cancer: I. the effect of castration, of estrogen and of androgen injection on serum phosphatases in metastatic carcinoma of the prostate. 1941. *J Urol* 2002 Jul; 168(1): 9–12.
87. Ibid.
88. Beatson, G. The treatment of cancer of the breast by oophorectomy and thyroid extract. *Br J Med* 1901 Oct. 19; 1145–48.
89. Ibid.
90. Huggins, C, et al. Inhibition of human mammary and prostatic cancers by adrenalectomy. *Cancer Research* 1952 Feb; 12: 134–141.
91. Huggins, C, et al. Studies on prostatic cancer: I. the effect of castration, of estrogen and of androgen injection on serum phosphatases in metastatic carcinoma of the prostate. 1941. *J Urol* 2002 Jul; 168 (1): 9–12.
92. Winkle, W. Estrogens and androgens in mammary cancer. *JAMA* 1949; 140: 1214–15.
93. Current status of hormone therapy of advanced mammary cancer. *JAMA* 1951; 146: 472–77.
94. Effects of intensive sex steroid hormone therapy in advanced breast cancer. *JAMA* 1953; 152: 1135–41.
95. Androgens and estrogens in the treatment of disseminated mammary carcinoma. *JAMA* 1960; 172: 135–47.
96. Winkle, W. Estrogens and androgens in mammary cancer. *JAMA* 1949; 140: 1214–15.
97. Huggins, C, et al. Inhibition of human mammary and prostatic cancers by adrenalectomy. *Cancer Research* 1952 Feb; 12: 134–141.
98. Lee, YH, et al. Aromatase inhibitors block natural sex change and induce male function in the protandrous black porgy. *Biol Reprod* 2002 Jun; 66 (6): 1749–54.

99. Gerardin, DC, et al. Reproductive changes in male rats treated perinatally with an aromatase inhibitor. *Pharmacol Biochem Behav* 2002 Jan–Feb; 71 (1–2): 301–5.
100. Wickman, S, et al. Inhibition of P450 aromatase enhances gonadotropin secretion in early and midpubertal boys: evidence for a pituitary site of action of endogenous E. *J Clin Endocrinol Metab* 2001 Oct; 86 (10): 4887–94.
101. Bouchardy, C, et al. Increased risk of malignant mullerian tumor of the uterus among women with breast cancer treated by tamoxifen. *J Clin Oncol* 2002 Nov 1; 20 (21): 4403.
102. Nolvadex: cancer warning added to tamoxifen label. *Nursing* 2002 Oct; 32 (10): 24.
103. Alwitry, A, et al. Tamoxifen maculopathy. *Arch Ophthalmol* 2002 Oct; 120 (10): 1402.
104. First results from the International Breast Cancer Intervention Study (IBIS-I): a randomised prevention trial. *Lancet* 2002 Sep 14; 360 (9336): 817–24.
105. McMillan, P, et al. Tamoxifen enhances choline acetyltransferase mRNA expression in rat basal forebrain cholinergic neurons. *Brain Res Mol Brain Res* 2002 Jun 30; 103 (1–2): 140–5.
106. Gao, X, et al. Tamoxifen abolishes estrogen's neuroprotective effect upon methamphetamine neurotoxicity of the nigrostriatal dopaminergic system. *Neuroscience* 2001; 103 (2): 385–94.
107. Huggins, C, et al. Extinction of experimental mammary cancer: 1. Estradiol-17b and progesterone. Proc. *Nat Acad Sci* 1962 March; 48: 379–386.
108. Ibid.
109. Ibid.
110. Gilman, A. The initial clinical trial of nitrogen mustard. *American Journal of Surgery* 1963; 105: 574–578.
111. Guyatt, G. Users' guide to the medical literature. *JAMA* 1993; 270: 2096–97.
112. *http://www.ncbi.nlm.nih.gov/entrez/query.fcgi.*
113. Lerner, Barron H. *The Breast Cancer Wars.* Oxford University Press, New York, NY, 2001. Page 176.
114. Ibid. Page 103.
115. Ibid. Page 72.
116. Ibid. Page 81.
117. Grant, R. Scientific Russian roulette. *CA* 1963; 1: 44–45.
118. Lerner, Barron H. *The Breast Cancer Wars.* Oxford University Press, New York, NY, 2001. Page 27.
119. Mertens, A, et al. Pulmonary complications in survivors of childhood and adolescent cancer. *Cancer* 2002; 95: 2431–2441.
120. Johnston, C. Radiation induced pulmonary fibrosis. *Radiation Research* 2002; 157: 256–265.
121. Lerner, Barron, H. *The Breast Cancer Wars.* Oxford University Press, New York, NY, 2001. Page 93.
122. Ibid. Page 94.
123. Daland, E. Untreated cases of breast cancer. *Surgery Gynecology Obstetrics* 1927; 44: 264–268.
124. Lewis, D, Rienhoff, W. A study of the results of operations for the cure of cancer of the

breast performed at Johns Hopkins Hospital from 1889–1931. *Annals of Surgery* 1932; 95: 336–400.

125. Lewis, Dean, and Reinhoff, William. A study of the results of operations for the cure of cancer of the breast performed at Johns Hopkins Hospital from 1889–1931. *Annals of Surgery* 1932; 95: 336–400.
126. Halsted, U. The results of operations for the cure of breast cancer performed at the John Hopkins Hospital from June 1889 to January 1894. *John Hopkins Hospital Reports* 1894–5; 4:1–60.
127. Lewis, D, et al. A study of the results of operations for the cure of cancer of the breast performed at the Johns Hopkins Hospital from 1889 to 1931. *Annals of Surgery* 1932; 95: 336–400.
128. Lerner, Barron, H. *The breast cancer wars.* Oxford University Press, New York, NY 2001. Pages 36–37.
129. Ibid. Pages 21–23.
130. Ibid. Pages 25–26.
131. Slaughter, F. *The new science of surgery.* J. Mesmer, New York, NY, 1946.
132. Kushner, R. *Breast cancer: a personal and investigative report.* Harcourt Brace Jovanovich, New York 1975. Page 27.
133. Warner, Nancy E. Lobular Carcinoma of the Breast. *Cancer* 1969; 23: 840–846.
134. Kushner, R. *Breast cancer: a personal and investigative report.* Harcourt Brace Jovanovich, New York, 1975. Page 27.
135. Lerner, Barron H. *The breast cancer wars.* Oxford University Press, New York, NY, 2001. Page 198.
136. Kushner, R. *Breast cancer: a personal and investigative report.* Harcourt Brace Jovanovich, New York, NY, 1975. Page 27.
137. Lerner, Barron H. *The breast cancer wars.* Oxford University Press, New York, NY, 2001. Page 243.
138. Moss, Ralph W. *Questioning chemotherapy.* Equinox Press, Brooklyn, NY, 1995. Page 59.
139. Braverman, A. Medical oncology in the 1990's. *Lancet* 1991; 337:901–902.
140. Braun, S, et al. Cytokeratin positive cells in the bone marrow and survival of patients w/ stage I, II, or III breast cancer. *N Engl J Med* 2000 Feb 24; 342(8): 525–33.
141. Baylor, John C. III. Mammography: a contrary view. *Annals of Internal Medicine* 1976; 84: 77–84.
142. Tomlinson, I, et al. The mutation rate and cancer. *Proc. Natl: Acad. Sci.* I, (USA) 1996 December; 93: 14800–14803.
143. Strauss, Bernard S. Hypermutability in carcinogenesis. *Genetics* 1998 April; 148: 1619–1626.
144. Simpson, A.J. The natural somatic mutation frequency and human carcinogenesis. *Adv Cancer Res* 1997; 71: 209–240.
145. Thornton, Hazel. Breast screening seems driven by belief rather than evidence. *British Journal of Medicine* 2002; 324: 677.
146. Rainey, PB. Evolutionary genetics: the economics of mutation. *Current Biology* 1999 May; 20 (10): R371–3.

147. Radiation-induced breast cancer. *Br Med J* 1977; 2: 191–92.
148. Frankenberger-Schwager, M, et al. Mutagenicity of low-filtered 30 kVp X-rays, mammography X-rays and conventional X-rays in cultured mammalian cells. *Int J Radiat Biol* 2002; 78: 781–9.
149. Kulldorff, M, et al. Breast cancer clusters in the northeast United States: a geographic analysis. *Am J Epidemiol* 1997 Jul 15; 146 (2): 161–70.
150. Timander, LM, et al. Breast cancer in West Islip, NY: a spatial clustering analysis with covariates. *Soc Sci Med* 1998 Jun; 46 (12): 1623–35.
151. Sharan, Shyam K, et al. Embryonic lethality and radiation hypersensitivity mediated by rad51 in mice lacking BRCA2. *Nature* 1997; April 24; 386.
152. Lerner, Barron H. *The Breast Cancer Wars.* Oxford University Press, New York, NY, 2001. Page 102.
153. Ibid. Page 107.
154. Ibid. Page 209.
155. Bailar, J. Mammography: a contrary view. *Ann Intern Med* 1976; 84: 77–84.
156. Radiation-induced breast cancer. *Br Med J* 1977; 2: 191–92.
157. Law, J. Variations in individual radiation dose in a breast screening programme and consequences for the balance between associated risk and benefit. *Br J Radiol* 1993; 66: 691–8.
158. Frankenberger-Schwager, M, et al. Mutagenicity of low-filtered 30 kVp X-rays, mammography X-rays and conventional X-rays in cultured mammalian cells. *Int J Radiat Biol* 2002; 78: 781–9.
159. Law, J, et al. Concerning the relationship between benefit and radiation risk, and cancer being detected and induced, in a breast cancer screening programme. *Br Journal of Radiology* 2002; 75: 678–684.
160. Frankenberg, D, et al. Enhanced neoplastic transformation by mammography x-rays. *Radiation Research* 2002; 157: 99–105.
161. Leon, A, et al. Study of radiation induced cancers in breast screening programme. *Radiat Prot Dosimetry* 2002; 93: 19–30.
162. Yaffe, M, et al. Breast cancer risk and measured mammographic density. *European Journal of Cancer Prevention* 1998; 7: 547–555.
163. Huang, J, et al. Risk of thyroid carcinoma in a female population after radiotheraphy for breast carcinoma. *Cancer* 2001; 92: 1411–1418.
164. Brody, J. Radiation benefits, risks in breast cancer debated. *New York Times* 1976 March 28.
165. Yalum, M.A. *A history of the breast.* Alfred A. Knopf, New York, NY, 1997. Pages 227–229.
166. Unnithan, J, et al. Contralateral breast cancer risk. *Radiotherm Oncol* 2001, Sept; 60 (3): 239–46.

CHAPTER SIX

1. Peto, J, et al. Prevalence of BRCA1 and BRCA2 gene mutations in patients with early-onset breast cancer. *J National Cancer Institute* 1999 June 2; 91 (11): 943–949.
2. Breast Cancer Linkage Consortium. Pathology of familial breast cancer: differences between breast cancers in carriers of BRCA1 or BRCA2 mutations and sporadic cases. *Lancet* 1997 May 24; 349: 1505–1510.

3. Mole, RH. Radiation-induced breast cancer. *Lancet* 1970 March 7; 332 (13): 524–525.
4. Tamplin, A, et al. Radiation-induced breast cancer. *Lancet* 1970 March 7; 332 (13): 297.
5. Gowen, L, et al. BRCA1 required for transcription-coupled repair of oxidative DNA damage *Science* 1998 August 14; 281: 1009–1012.
6. Blackwood, M, et al. BRCA1 and BRCA 2: from molecular genetics to clinical medicine. *J Clinical Oncology* 1998 May; 16 (5): 1969–1977.
7. Burke, W, et al. BRCA1 and BRCA2: a small part of the puzzle. *J National Cancer Institute* 1999 June 2; 91 (11): 904–905.
8. Nelson, L, et al. Prevalence of mutations in the BRCA1 gene among chinese patients with breast cancer. *J National Cancer Institute* 1999 May 19; 91 (10): 882–884.
9. Olsen, O, et al. Cochrane review on screening for breast cancer with mammography. *Lancet* 2001 October 20; 358: 1340–1342.
10. Sharan, S, et al. Embryonic lethality and radiation hypersensitivity mediated by Rad51 in mice lacking BRCA2. *Nature* 1997 April 24; 386: 804–809.
11. Radiation-induced breast cancer. *Br Med J* 1977 Jan 22; 1 (6055): 191–2.
12. Edwards, Rob. Mammogram "risk" for certain women. *New Scientist* 2002 Nov 9.
13. Olsen, Ole, et al. Cochrane review on screening for breast cancer with mammography. *Lancet* 2001; 358: 1340–42.
14. Jasen, P. Breast cancer and the language of risk 1750–1950. *Social History of Medicine* 2002; 15: 17–43.
15. Rigby, JE, et al. Can physical trauma cause breast cancer? *Eur J Cancer Prev* 2002 Jun; 11 (3): 307–11.
16. McElroy, JA, et al: Electric blanket or mattress cover use and breast cancer incidence in women 50-79 years of age. *Epidemiology* 2001, Nov; 12 (6): 613–7.
17. Unnithan, J, et al. Contralateral breast cancer risk. *Radiotherm Oncol* 2001, Sept; 60 (3): 239–46.
18. Poirier, L. The importance of screening for domestic violence in all women. *Nurse Pract* 1997 May; 22 (5): 105–8, 111–2, 115.
19. Threlfall, Anthony G, et al. Risk of breast cancer in women who attend the NHS breast screening programme: cohort study. *BMJ* 2001 Jul 21; 323 (7305): 140.
20. Ibid.
21. de Korvin, B, et al. Radiologic analysis of known-interval cancers after 2 years of organized screening for breast cancer in Ill-et-Vilaine. *J Radiol* 1998; 79: 379–86.
22. Radiation-induced breast cancer. *Br Med J* 1977 Jan 22; 1 (6055): 191–2.
23. Law, J. Variations in individual radiation dose in a breast cancer screening programme and consequence for the balance between associated risk and benefit. *Br J Radiol* 1993; 66: 591–8.
24. van der Houven van Oordt, CW, et al. The genetic background modifies the spontaneous and X-ray-induced tumor spectrum in the Apc1638N mouse model. *Genes Chromosomes and Cancer* 1999; 24: 191–8.
25. Miller, A, Howe, G, Sherman, G, et al. Mortality from breast cancer after irradiation during fluoroscopic examination in patients being treated for tuberculosis. *N Engl J Med* 1989; 321: 1285–9.

26. Ascroft, V. Adjuvant radiotherapy and risk of contralateral breast cancer. *J Natl Cancer Inst* 1992; 84: 1245–50.
27. Radiation-induced breast cancer. *Br Med J* 1977 Jan 22; 1 (6055): 91–2.
28. Hilreth, N, et al. The risk of breast cancer after irradiation of the thymus in infancy. *N Engl J Med* 1989; 321: 1281–4.
29. Familial breast cancer: collaborative reanalysis of individual data from 52 epidemiological studies including 58,209 women with breast cancer and 101, 986 women without the disease. *Lancet* 2001 Oct 27; 358 (9291): 1389–99.
30. Hemminki, K, et al. Attributable risks for familial breast cancer by proband status and morphology: a nationwide epidemiologic study from Sweden. *Int J Cancer* 2002 Jul 10; 100 (2): 214–9.
31. Radiation-induced breast cancer. *Br Med J* 1977 Jan 22; 1 (6055): 191–2.
32. Law, J. Variations in individual radiation dose in a breast cancer screening programme and consequence for the balance between associated risk and benefit. *Br J Radiol* 1993; 66: 691–8.
33. van der Houven van Oordt, CW, et al. The genetic background modifies the spontaneous and X-ray-induced tumor spectrum in the Apc 1638N mouse model. *Genes Chromosomes and Cancer* 1999; 24: 191–8.
34. Miller, A, Howe, G, Sherman, G, et al. Mortality from breast cancer after irradiation during fluoroscopic examination in patients being treated for tuberculosis. *N Engl J Med* 1989; 321: 1285–9.
35. Ascroft, V. Adjuvant radiotherapy and risk of contralateral breast cancer. *J Natl Cancer Inst* 1992; 84: 1245–50.
36. Radiation-induced breast cancer. *Br Med J* 1977 Jan 22; 1 (6055): 191–2.
37. Hilreth, N, et al. The risk of breast cancer after irradiation of the thymus in infancy. *N Engl J Med* 1989; 321: 1281–4.
38. Jasen, P. Breast cancer and the language of risk, 1750–1950. *Social History of Medicine* 2002; 15: 17–43.
39. Norford. *An Essay on the General Method of Treating Cancerous Tumors*. Pages 156–8.
40. Rigby, JE, et al. Can physical trauma cause breast cancer? *Eur J Cancer Prev* 2002 Jun; 11 (3): 307–11.
41. Van Netten, JP, et al. Physical trauma and breast cancer. *Lancet* 1994 Apr 16; 343 (8903): 978–9.
42. Kopans, DB. Physical trauma and breast cancer. *Lancet* 1994 May 28; 343 (8909): 1364–5.
43. Jasen, P. Breast cancer and the language of risk, 1750–1950. *Social History of Medicine* 2002; 15: 17–43.
44. Venkitaraman, A. Functions of BRCA1 and BRCA2 in the biological response to DNA damage. *J Cell Sci* 2001; 114: 3591–98.
45. Nieuwenhuis, B, et al. BRCA1 and BRCA2 heterozygosity and repair of X-ray induced DNA damage. *Int J Radiat Biol* 2002; 78: 285–95.
46. Bennett, L, et al. Mice heterozygous for a BRCA1 or BRCA2 mutation display distinct mammary gland and ovarian phenotype in response to diethylstibestrol. *Cancer Res* 2000; 60:3461–9.

47. Goelen, G, et al. High frequency of BRCA1/2 germline mutations in 42 Belgian families with a small number of symptomatic subjects. *J Med Genet* 1999; 36: 304–8.
48. Robson, M, et al. BRCA-associated breast cancer in young women. *J Clin Oncol* 1998; 16: 1642–9.
49. Venkitaraman, A. Functions of BRCA1 and BRCA2 in the biological response to DNA damage. *J Cell Sci* 2001; 114: 3591–98.
50. Nieuwenhuis, B, et al. BRCA1 and BRCA2 heterozygosity and repair of X-ray induced DNA damage. *Int J Radiat Biol* 2002; 78: 285–95.
51. Sharan, Shyam K, et al. Embryonic lethality and radiation hypersensitivity mediated by Rad51 in mice lacking BRCA2. *Nature* 1997 April 24; 386: 804–10.
52. Tang, NL, et al. Prevalence of mutations in the BRCA1 gene among chinese patients with breast cancer. *J Nat Cancer Inst* 1999 May 18; 91 (10): 882–56.
53. Burke, Wylie, et al. BRCA1 and BRCA2: a small part of the puzzle. *J Nat Cancer Inst* 1999 June 2; 91 (11): 904–5.
54. Blackwood, Anne M, et al. BRCA1 and BRCA2: from molecular genetics to clinical medicine. *J Clin Oncol* 1998 May; 16 (5): 1969–77.
55. Gowen, Lori C, et al. BRCA1 required for transcription-coupled repair of oxidative DNA damage. *Science* 1998 14 August; 281: 1009–12.
56. Breast Cancer Linkage Consortium. Pathology of familial breast cancer: differences between breast cancers in carriers of BRCA1 or BRCA2 mutations and sporadic cases. *Lancet*. 1997; 349: 1505–10.
57. Kulldorff, M, et al. Breast cancer clusters in the northeast United States: a geographic analysis. *Am J Epidemiol* 1997 Jul 15; 146 (2): 161–70.
58. Timander, LM, et al. Breast cancer in West Islip, NY: a spatial clustering analysis with covariates. *Soc Sci Med* 1998 Jun; 46 (12): 1623–35.
59. Lerner, Barron H. *The Breast Cancer Wars*. Oxford University Press, New York, NY, 2001. Pages 280–284.
60. Lynden, Patricia. Your breasts or your life? *American Health* 1997 June; 99: 29–31.
61. Kahn, Patricia. Coming to grips with genes and risk. *Science* 1996; 274: 496–498.
62. Parens, Erik. Glad and terrified: on the ethics of BRCA1 and BRCA2 testing. *Cancer Investigations* 1996; 14: 405–411.
63. Stolberg, Sheryl Gay. Concern among Jews is heightened as scientists deepen gene studies. *New York Times* 1998 April 22; A24.
64. Kolata, Gina. Bad genes: a cancer-causing mutation is found in European Jews. *New York Times* 1995 Oct 1; IV: 2.
65. Kessler, EJ. The secret shake-up in the shiduch. *Forward*, 1996 July 26; 11, 13.
66. Feychting, M, et al. Magnetic fields and breast cancer in Swedish adults residing near high-voltage power lines. *Epidemiology* 1998; 9: 392–7.
67. Forssen, U, et al. Occupational and residential magnetic field exposure and breast cancer in females. *Epidemiology* 2000; 11: 24–9.
68. Anisimov, V. The light-dark regimen and cancer development. *Neuroendocrinol Lett* 2002; 23 supp 112: 28–36.
69. Poole, G. The darkness at the end of the tunnel; summary and evaluation of an interna-

tional symposium on light, endocrine systems and cancer. *Neuroendocrinol Lett* 2002; 23 supp 12: 71–8.

70. Kushner, Harvey D. *Rose Kushner's If You've Thought About Breast Cancer.* Rose Kushner Breast Cancer Advisory Center, Kensington, Md., 2000.
71. Rose Kushner to Dr. Greenberg, November 8, 1975, Kushner Papers, box 6, correspondence folder, 1975.
72. Fisher, Bernard. Highlights of the NSABP Breast Cancer Prevention Trial. *Cancer Control* 1997; 4 (1): 78–86.
73. Lerner, Barron H. *The Breast Cancer Wars.* Oxford University Press, New York, NY, 2001. Page 263.
74. Ibid. Page 264.
75. Guerrieri-Gonzaga, A, et al. The Italian breast cancer prevention trial with tamoxifen; findings and new perspectives. *Ann N Y Acad Sci* 2001; 949: 113–22.
76. Veronesi, U, Maisonneuve, P, Costa, A, et al. Prevention of breast cancer with tamoxifen: preliminary findings from the Italian randomized trial among hysterectomised women. Italian Tamoxifen Prevention Study. *Lancet* 1998; 352: 93–7.
77. Powles, T. The Royal Marsden Hospital trial. Key points and remaining questions. *Ann N Y Acad Sci* 2001; 949: 109–12.
78. Nease, R, Ross, J. The decision to enter a randomized trial of tamoxifen for the prevention of breast cancer in healthy women: an analysis of the tradeoffs. *Am J Med* 1995; 99: 180–9.
79. Fisher, B. Endometrial cancer in tamoxifen-treated breast cancer patients: findings from the National Surgical Adjuvant Breast and Bowel (NSABP) B-14. *J Natl Cancer Inst* 1994; 86: 527–37.
80. Nephrew, K. Tamoxifen-induced proto-oncogene expression persists in uterine endometrial epithelium. *Endocrinol* 1996; 137: 219–24.
81. Horwitz, KB. Editorial: when tamoxifen turns bad. *Endocrinology* 1996; 136 (3): 821–3.
82. Anticancer drug under scrutiny as carcinogen. *Science* 1995; 270: 19.
83. Cover Story: Tamoxifen: Cancer causing drug approved for healthy women. *Life Extension* magazine. May 1999. *http://www.lef.org/magazine/mag99/may99-cover.html*
84. Ibid.
85. Fisher, B, et al. Tamoxifen for Prevention of Breast Cancer: Report of the National Surgical Adjuvant Breast and Bowel Project P-1 study. *Journal of the National Cancer Institute* 1998 Sept 16; 90 (18): 1371–88.
86. Ibid.
87. Holli, K, et al. Adjuvant trials of toremifene vs. tamoxifen: the European experience. *Oncology (Huntingt)* 1998 Mar; 12 (3 Suppl 5): 23–7. Review.
88. Powles, Trevor J. The Royal Marsden Hospital Trial: key points and remaining questions. *Annals New York Academy of Sciences* 2001; 949: 109–112.
89. Guerrieri-Gonzaga, Aliana, et al. The Italian Breast Cancer Prevention Trial with tamoxifen: findings and new prespectives. *Annals New York Academy of Sciences* 2001; 949: 113–122.

90. Fisher, BJ, et al. Long-term follow-up of axillary node-positive breast cancer patients receiving adjuvant tamoxifen alone: patterns of recurrence. *Int J Radiat Oncol Biol Phys* 1998 Aug 1; 42 (1): 117–23.
91. Berliere, M, Galant, C, Donnez, J. The potential oncogenic effect of tamoxifen on the endometrium. *Hum Reprod* 1999; 14: 1381–83.
92. Graham, DJ, et al. Thoughts on tamoxifen resistant breast cancer. Are coregulators the answer or just a red herring? *J Steroid Biochem Mol Biol* 2000 Nov 30; 74 (5): 255–9.
93. Curtis, RE, et al. Second cancers after adjuvant tamoxifen therapy for breast cancer. *J Natl Cancer Inst* 1996 Jun 19; 88 (12): 832–4.
94. Gottardis, M, Jordan, V. Development of tamoxifen stimulated growth of mcf-7 tumors in athymic mice after long-term antiestrogen administration. *Cancer Res* 1988; 48: 5183–87.
95. Freedman, G, Hanlon, A, Fowble, B, et al. Recursive partitioning identifies patients at high and low risk for ipsilateral tumor recurrence after breast-conserving surgery and radiation. *J Clin Oncol* 2002; 20: 4015–21.
96. Li, C, Malone, K, Weiss, N, et al. Tamoxifen therapy for primary breast cancer and risk of contralateral breast cancer. *J Natl Cancer Inst* 2001; 93: 1008–13.
97. IBIS investigators. First results from the international Breast Cancer Intervention Study (IBIS-I): a randomised prevention trial. *Lancet* 2002; 360: 317–24.
98. Engstrom, F, Levin, B, Moertel, C, et al. A phase II trial of tamoxifen in hepatocellular carcinoma. *Cancer* 1990; 65: 2641–3.
99. Dragan, Y, Fahey, S, Street, K, et al. Studies of tamoxifen as a promotor of hepatocarcinogenesis in female Fischer F344 rats. *Breast Cancer Res Treat* 1994; 31: 11–25.
100. Zhang, J, Jacob, T. Volume regulation in the bovine lens and cataract. *J Clin Invest* 1996; 97: 971–78.
101. Nilius, B, Prenen, J, Szucs, J, et al. Calcium-activated chloride channels in bovine pulmonary artery endothelial cells. *J Physiol (Lond)* 1997; 498: 381–96.
102. Zhang, J, Jacob, T, Valverde, M. Tamoxifen blocks chloride channels. A possible mechanism for cataract formation. *J Clin Invest* 1994; 94: 1690–7.
103. Mortimer, J, Boucher, L, Baty, J, et al. Effect of tamoxifen on sexual functioning in patients with breast cancer. *J Clin Oncol* 1999; 17: 1488–92.
104. Verrecchia, F, Herve, J. Reversible inhibition of gap junctional communication by tamoxifen in cultured cardiac myocytes. *Pflugers Arch* 1997; 434: 113–7.
105. Colls, BM, et al. Severe hypertriglyceridaemia and hypercholesterolaemia associated with tamoxifen use. *Clin Oncol (R Coll Radiol)* 1998; 10 (4): 270–1.
106. Loprinzi, C, Zahasky, K, Sloan, J. Tamoxifen-induced hot flashes. *Clin Breast Cancer* 2000; 1: 52–6.
107. Mourits, M, Bockermann, J, de Vries, E, et al. Tamoxifen effects on subjective and psychosexual wellbeing, in a randomised breast cancer study comparing high-dose and standard-dose chemotherapy. *Br J Cancer* 2002; 86: 1546–50.
108. Li, C, et al. Tamoxifen therapy for primary breast cancer and risk of ultralateral mast cancer. *Natl Cancer Inst* 2001; 93: 1008–13.

109. Freedman, G, Hanlon, A, Fowble, B, et al. Recursive partitioning identifies patients at high and low risk for ipsilateral tumor recurrence after breast-conserving surgery and radiation. *J Clin Oncol* 2002; 20: 4015–21.
110. Vogel, VG, et al. The study of tamoxifen and raloxifene: preliminary enrollment data from a randomized breast cancer risk reduction trial. *Clin Breast Cancer* 2002 Jun; 3 (2): 153–9.
111. *www.desaction.ie/.DES Action*, Ireland.
112. Goldstein, SR, et al. Adverse events that are associated with the selective estrogen receptor modulator levormeloxifene in an aborted phase III osteoporosis treatment study. *American J Obstet Gynecol* (Sept); 187 (3): 521–7.
113. Buzdar, A, et al. Tamoxifen and toremifene in breast cancer: comparison of safety and efficacy. *J Clin Oncol*, 1998 (Jan); 16 (1): 348–353.
114. Davies, AM, et al. Peroxidase activation of tamoxifen and toremifene resulting in DNA damage and covalently bound protein adducts. *Carcinogenesis* 1995; 16: 539–545.
115. Clarkson, TB. Raloxifene revisited. *Fert Steril* 2002 (Mar); 77 (3): 445–447.
116. Colls, BM, et al. Severe hypertriglyceridaemia and hypercholesterolaemia associated with tamoxifen use. *Clin Oncol (R Coll Radio)* 1998; 10 (4): 270–1.
117. Santen RJ, et al. Use of aromatase inhibitors in breast carcinoma. *Endocrine-Related Cancer* 1999; (6): 75–92.
118. Altan, Nihal, et al. Tamoxifen inhibits acidification in cells independent of the estrogen receptor. *Proc Natl Acad Sci* (USA) 1999 (Apr 13); 96 (8): 4432–7.
119. Pritchard, KI. Endocrine therapy for breast cancer. *Oncology* 2000 (Apr); 483–198.
120. Paige, LA, et al. Estrogen receptor (ER) modulators each induce distinct conformational changes in ER alpha and ER beta. *Proc Natl Acad Sci* (USA) 1999 Mar 30; 96 (7): 3999–4004.
121. Norris, JD, et al. Peptide antagonists of the human estrogen receptor. *Science* 1999 Jul 30; 285 (5428): 744–6.
122. Bates, NP, et al. An intron 1 enhancer element meditates oestrogen-induced suppression of ERBB2 expression. *Oncogene* 1997 Jul 24; 15 (4): 473–81.
123. Lerner, Barron H. *The breast cancer wars*. Oxford University Press, New York, NY, 2001. Page 104.
124. Ibid. Page 109.
125. DiLeo, A, et al. Predictive molecular markers in the adjuvant therapy of breast cancer: state of the art in the year 2002. *Int J Clin Oncol* 2002 Aug; 7 (4): 245–53. Review.
126. Medina-Franco, H, et al. Occult breast carcinoma presenting with axillary lymph node metastases. *Rev Invest Clin* 2002 May–Jun; 54 (3): 204–8.
127. American Cancer Society Statistics 2002.
128. Moss, Ralph W. *Questioning chemotherapy*. Equinox Press, Brooklyn, NY, 1995. Page 20.
129. Ibid. Page 27.
130. Cairns, J. The treatment of diseases and the war against cancer. *Sci AM* 1985; 253: 51–59.

131. Patterson, JT. *The dread disease.* Harvard University Press, Cambridge, MA, 1987.
132. DiLeo, A, et al. Predictive molecular markers in the adjuvant therapy of breast cancer: state of the art in the year 2002. *Int J Clin Oncol* 2002 Aug; 7 (4): 245–53. Review.
133. Medina-Franco, H, et al. Occult breast carcinoma presenting with axillary lymph node metastases. *Rev Invest Clin* 2002 May–Jun; 54 (3): 204–8.
134. American Cancer Society Statistics 2002.
135. Fossati, R, et al. Cytotoxic and hormonal treatment for metastatic breast cancer: a systematic review of published randomized trials involving 31,510 women. *J Clin Oncol* 1998 Oct; 16 (10): 3439–60. Review.
136. American Cancer Society statistics 2002.
137. Halsted, WS. The results of operations for the cure of cancer of the breast performed at the Johns Hopkins Hospital for June 1889 to January 1894. *Johns Hopkins Hospital Reports*; 4 (1894–1895): 1–60.
138. Moss, Ralph W. *Questioning chemotherapy.* Equinox Press, Brooklyn, NY, 1995. Page 44.
139. Ibid. Page 44.
140. Ibid. Page 84, 97.
141. Ibid. Page 60.
142. Miller, BA, et al. *SEER Cancer Statistics Review: 1973–1990* (NIH Pub No. 93-2789). NCI, Bethesda, MD, 1993.
143. Feinleib, M, et al. Some pitfalls in the evaluation of screening programs. *Arch Environ Health* 1969; 19: 412–415.
144. Hutchinson, GB, et al. Lead time gained by diagnostic screening for breast cancer. *JNCI* 1968; 41: 666–673.
145. The reporting of unsuccessful cases. *Boston Med Surg J* 1909; 263–264.
146. Feinstein, AR, et al. The Will Rogers phenomenon: stage migration and new diagnostic techniques as a source of misleading statistics for survival in cancer. *NEJM* 1985; 312: 1604–1608.
147. Moss, Ralph W. *Questioning chemotherapy:* Equinox Press, Brooklyn, NY, 1995. Pages 61–62.
148. Fossati, R, et al. Cytotoxic and hormonal treatment for metastatic breast cancer: a systematic review of published randomized trials involving 31,510 women. *J Clin Oncol* 1998 Oct; 16 (10): 3439–60. Review.
149. Moss, Ralph W. *Questioning chemotherapy.* Equinox Press, Brooklyn, NY, 1995. Pages 61–66.
150. Feinstein, AR, et al, The Will Rogers phenomenon: stage migration and new diagnostic techniques as a source of misleading statistics for survival in cancer. *NEJM* 1985; 312: 1604–1608.
151. Dickersin, K, et al. Publication bias and clinical trials. *Controlled Clin Trials* 1987; 8: 343–353.
152. Dickersin, K, et al. Publication bias: the problem that won't go away. In *Doing More Good than Harm: The Evaluation of Health Care Interventions. New York Annals of the NYAS* 1993: 135–148.

153. Moss, Ralph W. *Questioning chemotherapy.* Equinox Press, Brooklyn, NY, 1995. Pages 43–46.
154. Slevin, ML. et al. *Randomized trials in cancer.* Raven Press, Philadelphia, PA, 1986.
155. Gehan, EA, et al. *Statistics in Medical Research: Developments in Clinical Trials.* Plenum, New York, NY, 1994.
156. U.S. Congress, Office of Technology Assessment. *The Impact of Randomized Clinical Trials on Health Policy and Medical Practice.* Washington, DC, 1983.
157. Moss, Ralph W. *Questioning chemotherapy.* Equinox Press, Brooklyn, NY, 1995. Page 45.
158. Liel, Y. Preparation for radioactive iodine administration in differentiated thyroid cancer patients. *Clin Endocrinol (Oxf)* 2002 Oct; 57 (4): 523–7.
159. Advisory Committee on Human Radiation Experiments (ACHRE) Final Report. *http://tis.eh.doe.gov/ohre/roadmap/achre/intro=_1.html.*
160. Radioactivity History for Radioactive Century and 20 Years of LAPP. *http://wwwlapp.in2p3.fr/centenaire/rada.html.*
161. Advisory Committee on Human Radiation Experiments (ACHRE) Final Report. *http://tis.eh.doe.gov/ohre/roadmap/achre/intro=_1.html.*
162. Ibid.
163. Marie Curie Bio: A Nobel Prize Pioneer at the Pantheon. *www.france.diplomatie.fr/label=_france/english/sciences/curie/marie.html.*
164. Ibid.
165. Ibid.
166. Ibid.
167. Ibid.
168. Izzo, Louis M. History of Nuclear Medicine. *http://www.uvm.edu/;sllizzo/NMTS51/history.htm.*
169. Brenner, Daid J. Radiation biology in brachytherapy. *J Surgical Oncol* 1997; 65: 66–70.
170. Bell, AG. The uses of radium. *Am Med* 1903; 6: 261.
171. Gratzer, Walter. *A bedside nature, genius and eccentricity in science 1869–1953.* WH Freeman, New York, NY, 1998.
172. Oak Ridge Associated Universities' Health Physics Historical Instrumentation Museum. *http://www.orau.com/ptp/collection/shoefittingfluor/shoe.htm.*
173. Moss, Ralph W. *Questioning Chemotherapy.* Equinox Press, Brooklyn, NY, 1995. Pages 15–20.
174. Ibid. Page 16.
175. Ibid. Page 16.
176. Shimkin, MB. *Contrary to nature* (DHEW Publication No. NIH 79–720). National Cancer Institute Bethesda, MD, 1979.
177. Moss, Ralph W. *Questioning chemotherapy.* Equinox Press, Brooklyn, NY, 1995. Page 16.
178. Adair, FE, et al. Experimental and clinical studies on treatment of cancer by dichloroethylsulfide (mustard gas). *Ann Surg* 1931; 93: 190.
179. Chemical Heritage Foundation. Cancer Chemotherapy—A Timeline. *http://www.chemheritage.org/EducationalServices/pharm/chemo/readings/timeline.htm.*

180. Moss, Ralph W. *Questioning chemotherapy.* Equinox Press, Brooklyn, NY, 1995. Page 15.
181. Pack, GT, Livingston, EM. *Treatment of cancer and allied diseases, by 147 international authors.* Paul B. Hoeber, New York, NY, 1940.
182. Moss, Ralph W. *Questioning chemotherapy.* Equinox Press, Brooklyn, NY, 1995. Page 15.
183. Rinsky, RA, et al. Benzene and leukemia. *NEJM* 1987; 316: 1004.
184. Moss, Ralph W. *Questioning chemotherapy.* Equinox Press, Brooklyn, NY, 1995. Page 15.
185. Ibid.
186. Ehrlich, P. *The collected papers of Paul Ehrlich*. F. Himmelweit, ed. Pergamon, London, 1956.
187. Golomb, FM. Agents used in cancer chemotherapy. *Am J Surg* 1963; 105: 579–590.
188. Moss, Ralph W. *Questioning chemotherapy.* Equinox Press, Brooklyn, NY, 1995. Page 16.
189. Ibid. Page 17.
190. Ibid.
191. Ibid.
192. Gilman, A. The initial clinical trial of nitrogen mustard. *Am J Surg* 1963; 105: 574–578.
193. Moss, Ralph W. *Questioning chemotherapy.* Equinox Press, Brooklyn, NY, 1995. Page 17.
194. Ibid.
195. Gilman, A. The initial clinical trial of nitrogen mustard. *Am J Surg* 1963; 105: 574–578.
196. Moss, Ralph W. *Questioning chemotherapy.* Equinox Press, Brooklyn, NY, 1995. Pages 17–18.
197. Patterson, JT. *The dread disease*. Harvard University Press, Cambridge, MA, 1987.
198. Ibid.
199. Moss, Ralph W. *Questioning chemotherapy.* Equinox Press, Brooklyn, NY, 1995. Page 16.
200. Gilman, A. The initial clinical trial of nitrogen mustard. *Am J Surg* 1963; 105: 574–578.
201. Fossati, R, et al. Cytotoxic and hormonal treatment for metastatic breast cancer: a systemic review of published randomized trials involving 31,510 women. *J Clin Oncol* 1998; 16: 3439–60.
202. Moss, Ralph W. *Questioning chemotherapy.* Equinox Press, Brooklyn, NY, 1995. Page 172.
203. Ibid. Page 22.
204. Ibid. Page 23.
205. Ibid. Page 19.
206. Hill, DL. *A review of cyclophosphamide.* Thomas, Springfield, IL, 1975.
207. Moss, Ralph W. *Questioning chemotherapy.* Equinox Press, Brooklyn, NY, 1995. Page 20.
208. Patterson, JT. *The dread disease*. Harvard University Press, Cambridge, MA, 1987.
209. Moss, Ralph W. *Questioning chemotherapy.* Equinox Press, Brooklyn, NY, 1995. Page 20.
210. Hill, DL. *A review of cyclophosphamide.* Thomas, Springfield, IL, 1975.
211. Moss, Ralph W. *Questioning chemotherapy.* Equinox Press, Brooklyn, NY, 1995. Page 20.
212. Greenberg, DS. Medicine and public affairs. "Progress" in cancer research—don't say it isn't so. *N Engl J Med* 1975 Mar 27; 292 (13): 707–8.
213. Sherman, AI. Progesterone caproate in the treatment of endometrial cancer. *Obstet Gynecol* 1966 Sept; 28 (3): 309–14.
214. DeVivo, I, et al. A functional polymorphism in the promoter of the progesterone receptor

gene associated with endometrial cancer risk. *Proc Natl Acad Sci* (USA) 2002 Sep 17; 99 (19): 12263–8.

215. Dai, D, et al. Progesterone inhibits human endometrial cancer cell growth and invasiveness: down-regulation of cellular adhesion molecules through progesterone B receptors. *Cancer Res* 2002 Feb 1; 62 (3): 381–6.
216. DeVivo, I, et al. A functional polymorphism in the promoter of the progesterone receptor gene associated with endometrial cancer risk. *Proc Natl Acad Sci* (USA) 2002 Sep 17; 99 (19): 12263–8.
217. Fujimoto, J, et al. Progestins suppress estrogen-induced expression of vascular endothelial growth factor (VEGF) subtypes in uterine endometrial cancer cells. *Cancer Lett* 1999 Jul 1; 141 (1–2): 63–71.
218. Hiemke, C, et al. Antioestrogen inhibition of oestradiol-induced alterations in hypothalamic noradrenaline turnover. *J Endocrinol* 1985 Jul; 106 (1): 37–42.
219. Ishiwata, I, et al. Effects of progesterone on human endometrial carcinoma cells in vivo and in vitro. *J Natl Cancer Inst* 1978 May; 60 (5): 947–54.
220. Saegusa, M, et al. Down-regulation of bcl-2 expression is closely related to squamous differentiation and progesterone therapy in endometrial carcinomas. *J Pathol* 1997 Aug; 182 (4): 429–36.
221. Boman, K, et al. The influence of progesterone and androgens on the growth of endometrial carcinoma. *Cancer* 1993 Jun 1; 71 (11).
222. Saegusa, M, et al. Progesterone therapy for endometrial carcinoma reduces cell proliferation but does not alter apoptosis. *Cancer* 1998 July 1; 83 (1).
223. Sherman, AI. Progesterone caproate in the treatment of endometrial cancer. *Obstet Gynecol* 1966 Sep; 28 (3): 309–14.
224. Jasen, P. Breast cancer and the language of risk, 1750–1950. *Social History of Medicine* 2002; 15: 17–43.
225. Ibid.
226. Ibid.
227. Yalom, Marilyn. *A history of the breast*. Alfred A. Knopf, New York, NY, 1997. Page 217.
228. Ibid.
229. Lerner, Barron H. *The breast cancer wars*. Oxford University Press, New York, NY, 2001. Page 163.
230. Jasen, P. Breast cancer and the language of risk, 1750–1950. *Social History of Medicine* 2002; 15: 17–43.
231. Rodman. *A practical explanation of cancer*. Pages 6, 19, 9–10, 56–9, 66–70.
232. Jasen, P. Breast cancer and the language of risk, 1750–1950. *Social History of Medicine* 2002; 15: 17–43.
233. Walshe. *The Nature and Treatment of Cancer*. Page 154.
234. Wiley, TS, et al. *Lights out: sleep, sugar, and survival.* Pocket Books, New York, NY, 2000.
235. Yalom, Marilyn. *A history of the breast*. Alfred A. Knopf, New York, NY, 1997. Page 141.
236. Baumslag, Naomi, et al. *Milk, money and madness: The culture and politics of breastfeeding*. Bergin and Garvey, Westport, CT, 1995.

237. Palmer, Gabrielle. *The politics of breast-feeding*. Pandora, London, 1988.
238. Baby Milk Action. Briefing Paper. History of the Campaign. *www.babymilkaction.org*.
239. Fomon, S. Infant feeding in the 20th century: formula and beikost. *J Nutr* 2001 Feb; 131 (2): 409S–20S.
240. Jasen, P. Breast cancer and the language of risk, 1750–1950. *Social History of Medicine* 2002; 15: 27.
241. Ibid. pages 17–43.
242. Norford, W. *An essay on the general method of treating cancerous tumors*. London, 1753. Page 30.
243. Jasen, P. Breast cancer and the language of risk, 1750–1950. *Social History of Medicine* 2002; 15: 17–43.
244. Ibid.
245. Ibid.
246. Ibid.
247. Ibid.
248. Singer, Sydney Ross. *Dressed to kill: The link between breast cancer and bras*. ISCD Press, New York, NY, 2002.
249. Jasen, P. Breast cancer and the language of risk, 1750–1950. *Social History of Medicine* 2002; 15: 17–43.
250. Ibid.
251. Jasen, P. Breast cancer and the language of risk, 1750–1950. *Social History of Medicine* 2002; 15: 34.
252. Jasen, P. Breast cancer and the language of risk, 1750–1950. *Social History of Medicine* 2002; 15: 17–43.
253. Yalom, M. *A history of the breast*. Alfred A. Knopf, New York, NY, 1997.
254. Stuber, Irene. Women of Achievement and Herstory. May 6, 2000. *http://www.undelete.org/woa/woa05-06.html*.
255. Lerner, Barron H. *The breast cancer wars*. Oxford University Press, New York, NY, 2001. Page 177.
256. Kushner, Rose. *Breast Cancer: A personal and an investigative report*. Harcourt Brace Jovanovich, New York, NY, 1975. Page 27.
257. De Moulin, D. *A short history of breast cancer*. The Hague, 1983. Page 33.
258. Jasen, P. Breast cancer and the language of risk, 1750–1950. *Social History of Medicine* 2002; 15: 22.
259. Moss, Ralph W. *Questioning chemotherapy*. Equinox Press, Brooklyn, NY, 1995. Page 71.
260. Perry, M, ed. *The chemotherapy source book*. Williams & Wilkins, Baltimore, MD, 1997. Pages 506–507, 1137.
261. Conversations with Julie Taguchi, M.D.
262. Harris, J, et al. *Diseases of the breast*. Lippincott-Raven, New York, NY, 1996.
263. Horwitz, KB. Editorial: when tamoxifen turns bad. *Endocrinology* 1995; 136 (3): 821–3.
264. Conversations with Julie Taguchi, M.D.
265. Takimoto, GS, et al. Tamoxifen resistant breast cancer: coregulators determine the direc-

tion of transcription by antagonist-occupied steroid receptors. *J Steroid Biochem Mol Biol* 1999 Apr–Jun; 69 (1–6): 45–50.

266. Graham, DJ, et al. Thoughts on tamoxifen resistant breast cancer. Are coregulators the answer or just a red herring? *J Steroid Biochem Mol Biol* 2000, 30 Nov; 74 (5).
267. Curtis, RE, et al. Second cancers after adjuvant tamoxifen therapy for breast cancer. *J Natl Cancer Inst* 1996 Jun 19; 88 (12): 832–4.
268. Tamoxifen Statistics. Table 1. J Natl Cancer Inst, Volume 88, Number 12, June 19, 1996.
269. Microsoft word, 1998. Thesaurus.
270. *http:dictionary.cambridge.org/define.asp? key=palliative&1+0.* Cambridge International Dictionary.

CHAPTER SEVEN

1. National vital statistics report 2002; 50: 13–26.
2. American Heart Association; 2002; Women, Heart disease and stroke statistics.
3. American Heart Association 2002; Baby boomers and cardiovascular diseases.
4. Grady, D, et al. Cardiovascular disease outcomes during 6.8 years of hormone therapy (HERS II), *JAMA* 2002; 288: 49–57.
5. American Heart Association. Facts about women and cardiovascular diseases 2002; 1–2.
6. Brochier, M, Arwidson, P. Coronary heart disease risk factors in women. *Eur Heart J* 1998; 19 (A): 45–52.
7. Carlsson, C, Stein, J. Cardiovascular disease and the aging women: overcoming barriers to lifestyle changes. *Curr Womens Health rep* 2002; 266–72.
8. Schenck-Gustafsson, K. Risk factors for cardiovascular disease in women. *Eur Heart J* 1996; 17: 2–8.
9. Jousilahti, P, Vartianinen, E, Tuomelilehto J, et al. Sex, age, cardiovascular risk factors, and coronary heart disease. *Circulation* 1999; 99: 1165–72.
10. National vital statistics report 2002; 50: 13–26.
11. Vakili, B, Kaplan, R, Brown, D. Sex-based differences in earely mortality of patients undergoing primary angioplasty for first acute myocardial infarction. *Circulation* 2001; 104: 3034–8.
12. Grady, D, Herrington, D, Bittnere, V, et al. cardiovascular disease outcomes during 6.8 years of hormone therapy: Heart and Estrogen/progestin replacement study follow-up (HERS II). *JAMA* 2002; 288: 49–57.
13. McDonough, P. The randomized world is not without imperfection: reflections on the women's health initiative study. *Fertil Steril* 2002; 78: 951–6.
14. Derry, P. Time trends in the HERS secondary prevention trial: much ado about nothing. *A Am Med Womens Assoc* 2002; 57: 215–6.
15. Kawano, H, Motoyama, T, Hirai, N, et al. Estradiol supplementation suppresses hyperventilation-induced attacks in postmenopausal women with variant angina. *J Am Coll Cardiol* 2001; 37: 735–40.
16. Hayward, C, Webb, C, Collins, P. Effect of sex hormones on cardiac mass. *Lancet* 2001; 357: 1354–6.

17. Miettinen, Tatu A, et al. Cholesterol-lowering therapy in women and elderly patients with myocardial infarction or angina pectoris. *Circulation*. 1997; 96: 4211–4218.
18. Pinney, S, Rabbani, L. Myocardial infarction in patients with normal coronary arteries: proposed pathogenesis and predisposing risk factors. *J Thromb Thrombolysis* 2001; 11: 11–7.
19. Menstrual cyclic variation of myocardial ischemia in premenopausal women with variant angina. *Ann Intern Med* 2001; 135: 977–81.
20. Jeppesen, J, Schaaf, P, Jones, C, et al. Effects of low-fat, high-carbohydrate diets on risk factors for ischemic heart disease in postmenopausal women. *Am J Clin Nutr* 1997; 65: 1027–33.
21. Sesso, H, Paffenbarger, R, Ha, T, et al. Physical activity and cardiovascular disease risk in middle-aged and older women. *Am J Epidemiol* 1999; 150: 408–16.
22. Schwartz, D, Penckofer, S. Sex differences and the effects of sex hormones on homeostasis and vascular reactivity. *Heart Lung* 2001; 30: 401–26.
23. National vital statistics report 2002; 50: 13–26.
24. Ibid.
25. American Heart Association; 2002; Women, heart disease and stroke statistics.
26. Fletcher, S, Colditz, G. Failure of estrogen plus progestin therapy for prevention. *JAMA* 2002; 288: 1–17.
27. *http://216.110.171.197/02/09/womenshealth902.html.*
28. *http://www.hhponline.com/Stevens/HHPPub.nsf/frame?open&redirect=http://www.hhponline.com/stevens/hhppub.nsf/PubNews/6272BD5A5CDDFEF286256C9C0055DAB8?Opendocument.*
29. Fletcher, S, Colditz, G. Failure of Estrogen plus progestin therapy for prevention. *JAMA* 2002; 288: 1–17.
30. Skegg, CG. Hormone therapy and heart disease after the menopause. *Lancet* 2001; 358: 1196–7.
31. Kolata, Gina, et al. Menopause without pills: rethinking hot flashes. *New York Times* 2002 November 10; Section 1, Page 1.
32. Effects of estrogen or estrogen/progestin regimens on heart disease risk factors in postmenopausal women. The postmenopausal estrogen/progestin interventions (PEPI) trial. The writing group for the PEPI trial. *JAMA* 1995; 273: 199–208.
33. Ibid.
34. Ibid.
35. Ibid.
36. Grady, D, Rubin, S, Petitti, et al. Hormone therapy to prevent disease and prolong life in postmenopausal women. *Ann Intern Med* 1992; 117: 1016–37.
37. Chlebowski, R. Reducing the risk of breast cancer. *N Engl J Med* 2000; 343: 191–8.
38. Stampfer, M, Colditz, G, Willett, W, et al. Postmenopausal estrogen therapy and cardiovascular disease. Ten-year follow-up from the nurses health study. *N Engl J Med* 1991; 325: 756–62.
39. Sherman, AI. Progesterone Caproate in the Treatment of Endometrial Cancer. *Obstet Gynecol*. 1996 Sep; 28 (3): 309–14.

40. Fujimoto, J, Sakaguchi, H, Hirose, R, et al. Progestins suppress estrogen-induced expression of vascular endothelial growth factor (VEGF) subtypes in uterine endometrial cancer cells. *Cancer lett* 1999; 141: 63–71.
41. Poulter, N, Chang, C, Farley, TM et al. Risk of cardiovascular diseases associated with oral progestagen preparations with therapeutic indications. *Lancet* 1999; 354: 1610–11.
42. World health organization collaborative study of cardiovascular disease and steroid hormone contraception (WHOCS). A multinational study of cardiovascular disease and steroid hormone contraceptives. *J Clin Epidemiol* 1995; 48: 1513–47.
43. WHOCS. Cardiovascular disease and use of oral progestogen. *Contraception* 1998; 57: 315–24.
44. WHOCS. Venous thromboembolic disease and prostagen. *Lancet* 1995; 346: 1575–82.
45. WHOCS. Ischaemic stroke and stroke risk by prostagens. Results of an international multicentre, case-control study. *Lancet* 1996; 348: 498–510.
46. Hulley, S, Grady, D, Bush, T, et al. Randomized trial of estrogen plus progestin for secondary prevention of coronary heart disease in postmenopausal women, Heart and estrogen/progestin replacement study (HERS) research group. *JAMA* 1998; 280: 605–13.
47. Poulter, N, Chang, C, Farley, TM et al. Risk of cardiovascular diseases associated with oral progestagen preparations with therapeutic indications. *Lancet* 1999; 354: 1610–11.
48. World health organization collaborative study of cardiovascular disease and steroid hormone contraception (WHOCS). A multinational study of cardiovascular disease and steroid hormone contraceptives. *J Clin Epidemiol* 1995; 48: 1513–47.
49. WHOCS. Cardiovascular disease and use of oral progestogen. *Contraception* 1998; 57: 315–24.
50. WHOCS. Venous thromboembolic disease and prostagen. *Lancet* 1995; 346: 1575–82.
51. WHOCS. Ischaemic stroke and stroke risk by prostagens. Results of an international multicentre, case-control study. *Lancet* 1996; 348: 498–510.
52. WHOCS. Acute myocardial infarction and prostagens. *Lancet* 1997; 349: 1202–9.
53. Skegg, CG. Hormone therapy and heart disease after the menopause. *Lancet* 2001, 358: 1196–7.
54. Heald, A, Selby, P, White, A, et al. Progestins abrogate estrogen-induced changes in the insulin-like growth factor axis. *Am J Obstet Gynecol* 2000; 183: 593–600.
55. Christ, M, et al. Attenuation of heart-rate variability in postmenopausal women on progestin-containing hormone replacement therapy. *Lancet* 1999 Jun 5; 353 (9168): 1939–40.
56. Farley, T, Meirik, O, Chang, C, et al. Effect of different progestagens in low estrogen oral contraceptives on venous thromboembolic disease. *Lancet* 1995; 346: 1582–8.
57. Kawano, H, Motoyama, T, Hirai, N, et al. Effect of medroxyprogesterone acetate plus estradiol on endothelium-dependent vasodilation in postmenopausal women. *Am J Cardiol* 2001; 87: 238–49.
58. van Baal, W, Emeis, J, Mooren, M, et al. Impaired procoagulant-anticoagulant balance during hormone replacement therapy? A randomised, placebo-controlled 12-week study. *Thromb Haemost* 2000; 83: 29–34.
59. Shilipak, M, Simon, J, Vittinghoff, E, et al. Estrogen and progestin, lipoprotein and the risk of recurrent coronary heart disease events after menopause. *JAMA* 2000; 283: 1845–52.

60. Miyagawa, K, Rosch, J, Stanczyk, E, et al. Medroxyprogesterone interferes with ovarian steroid protection against coronary vasospasm. *Nat Med* 1997; 3: 324–7.
61. Rosano, G, Fini, M. Comparative cardiovascular effects of different progestins in menopause. *Int J Fertil Womens Med* 2001; 46: 248–56.
62. Fujimoto, J, Sakaguchi, H, Hirose, R, et al. Progestins suppress estrogen-induced expression of vascular endothelial growth factor (VEGF) subtypes in uterine endometrial cancer cells. *Cancer lett* 1999; 141: 63–71.
63. Resano, G, et al. Prospective physiology of natural progesterone. *J Am Coll Cardiol* 2000; 36: 154–9.
64. Writing group for the women's health initiative investigators. Risks and benefits of estrogen plus progestins in healthy postmenopausal women: principal results from the women's health initiative randomized controlled trial. *JAMA* 2002; 288: 321–33.
65. Webb, C, Ghatei, M, McNeill, J, et al. 17beta-estradiol decreases endothelin-1 levels in the coronary circulation of postmenopausal women with coronary artery disease. *Circulation* 2000; 102: 1617–22.
66. Alpastan, M, et al. Short-term estrogen effects on heart rhythm. *J Am Coll Cardiol* 1997; 30: 1466–71.
67. Williams, J, Adams, M. Short-term administration of estrogen and vascular responses to atheresclerotic coronary arteries. *J Am Coll Cardiol* 1992; 20: 452–57.
68. Reis, SE, et al. Ethinyl estradiol acetylcholine in postmenopausal women. *Circulation* 1994 Jan; 89 (1): 52–60.
69. Gilligan, D, Quyyumib, A, Cannon, R, et al. Effects of physiological levels of estrogen on coronary function in postmenopausal women. *Circulation* 1994; 89: 2445–51.
70. Collins, R, Rosano, G, Sarrel, P, et al. Estradiol 17beta attenuates acetylcholine-induced coronary arterial constriction in women but not men with coronary heart disease. *Circulation* 1995; 92: 24–30.
71. Hishikawa, K, Nakaki, T, Masruno, T, et al. Up-regulation of nitric oxide synthase by estradiol in human aortic endothelial cells. *FEBS lett* 1995; 360: 291–93.
72. Webb, C, Rosano, G, Collins, P. Oestrogen improves exercise-induced myocardial ischaemia in women. *Lancet* 1998; 351: 1556–57.
73. Sullivan, J, Vander, Z, Lemp, G, et al. Postmenopausal estrogen use and coronary artherosclerosis. *Ann Intern Med* 1988; 108: 358–63.
74. Xiao, C, Goff, A. Hormonal regulation of oestrogen and progesterone receptors in cultured bovine endometrial cells. *J Reprod Fertil* 1999; 115: 101–9.
75. Malet, C, Spritzer, P, Guillaumin, D, et al. Progesterone effect on cell growth, ultrastructurel aspect and estradiol receptors of normal human breast epithelial cells in culture. *J Steroid Biochem Mol Biol* 2000; 73: 171–81.
76. Stubbs, PJ, Laycock, J, Zadeh, J, et al. Circulating stress hormone and insulin concentrations in acute coronary syndromes: identification of insulin resistance on admission. *Clin Sci (Lond)* 1999; 96: 589–95.
77. Keltikangas, L, Ravaja, N, Raikkonen, K, et al. Relationships between the pituitary-adrenal hormones, insulin, and glucose in middle-aged men: moderating influence of psychological stress. *Metabolism* 1998; 47: 1440–9.

78. Altun, A, Yaprak, M, Aktoz, M, et al. Impaired nocturnal synthesis of melatonin in patients with cardiac syndrome X. *Neurosci Lett* 2002; 327: 143–5.
79. Sewerynek, E. Melatonin and the cardiovascular system. *Neuroendocrinol Lett* 2002; 1: 79–83.
80. Buck, M, Squire, T, Andrews, M. Coordinate expression of the PDK4 gene: a means of regulating fuel selection in hibernating mammal. *Physiol Genomics* 2002; 8: 5–13.
81. Andrews, M, Squire, T, Bowen, S, et al. Low-temperature carbon utilization is regulated by novel gene activity in the heart of a hibernating mammal. *Proc Natl Acad Sci* (USA) 1998; 95: 8392–7.
82. Bradbury, J. How hibornators might one day solve medical problems. *Lancet* 2001; 358: 1164.
83. Ahlersova, A, Ahlers, I, Garlatiova, E, et al. Influence of the seasons on the circadian rhythm of blood glocose and tissue glycogen in male Wistar rats. *Physiol Bohemoslov* 1982; 31: 45–55.
84. Belke, D, Wang, L, Lopaschuk, G. Acetyl-CoA carboxylase control of fatty acid oxidation in hearts from hibernating Richardson's ground squirrels. *Biochim Biophys Acta* 1998; 1391: 25036.
85. Bauer, V, Squire, T, Lowe, M, et al. Expression of a chimeric retroviral-lipase mRNA confers enhanced lipolysis in a hibernating mammal. *Am J Physiol Regul Integr Comp Physiol* 2001; 281: R1186–92.
86. Holness, M, Smith, N, Bulmer, K, et al. Evaluation of the role of peroxisome-proliferator-activated receptor alpha in the regulation of cardiac pyruvate dehydrogenase kinase 4 protein expression in response to starvation, high-fat feeding and hyperthyrodism. *Biochem J* 2002; 364: 687–94.
87. Wiley, TS. *Lights Out: Sleep, sugar, and survival.* Pocket, 2000.
88. Wynn, A, et al. The effects of food shortage on human reproduction. *Nutr Health* 1993; 9: 43–52.
89. de Simone, G, et al. Influence of obesity on left ventricular midwall mechanics in arterial hypertension. *Hypertension* 1996; 28: 276–83.
90. Hermsmeyer, K, Miyagawa, K, Kelley, S, et al. Reactivity-based coronary vasospasm independent of atherosclerosis in rhesus monkeys. *J Am Coll Cardiol* 1997; 29: 671–80.
91. Minshall, R, Miyagawa, K, Chadwick, C, et al. In vitro modulation of primary coronary vascular muscle cell reactivity by ovarian steroid hormones. *FASEB J* 1998; 121: 1419–29.
92. Kaski, JC, et al. Spontaneous coronary artery spasm in variant angina is caused by a local hyperreactivity to a generalized constrictor stimulus. *J Am Coll Cardiol* 1989 Nov 15; 14 (6): 1456–63.
93. Maseri, A. Coronary artery spasm and vasoconstriction. *Circulation* 1990; 81: 1983–90.
94. Hermsmeyer, K, Minshall, R. Estrogen and progesterone protective actions on coronary arteries. *Nat Med* 1997; 3: 324–27.
95. Orino, A. Vascular smooth cells and vasospasm. *Biochem Biophys Res Commun* 1993; 195: 730–36.
96. Kloner, R, et al. Consequence of brief ischemia: stunning, preconditioning, and their clinical implications: part 2. *Circulation* 2001; 104: 3158–67.

97. Hearse, D. Oxygen deprivation and early myocardial contractile failure: a reassessment of the possible role of adenosine triphosphate. *Am J Cardiol* 1979;44: 1115–21.
98. Rysommuti, S, et al. Excess dietary glucose alters renal function before increasing arterial pressure and inducing insulin resistance. *Am J Hypertens* 2002; 15: 773–9.
99. Burg, M. Molecular basis of osmotic regulation. *Am J Physiol* 1995; 268 (6Pt2): F983–96.
100. Brands, M, et al. Chronic intravenous glucose infusion causes moderate hypertension in rats. *Am J Hypertens* 2000; 13: 99–102.
101. Andrews, M, et al. Low-temperature carbon utilization is regulated by novel gene activity in the heart of a hibernating mammal. *Proc Natl Acad Sci* (USA) 1998; 95: 8392–97.
102. Dargie, H, Byrne, J. Pathophysiological aspects of the renin-angiotensin-aldosterone system in acute myocardial infraction. *J Cardiovasc Risk* 1995; 2: 389–95.
103. Launay, J, Herve, P, Poec, K, et al. Function of the serotonin 5-hydroxytryptamine 2B receptor in pulmonary hypertension. *Nat Med* 2002; 8: 1129–35.
104. Blaufarb, I, Sonnenblick, E. The renin-angiotensin system in the left ventricular remodeling. *Am J Cardiol* 1996; 77: 8C–16C.
105. Voors, A, Kingma, J, Glist, W. Drug differences between ACE inhibitors in experimental settings and clinical practice. *J Cardiovasc Risk* 1995; 2: 413–22.
106. Tin, L. Hypertension, left ventricular hypertrophy, and sudden death. *Curr Cardiol Rep* 2002; 4: 449–57.
107. Slama, M, Sisic, D. Diastolic dysfunction in hypertension. *Curr Opin Cardiol* 2002; 17: 368–73.
108. Williams, D. Pharmacokinetic-pharmacodynamic drug interactions with HMG-CoA reductase inhibitors. *Clin Pharmacokinet* 2002; 41: 343–70.
109. Husten, L. Receptor offer clues to how "Good" cholesterol works. *Science* 1997; 278: 1228.
110. Nebert, D, Russell, D. Clinical importance of the cytochromes P450. *Lancet* 2002; 360: 1155–62.
111. Robert, L. Aging of the vascular-wall and atherosclerosis. *Exp Gerontol* 1999; 34: 491–501.
112. Corti, M, Barbato, G, Baggio, G. Lipoprotein alternations and atherosclerosis in the elderly. *Curr Opin Lipidol* 1997; 4: 236–41.
113. Lewis, S. Cholesterol and coronary heart disease in women. *Cardiol Clin* 1998; 16: 9–15.
114. Lange, Y, Chin, J. The fate of cholesterol exiting lysosomes. *J Biol Chem* 1997; 272: 17018–17022.
115. Butler, J, Mackie, J, Goldin, E, et al. Progesterone blocks cholesterol translocation from lysosomes. *J Biol Chem* 1992; 267: 23797–805.
116. Mazzone, T, Krishna, M, Lange, Y. Progesterone blocks intracellular translocation of free cholesterol derived cholesteryl ester in macrophages. *J Lipid Res* 1995; 36: 544–51.
117. Freedman, D. The importance of body fat distribution in early life. *Am J Med Sci* 1995; 310: 72–6.
118. Vega, G, Grundy, S. Effects of statins on metabolism of apo-containing lipoproteins in hypertriglyceridemic patients. *Am J Cardiol* 1998; 81: 36–42.
119. McCormick, S, Frye, S, Eskin, S, et al. Microarray analysis of shear stressed endothelial cells. *Biorheology* 2003; 40: 5–11.

120. Ingber, D. Mechanical signaling and the cellular response to extracellular matrix in angiogenesis and cardiovascular physiology. *Circ Res* 2002; 91: 877–87.
121. Ferrero, E, et al. Regulation of endothelial cell shape and barrier function by chromogranin A. *Ann N Y Acad Sci* 2002; 971: 355–8.
122. Haas, T. Molecular control of capillary growth in skeletal muscle. *Can J Appl Physiol* 2002; 27: 491–515.
123. Chavakis, E, et al. Regulation of endothelial cell survival and apoptosis during angiogenesis. *Artherioscler Thromb Vasc Biol* 2002; 22: 887–93.
124. Lee, J. Microtubule-actin interactions may regulate endothelial integrity and repair. *Cardiovasc Pathol* 2002; 11: 135–40.
125. Bernoud, N, et al. Astrocytes are mainly responsible for the polyunsaturated fatty acid enrichment in blood-brain barrier endothelial cells in vitro. *J Lipid Res* 1998; 39: 1816–24.
126. Delton-Vandenbroucke, I, et al. Polyunsaturated fatty acid metabolism in retinal and cerebral microvascular endothelial cells. *J Lipid Res* 1997; 38: 147–59.
127. Hough, J, et al. Effect of 17 beta estradiol on aortic cholesterol content and metabolism in cholesterol-fed rabbits. *Arteriosclerosis* 1986; 6: 57–63.
128. Krasinski, K, et al. Estradiol accelerates functional endothelial recovery after arterial injury. *Circulation* 1997; 95: 1768–72.
129. DeLarue, F, et al. Estrogens modulate bovine vascular endothelial cell permeability and HSP 25 expression concomitantly. *Am J Physiol* 1998 (Heart Circ. Physiol 44): H1011–15.
130. Hodkin, J, et al. Estrogen receptor alpha is a major mediator of 17 beta-estradiol's atheroprotective effects on lesion in Apoe-/-mice. *J Clin Invest* 2001; 107: 333–40.
131. Levin, E. Estrogen receptor-beta and the cardiovascular system. *Trends Endocrinol Metab* 2002; 13: 184–85.
132. Chen, Z, et al. Estrogen receptor alpha mediates the nongenomic activation of endothelial nitric oxide synthetase by estrogen. *J Clin Invest* 1999; 103: 401–6.
133. Nasr, A, et al. Estrogen replacement therapy and cardiovascular protection: lipid mechanisms are the tip of an iceberg. *Gynecol Endocrinol* 1998; 12: 43–59.
134. Tomita, T, et al. Inhibition of cholesterylester accumulation by 17 beta-estradiol in macrophages through activation of neutral cholesterol esterase. *Biochim Biophys Acta* 1996; 1300: 210–8.
135. Fernstrom, MH, et al. Brain tryptophan concentrations and serotonin synthesis remain responsive to food consumption after ingestion of sequential meals. *Am J Clin Nutr* 1995; 61: 312–9.
136. Urbich, C, et al. Shear stress-induced endothelial cell migration involves integrin signaling via fibronectin receptor subunits alpha(5) and beta(1). *Arterioscler Thromb Vasc Biol* 2002; 22: 69–75.
137. Gotlieh, A. The endothelial cytoskeleton: organization in normal and regenerating endothelium. *Toxicol Pathol* 1990; 18: 603–17.
138. Kiosses, W, et al. Rac recruits high-affinity integrin alphaVBeta3 to lamellipodia in endothelial cell migration. *Nat Cell Biol* 2001; 3: 316–20.

139. Li, S, et al. The role of the dynamics of focal adhesion kinase in the mechanotaxis of endothelial cells. *Proc Natl Acad Sci (USA)* 2002; 99: 3546–51.
140. Parker, K, et al. Directional control of lamellipodia extension by constraining cell shape and orienting cell tractional forces. *FASEB J* 2002; 16: 1195–204.
141. Caulin-Glaser, T, et al. Effect of 17beta-estradiol on cytokine-induced endothelial cell adhesion molecule expression. *J Clin Invest* 1996; 98: 36–42.
142. Nakai, K, et al. Estradiol-17 beta regulates the induction of VCAM-1 mRNA expression by interleukin-1 beta in human umbilical vein endothelial cells. *Life Sci* 1994; 54: PL21–7.
143. Cid, M, et al. Estradiol enhances leukocyte binding to tumor necrosis factor (TNF)-stimulated endothelial cells via an increase in TNF-induced adhesion molecules E-selectin, intracellular adhesion molecule type 1, and vascular cell adhesion molecule 1. *J Clin Invest* 1994; 93: 17–25.
144. Weidinger, F, et al. Hypercholesterolemia enhances macrophage recruitment and dysfunction of regenerated endothelium after balloon injury of the rabbit iliac artery. *Circulation* 1991; 84:755–67.
145. Cybulsky, M, et al. Endothelial expression of a mononuclear leukocyte adhesion molecule during atherogenesis. *Science* 1991; 251: 788–91.
146. Geng, Y, et al. Progression of atheroma: a struggle between death and procreation. *Arterioscler Thromb Vasc Biol* 2002; 22: 1370–80.
147. Ng, M, et al. Sex-related differences in the regulation of macrophage cholesterol metabolism. *Curr Opin Lipidol* 2001; 12: 505–10.
148. McCrohon, J, et al. Estrogen and progesterone reduce lipid accumulation in human monocyte-derived macrophages. A Sex-specific effect. *Circulation* 1999; 100: 2319–25.
149. Marchien, W, et al. Hormone replacement therapy and plasma homocysteine levels. *Obstet Gynecol* 1999; 94: 485–91.
150. Dimitrova, K, et al. Estrogen and homocysteine. *Cardiovasc Res* 2002; 53: 577–88.
151. Chambliss, K, et al. Estrogen modulation of endothelial nitric oxide synthase. *Endocrin Rev* 2002; 23: 665–86.
152. Jayachandran, M, et al. Temporal effects of 17beta-estradiol on caveolin-1 mRNA and protein in bovine aortic endothelial cells. *Am J Physiol Circ Physiol* 2001, 281: H1327–33.
153. Minshall, R, et al. In vitro modulation of primate coronary vascular muscle cell reactivity by ovarian steroid hormones. *FASEB J* 1998; 12: 1419–29.
154. Nasr, A, et al. Estrogen replacement therapy and cardiovascular protection: lipid mechanisms are the tip of an iceberg. *Gynecol Endocrinol* 1998; 12: 43–59.
155. Christ, M, et al. Cardiovascular steroid actions: swift swallows or sluggish snails? *Cardiovasc Res* 1998; 40: 34–44.
156. van Eickels, M, et al. 17beta-estradiol attenuates the development of pressure-overload hypertropy. *Circulation* 2001; 104: 1419–23.
157. Rosano, G, et al. Natural progesterone, but not medroxyprogesterone acetate, enhances the beneficial effect of estrogen on exercise-induced myocardial ischemia in postmenopausal women. *J Am Coll Cardiol* 2000; 36: 2154–9.
158. Cicinelli, E, et al. Twice-weekly transdermal estradiol and vaginal progesterone as contin-

uous combined hormone replacement therapy in postmenopausal women: a 1-year prospective study. *Am J Obstet Gynecol* 2002; 187: 556–60.

159. Minshall, R, et al. Ovarian steroid protection against coronary artery hyperreactivity in Rhesus Monkeys. *J Clin Endocrinol Metab* 1998; 83: 649–59.
160. Ibid.
161. Ibid.
162. Paris, J, et al. Nomegestrol acetate and vascular reactivity. *Steroids* 200; 65: 621–7.
163. Miyagawa, K, et al. Medroxyprogesterone interferes with ovarian steroid protection against coronary vasospasm. *Nat Med* 1997; 3: 324–7.
164. Rosano, G, et al. Comparative cardiovascular effects of different progestins in menopause. *Int Fertil Womens Med* 2001; 46: 248–56.
165. Fahraeus, L, et al. L-norgestrel and progesterone have different influences on plasma lipoproteins. *Eur J Clin Invest* 1983; 13: 447–53.
166. Nilsen, J, et al. Impact of progestins on estradiol potentiation of the glutamate calcium response. *Neuroreport* 2002; 13: 825–30.
167. Linn, E. Clinical significance of the androgenicity of progestins in hormonal therapy of women. *Clin Ther* 1990.
168. Alexander, K, et al. Initiation of hormone replacement therapy after acute myocardial infaction is associated with more cardiac events during follow-up. *J Am Coll Cardiol* 2001; 38: 1–7.
169. Brache, V, et al. Nonmenstrual adverse events during use of implantable contraceptives for women: data from clinical trials. *Contraception* 2002; 65: 63–74.
170. Hague, S, et al. In-vivo angiogenesis and progestogens. *Hum Reprod* 2002; 17: 786–93.
171. Pokieser, W, et al. Clear cell carcinoma arising in endometriosis of the rectum following progestin therapy. *Pathol Res Pract* 2002; 198: 121–4.
172. Affandi, B. Long-acting progestogens. *Best Bract Res Clin Obstet Gynaecol* 2002; 16: 169–79.
173. Krikun, G, et al. Abnormal uterine bleeding during progestin-only contraception may result from free radical-induced alterations in angiopoietin expression. *Am J Pathol* 2002; 161: 979–86.
174. Zhou, Y, et al. Regulation of estrogen receptor protein and messenger ribonucleic acid by estradiol and progesterone in rat uterus. *J Steroid Biochem Mol Biol* 1993; 46: 687–98.
175. Korach, K. Estrogen receptor knock-out mice: molecular and endocrine phenotypes. *J Soc Gynecol Investig* 2000; 7(1 suppl): S16–7.
176. Ariazi, E, et al. Estrogen-related receptor alpha and estrogen-related receptor gamma associate with unfavorable and favorable biomarkers, respectively, in human breast cancer. *Cancer Res* 2002; 62: 6510–8.
177. Nicholson, R, et al. Modulation of epidermal growth factor receptor in endocrine-resistant, estrogen-receptor-positive breast cancer. *Ann N Y Acad Sci* 2002; 963: 104–15.
178. Galloway, C, et al. Anti-tumor necrosis factor receptor and tumor necrosis factor agonist activity by an anti-idiotypic antibody. *Eur J Immunol* 1992; 22: 3045–8.
179. Lim, I. Generation and characterization of anti-idiotypic antibodies recognizing the

interferon-alpha receptor: implications for ligand-receptor interactions. *J Interferon Res* 1993; 13: 295–301.

180. Crone, S, et al. ErbB2 is essential in the prevention of dilated cardiomyopathy. *Nat Med* 2002; 8: 459–64.
181. Kjekshus, J, et al. Reducing the risk of coronary events: evidence from the Scandinavian simvastatin survival study (4S). *AM J Cardiol* 1995 Sep 28; 76 1995 (9).
182. Gilbert, Tom. Low Cholesterol and Heart Problems. The Doctor Will See You Now, website. May 18, 2000.
183. http://www.thedoctorwillseeyounow.com/news/heart/0500/chol.shtml
184. Slung, A, et al. Changes in lipoprotein levels during the treatment with simvastatin. *Eur J Clin Pharmacol* 1992; 43: 369–73.
185. McNamara, DJ. Cholesterol intake and plasma cholesterol: an update. *J Am Coll Nutr* 1997; 16: 530–4.
186. Dobiasova, M, et al. High-density lipoprotein subclasses and esterification rate of cholesterol in children: effect of gender and age. *Acta Paediatr* 1998; 87: 918–23.
187. King, S, et al. An essential component in steroid synthesis, the steroidogenic acute regulatory protein, is expressed in discrete regions of the brain. *J Neurosci* 2002; 22: 10613–20.
188. Inoue, T, et al. Progesterone production and actions in the human central nervous system and neurogenic tumors. *J Clin Endocrinol Metab* 2002; 87: 5325–31.
189. Owen, K, et al. Toxicity of a novel HMG-CoA reductase inhibitor in the common marmoset (Callithrix jacchus). *Hum Exp Toxicol* 1994; 13: 357–68.
190. Mitter, D, et al. The synaotophysin/synaptobrevin interaction critically depends on the cholesterol content. *J Neurochem* 2003; 84: 35–42.
191. Fassbinder, K, et al. Effects of statins on human cerebral cholesterol metabolism and secretion of Alzheimer amyloid peptide. *Neurology* 2002; 59: 1257–8.
192. Chong, P. Lack of therapeutic interchangeability of HMG-CoA reductase inhibitors. *Ann Pharmacother* 2002; 36: 1907–17.
193. Bolego, C, et al. Safety considerations for statins. *Curr Opin Lipidol* 2002; 13: 637–44.
194. Newman, T, et al. Carcinogenicity of lipid-lowering drugs. *JAMA* 1996; 275: 55–60.
195. Jackson, P, et al. Statins for primary prevention: at what coronary risk is safety assured? *Br J Clin Pharmacol* 2001; 52: 439–46.
196. Gotto Jr, A, et al. Pleitropic effects of statins: do they matter? *Curr Opin Lipidol* 2001; 12: 391–4.
197. Decensi, A, et al. Effect of transdermal estradiol and oral conjugated estrogen on C-reactive protein in retrinoid-placebo trial in healthy women. *Circulation* 2002; 106: 1224–8.
198. De Meeus, J, et al. C-reactive protein levels at the onset of labour and at day 3 post partum in normal pregnancy. *Clin Exp Obstet Gynecol* 1998; 25: 9–11.

CHAPTER EIGHT

1. Garber, K. An end to Alzheimer's? *Technology Review*, 2001 March 70.
2. Shenk, D. *The forgetting: Alzheimer's portrait of an epidemic*. Doubleday, 2002.

3. Halpern, S. Heart of the darkness. *The New York Review of Books* 2002; 49: 16–22.
4. National Vital Statistic report, 2002; vol50#15
5. Monks, A, et al. Estrogen-inducible progesterone receptors in the rat lumbar spinal cord: Regulation by steroids and fluctuation across the estrous cycle. *Horm Behav* 2001; 17187–21
6. Murphy, D, et al. Brain-derived neurotropic factor mediates estradiol-induced dendritic spine formation in hippocampal neurons. *Proc Natl Acad Sci (USA)* 1998; 95: 11412–17.
7. Smith, Y, et al. Neuroimaging of aging estrogen effects on central nervous system physiology. *Fertil Steril* 2001; 76: 651–9.
8. McEwen, B. The molecular and neuroanatomical basis for estrogen effects in the central nervous system. *J Clin Endocrinol Metab* 1999; 84: 1790–7.
9. Mimitrova, K, et al. 17-beta-estradiol preserves endothelial viability in an in vitro model of homocysteine-induced oxidative stress. *J Cardiovasc Pharmacol* 2002; 39; 347–53.
10. Grodley, K, et al. Low concentrations of estradiol reduce beta-amyloid (25–35)-induced toxicity, lipid peroxidation and glucose utilization in human SK-N-SH neuroblastoma cells. *Brain Res* 1997; 778: 158–65.
11. McEwen, B, et al. Tracking the estrogen receptor in neurons: Implication for estrogen-induced synapse formation. *Proc Natl Acad Sci (USA)* 2001; 98: 7093–7100.
12. Levin-Allerhand, J, et al. Brain region-specific up-regulation of mouse apolipoprotein E by pharmacological estrogen treatments. *J Neurochem* 2001: 79: 796–803.
13. Bi, R, et al. Cyclic changes on estradiol regulate synaptic plasticity through the Map kinase pathway. *Proc Natl Acad Sci (USA)* 2001; 98: 13391–5.
14. Wise, P, et al. Estradiol is a protective factor in the adult and aging brain: understanding of mechanisms derived from in vitro and in vitro studies. *Brain Res Rev* 2001; 37: 313–19.
15. Mong, J, et al. Steroid-induced developmental plasticity in hypothalamic astrocytes: implications for synaptic pattering. *J Neurobiol* 1999; 40: 602–19.
16. Solum, D, et al. Estrogen regulates the development of brain-derived neurotrophic factor mRNA in the rat hippocampus. *J Neurosci* 2002; 22: 2650–9.
17. Hosli, E, et al. Histochemical and electrophysiological evidence for estrogen receptors on cultures astrocytes: colocalization with cholinergic receptors. *In J Dev Neuroscience* 2000; 18: 101–11.
18. Fitzpatrick, J, et al. Estrogen-mediated neuroprotection against beta-amyloid toxicity requires expression of estrogen receptor alpha or beta and activation of the MAPK pathway. *J Neurochem* 2002; 82: 674–82.
19. Zhang, I, et al. Estrogen protects against beta-amyloid neurotoxicity in rat hippocampal neurons by activation of Akt. *Neuroreport* 2001; 121: 1919–23.
20. Jung-Testas, I, et al. Progesterone as a neurosteroid: synthesis and actions in rat glial cells. *J Steroid Biochem Mol Biol* 1999; 69: 97–107.
21. Jung-Testas, I, et al. Actions of steroid hormones-and growth factors on glial cells of the central and peripheral nervous system. *J Steroid Biochem Mol Biol* 1994; 48: 145–54.
22. Akwa, V, et al. Neurosteroids: biosynthesis, metabolism and function of pregnenolone and dehydroepiandrosterone in the brain. *J Steroid Biochem Mol Biol* 1991; 40: 71–81.

23. Jung-Testas, I, et al. Estrogen-inducible progesterone receptor in primary cultures of rat glial cells. *Exp Cell Res* 1991; 193: 12–9.
24. Murphy, D, et al. Progesterone prevents estradiol-induced dendritic spione formation in cultured hippocampal neurons. *Neuroendocrinol* 2000; 72: 133–43.
25. Griffin, L. Selective serotonin reuptake inhibitors directly alter activity of neurosteroidogenic enzymes. *Proc Natl Acad Sci (USA)* 1999; 96: 13512–17.
26. Matsui, D, et al. Transcriptional regulation of the mouse steroid 5alpha-reductase type II gene by progesterone in brain. *Nucleic Acid Res* 2002; 30: 1387–93.
27. Petersen, S, et al. Progesterone increases levels of my-opioid receptor mRNA in the preoptic area and arcurate nucleus of ovariectomized, estradiol-treated female rats. *Mol Brain Res* 1997; 52: 32–37.
28. Lee, D, et al. Progesterone modulation of D5 expression in hypothalamic ANP the role of estrogen. *Mol Psychiatry* 2001; 6: 112–7.
29. Quadros, P, et al. Sex differences in progesterone receptor expression: a potential mechanism for estradiol-mediated sexual differentiation. *Endocrinol* 2002; 143: 3727–39.
30. Hilschmann, N, et al. The immunoglobulin-like genetic predetermination of the brain: the protocadherins, blueprint of the neuronal network. *Naturwissenschaften* 2001; 88: 2–12.
31. Catala, M. Embryonic and fetal development of structures associated with the cerebrospinal fluid in man and other species. Part I: The ventricular system, minenges and choroid plexuses. *Arch Anat Cytol Pathol* 1998; 46: 153–69.
32. Quigley, I, et al. Pigment pattern formation in Zebrafish: a model for developmental genetics and evolution of form. *Microsc Res Tech* 2001; 58: 442–55.
33. Kennea, N, et al. Neural stem cells. *J Pathol* 2002; 197: 536–50.
34. O'Rourke, M, et al. Twist functions in mouse development. *Int J Dev Biol* 2001; 46: 401–13.
35. Lightman, S, et al. New genomic avenues in behavioral neuroendocrinology. *Eur J Neurosci* 2001; 16: 369–72.
36. Loh, Y, et al. Mechanism of sorting proopiomelanocortin and proenkephalin to the regulated secretory pathway of neuroendocrine cells. *Ann N Y Acad Sci* 2002; 971: 416–25.
37. Haddad, J, et al. Cytokines and neuro-immune-endocrine interactions: a role for the hypothalamic-pituitary-adrenal revolving axis. *J Neuroimmunol* 2002; 133: 1–19.
38. Laslop, A, et al. Neuropeptides and chromogranins: sessions overview. *Ann N Y Acad Sci* 2000; 971: 294–9.
39. Hamilton, N. Interaction of steroids with the GABA(A)receptor. *Curr Top Med Chem* 2002; 2: 887–902.
40. Gibbs, TT, et al. Dueling enigmas: neurosteroids and sigma receptors in the limelight. *Sci STKE* 2000; 2000 (60): PE1.
41. Tasker, J. Coregulation of ion channels by neurostereoids and phosphorylation. *Sci STKE* 2000; 2000 (59): PE1.
42. Mellon, S, et al. Neurosteroids: biochemistry and clinical significance. *Trends Endocrinol Metab* 2002; 13: 35–43.
43. Wang, P, et al. Effects of estrogen on recognition, mood, and cerebral blood flow in AD; a controlled study. *Neurology* 2000; 54: 2061–6.

44. Oda, T, et al. Cytotoxicity of estradiol. Equilin, equilenin, and their derivatives on Chinese hamsters V79 cells. *Drug Chem Toxicol* 2001; 25: 765–82.
45. Zhang, F, et al. Equine estrogen metabolite 4-hydroxyequilenin induces DNA damage in the rat mammary tissues: formation of single-strand breaks, apurinic sites, stable adducts, and oxidative bases. *Chem Res Toxicol* 2001; 14: 1654–9.
46. Zhang, F, et al. Synthesis and reactivity of the catechol metabolites from the equine estrogen, 8, 9-dehydroestrone. *Chem Res Toxicol* 2001; 14: 754–63.
47. Bethea, C, et al. Ovarian steroid action in the serotonin neural system of macaques. *Novartis found Symp* 2000; 230: 112–30.
48. Magnaghi, V, et al. Neuroactive steroids and peripheral proteins. *Brain Res Brain Res Rev* 2001; 37: 360–71.
49. Melcai, R, et al. Formation and effects of neuroactive steroids in the central and peripheral nervous system. *Int Rev Neurobiol* 2001; 46: 145–76.
50. Mercier, G, et al. Early activation of transcription factor expression in Swann cells by progesterone. *Brain Res Mol Brain Res* 2001; 97: 137–48.
51. McEwen, B. Clinical Review 108. The molecular and neuroanatomical basis for estrogen effects in the central nervous system. *J Clin Endocrinol Metab* 1999; 84: 17.
52. Ibid.
53. Warner, M, et al. Cytochrome P450 in the brain neuroendocrine functions. *Front Neuroendocrinol* 1995; 3: 224–36.
54. Meinhardt, U, et al. The essential role of the aromatase/p450arom. *Semin Reprod Med* 2002 Aug; 20 (3): 277–84.
55. Balthazart, J, et al. Rapid and Reversable Inhibition of Brain Aromatase Activity. *Journal of Neuroendocrinology* 2001; 13: 63–73.
56. Balthazart, J, et al. Phosphorylation processes mediate rapid changes of brain aromatase activity. *J steroid Biochem Mol Biol* 2001; 79: 261–77.
57. Honda, SI, et al. Characterization and purification of a protein binding to the cis-acting element for brain-specific exon 1 of the mouse aromatase gene. *J Steroid Biochem Mol Biol* 2001 Dec; 79 (1–5): 255–60.
58. Michalak, S, et al. Cholestrerol synthesis in the rat brain in course of late development as determined by 3-hydroxy-3-methylglutaryl CoA reductase activity. *Folia Neuropathol* 1996; 34: 7–10.
59. Kovacs, W, et al. Putrification of brain peroxisomes and localization of 3-hydroxy-3methyl coenxyme A reductase. *Bur J Biochem* 2001; 268: 4850–9.
60. Roher, A. Beta peptides and reduced cholesterol and myelin proteins characterize white matter degeneration in Alzheimer's disease. *Biochemistry* 2002; 41: 11080–90.
61. Islam, E, et al. Inhibition of rat brain prostaglandin D synthetase by 3-hydroxymethylglutamyl coenzyme reductase inhibitors. *Biochem Int* 1990; 22: 601–5.
62. Shefer, S, et al. Is there a relationship between 3-hydroxy-3-methylglutamyl coenzyme a reductase activity and forebrain pathology in the PKU Mouse? *J Neurosci Res* 2000; 61: 549–63.
63. Michikawa, M, et al. Inhibition of cholesterol production but not nonsterol isoprenoid products induces neuronal cell death. *J Neurochem* 1999; 72: 2278–85.

64. Choi, J. Lovastatin-induced proliferation inhibition and apoptosis in C6 glial cells. *J Pharmacol Exp Ther* 1999; 2898: 572–9.

65. Corsini, A, et al. Relationship between mevalonate pathway and arterial myocyte proliferation: in vitro studies with inhibitors of HMGF-CoA reductase. *Atherosclerosis* 1993; 101: 117–25.

66. Nishio, E, et al. 3-hydroxy-3-methulglumamyl coenzyme A reductase inhibitor impairs cell differentiation cultured adipogenic cells (3T3-L). *Euro J Pharmacol* 1996; 301: 203–6.

67. Choi, J. Lovostatin induces apopotosis of spontaneously immortalized rat brain neuroblasts: involvement of nonsterol isoprenoid cells (3T3). *Eur J Pharmacol* 2001; 408:2–6.

68. Michikawa, M, et al. Apolipoprotein E4 induces neuronal cell death unnovo cholesterol synthesis. *J Neurosci Res* 1998; 54: 58–67.

69. Koudinavo, N, et al. Alzheimer's abetal2-40 peptide modulates lipid synthesis in neuronal cultures and intact rat fetal brain under normoxic and oxidative stress conditions. *Neurochem Res* 2000; 25: 653–60.

70. Michikawa, M, et al. Inhibition of cholesterol production but not of nonsterol isoprenoid products induces neuronal cell death. *J Neurochem* 1999 Jun; 72 (6): 2278–85.

71. Ibid. Inhibition of cholesterol production but not of nonsterol isoprenoid products induces neuronal cell death. *J Neurochem* 1999; 72: 2278–85.

72. Owen, K, et al. Toxicity of a novel HMG-CoA reductase inhibitor in the common masrmoset (Callithrix jacchus). *Hum Exp Toxicol* 1994; 13: 357–68.

73. Ness, G. Developmental regulation of the expression of genes encoding proteins involved in cholesterol homeostasis. *M J MED GENET* 1994; 50: 355–7.

74. Mitchalak, S, et al. Cholesterol synthesis in rat brain in course of late development as determined by 3-hydroxy-3-methylglutaryl CoA reductase.

75. Xu, G, et al. Relationship between abnormal cholesterol synthesis and retarded learning in rats. *Metabolism* 1998; 47: 878–82.

76. Garcia-Peregrin, E. Contribution of brain and liver to the biosynthesis of cholesterol during the postnatal development of the chicken. *Rev Esp Fisiol* 1982; 38: 247–50.

77. Zhang, L, et al. Sex-related differences in MAPKs activation in rat astrocytes: effects of estrogen on cell death. *Brain Res Mol Brain Res* 2002; 103: 1–11.

78. McMillan, PJ, et al. Tamoxifen enhances choline acetyltransferase mRNA expression in rat basal forebrain cholinergic neurons. *Brain Res Mol Brain Res* 2002; 103: 140–5.

79. Meinhardt, U, et al. The aromatase cytochrome P-450 and its clinical impact. *Horm Res* 2002; 57: 145–52.

80. Jordan, C. Steroid hormone receptors after aromatase inhibition. *J Steroid Biochem Mol* Biol 1998; 65: 123–9.

81. Jordan, C. Glia as mediators of steroid hormone action on the nervous system. An overview. *J Neurbiol* 1999; 40: 434–45.

82. Blaschuk, OW, et al. E-cadherin, estrogens and cancer: is there a connection? *Can J Oncol* 1994 Nov; (4): 291–301. Review.

83. Bakarat-Walter, D. Differential effect of thyroid hormone deficiency on the growth of calretinin-expressing neurons in rat spinal cord and dorsal root ganglia. *J Comp Neurol* 2000 Oct 30; 426 (4): 519–33.

84. Hawkinson, JE, et al. Correlation of neuroactive steroid modulation of [355]t-butylbicyclophosphorothionate and [3H] flunitrazepam binding and gamma-aminobutyric acid A receptor function. *Mer Pharm* 1994 Nov; 46(5): 977-85.
85. Zinder, O, et al. Neuroactive steroids: their mechanism of action and their function in the stress response. *Acta physiol Scand* 1999; 167: 181–8.
86. Monks, DA, et al. Estrogen-inducible progesterone receptors in the rat lumbar spinal cord: regulation by ovarian steroids and fluctuations across the estrous cycle. *Horm Behav* 2001; 40: 1717–22.
87. *http://www.cizstarnet.com/health/womens/021108motherhood.shtml.*
88. Mercier, G, et al. Early activation of transcription factor expression in Swann cells by progestereone. *Brain Res Mol Brain Res* 2001; 97: 137–48.
89. Gago, N, et al. Progesterone and the oligodendroglial lineage: stage-dependent biosynthesis and metabolism. *Glia* 2001; 36: 295–308.
90. Schumacher, M, et al. Progesterone synthesis and myelin formation in pereipheral nerves. *Brain Res Brain Rev* 2001; 37: 343–59.
91. Fields, R, et al. New Insight into Neuron-Glia Communication. *Science* 2002; 298: 556–62.
92. Minigar, A, et al. The role of macrophage/microglia and astrocytes in the pathogenesis of three neurological disorders: HIV-associated dementia, Alzheimer disease, multiple sclerosis. *J Neurol Sci* 2002; 202: 13–23.
93. Fields, R, et al. New Insight into Neuron-Glia Communication. *Science* 2002; 298: 556–62.
94. Minagar, A, et al. The role of macrophage/microglia and astrocytes in the pathogenesis of the three neuroligical odiseasaes: HIV-associated dementia, Alzheimer disease, multiple sclerosis. *J Neurol Sci* 2002; 202: 13–23.
95. Blake, C. Effects of estrogen and progesterone on luteinizing hormone release on ovariectomized rats. *Endocrinology* 19977; 101: 1122–1129.
96. Jacobson, W, et al. Decreased in mediobasal hypothalamic and preoptic area opoid binding are associated with the progesterone-induced luteinizing hormone surge. *Endocrinology* 1989; 124: 199–206.
97. Krey, L, et al. The estrogen-induced advance in the cyclic LH surge in the rat: dependency on ovarian progesterone secretion. *Endocrinology* 1973; 93: 385–390.
98. Petersen, SL, et al. Differential effects of estrogen and progesterone on levels of POMC mRNA levels in the arcuate nucleus: relationship to the timing of LH surge release. *J Neuroendocrinol* 1993; 5: 643–48.
99. Sar, M, et al. Neurons of the hypothalamus concentrate (3H) progesterone or its metabolites. *Science* 1973 Dec 21; 182 (118): 1266–8.
100. Weiland, N, et al. Aging abolishes the estradiol-induced suppression and diurnal rhythm of propiomelanocortin gene expression in the arcuate nucleus. *Endocrinology* 1990; 131: 2959–64.
101. Chowen, JA, et al. Sexual dimorphisms and sex steroid modulation of glial fibrillary acidic protein messenger RNA and immunoreactivity levels in the hypothalamus. *Neuroscience* 1995; 69: 519–32.

102. Day, JR, et al. Gonadal steroids regulate the expression of glial fibrillary acidic proteins in the adult male rat hippocampus. *Neuroscience* 1993, 55: 435–43.

103. Del Cerro, S, et al. Neuroactive steroids regulate astroglia morphology in hyppocampal cultures from adult rat. *Glia* 1995; 14: 65–71.

104. Duenas, M, et al. Interaction of insulin-like growth factor-I and estradiol signaling pathways on hypothalamic neuronal differentiation. *Neuroscience* 1996; 74: 531–39.

105. Fernandez-Galaz, MC, et al. Role of astroglia and insulin like growth factor-I in gonadal hormone dependent synaptic plasticity. *Brain Res bull* 1997; 44: 525–31.

106. Frankfurt, M, et al. Estrogen increases axodendritic synapses in the VMN of rats after ovarietectomy. *Neuroreport* 1991; 380–2.

107. Friend, KE, et al. Specific modulation of estrogen receptor mRNA isoforms in rat pituitary throughout the estrous cycle and in response to steroid hormones. *Mol Cell Endocrinol* 1997; 131: 147–55.

108. Garcia-Segura, M, et al. Gonadal hormones as promotors of structural synaptic plasticity: cellular mechanism. *Prog Neurobiol* 1994; 44: 279–307.

109. Gu, Q, et al. 17 beta-Estradiol potentiates kainate-induced currents via activation of the cAMP cascade. *J Neurosci* 1996 Jun 1; 16 (11): 3620–9.

110. Jung-Testa, I, et al. Demonstration of steroid hormone receptors and steroid action in primary cultures of rat glial cells. *Mol Biol* 1992; 41: 621–31.

111. Murphy, DD, et al. Estradiol increases dendritio spine density by reducing GABA neurotransmission in hippocampal neurons. *J Neuroscience* 1998; 18: 2550–82.

112. Stone, et al. Directional transcription regulation of glial fibrillary acidic proteins by estradiol in vivo and in vitro. *Endocrinology* 1998; 139: 3202–9.

113. Garcia-Segura, LM, et al. Estradiol promotion of changes in the morphology of astroglia growing in culture depends depends on the expression of polysialic acid of neural membranes. *Glia* 1995; 13: 209–16.

114. Garcia-Segura, LM, et al. Gonadal hormone regulation of fibrillary acidic protein immunoreactivity and glial ultrastructure in the rat neuroendocrine hypothalamus. *Glia* 1994; 10: 59–69.

115. Naftolin, A, et al. Neuronal membrane remodeling during the oestrus cycle: a freeze-freacture study in the arcuate nucleus of the rat hypothalemus. *J Neurocytol* 1988; 17: 377–83.

116. Garcia-Segura, LM, et al. Astrocytic shape and glial fabrially acidic protein immunoreactivity are modified by estradiol in primary rat hypothalamic cultures. *Dev Brain Res* 1989; 456: 357–63.

117. Hatton, P, et al. Function-related plasticity in hypothalamus. *Ann Rev Neurosci* 1997; 20: 375–97.

118. Hyden, H, et al. Satellite cells in the nervous system. *Sci Am* 1961; 205: 62–70.

119. Langub, MC, et al. Estrogen receptor immunoreactive glia, endothelia and ependyma in guinea pig preoptic area and median eminence: electron microscopy. *Endocrinology* 1992; 130: 364–72.

120. Mong, JA, et al. Estrogen mediates the hormonal responsiveness of arcuate astrocytes in neonatal rats. *Soc Neurosci* 1998; Abstr 24: 220–5.

121. Perducz, A, et al. Estradiol induces plasticity of GABAergic synapses in the hypothalamus. *Neuroscience* 1993; 53: 395–401.

122. Perez, S, et al. The role of estradiol and progesterone in phased synaptic remodeling of the rat arcuate nucleus. *Brain Res* 1993; 6508: 38–44.
123. Santagati, S, et al. Estrogen receptor is expressed in different types of glial cells in culture. *J Neurochem* 1994; 63: 2058–64.
124. Shughrue, A, et al. Comparative distribution of estrogen receptor alpha and—beta mRNA in the rat central nervous system. *J Comp Neurol* 1997; 388: 507–25.
125. Sison, F, et al. A potential influence of ovarian cycle day on the presence of polysialic acid neutral cell adhesion molecule (PSA-NCAM) in the rat hypothalamus. *Soc Neurosci* 1997; Abstr 23: 770–4.
126. Torres-Aleman, I, et al. Estradiol promotes cell shape changes and glial fibrillary acidic protein redistribution in hypothalamic astrocytes in vitro: a neuronal-mediated effect. *Glia* 1992; 6 (3): 180–7.
127. Wooley, P, et al. Estradiol mediates fluctuation in hyppocampal synapse density during the estrous cycle in adult rat. *J Neurosci* 1992; 12: 2449–54.
128. Wooley, P, et al. Estradiol regulates hippocampal dendritic spine density via an N-methyl-D-aspartate receptor mechanism. *J Neurosci* 1994; 14: 7680–87.
129. Wooley, P, et al. Estradiol increases the frequency of multiple synapse boutons in the hippocampal cal region of the adult female rat. *J Comp Neurol* 1996; 373: 108–17.
130. Wooley, P, et al. The molecular and neuroanatomical basis for estrogen effects in the central nervous system. *J Clin Endocrinol Metab* 1999; 84: 1790–7.
131. Jordan C. Glia as mediaters of steroid hormone action on the nervous system. An overview. *J Neurobiol* 1999; 40: 434–45.
132. Temburni, MK, et al. Receptor Targeting and Heterogeneity at interneuronal nicotinic cholinergic synapses *in vivo*. *Journal of Physiology* 2000; 525.1: 21–29.
133. Quattrocki, E, et al. Biological Aspects of the Link Between Smoking and Depression. *Harvard Rev Psychiatry* 2000 September; 99–110.
134. Mong, JA, et al. Steroid-induced developmental plasticity in hypothalamic astrocytes: implications for synaptic pattering. *J Neurobiol* 1999; 40: 602–19.
135. Hilschmann, G, et al. The immunoglobulin-like genetic predetermination of the brain: the protocadherins, blueprint of the neuronal network. *Naturwissenschaften* 2001; 88: 2–12.
136. Bakarat-Walter, I, et al. Role of thyroid hormones and their receptors in pereipheral nerve regeneration. *J Neurobiol* 1999; 40: 541–59.
137. Valera, S, et al. Progesterone modulates a neuronal nicotinic acetylcholine receptor. *Proc Natl Acad Sci* (USA) 1992; 89: 9949–53.
138. Changeux, J. The TIBS lecture; the nicotinic acetylcholine receptor: an allosteric protein prototype of ligand-gated ion channels. *Trends Pharmacol Sci* 1990; 11: 485–92.
139. Smith, SS. Progesterone administration attenuates excitatory amino acid responses of cerebellar Purkinje cells. *Neuroscience* 1991; 42 (2): 309–20.
140. Bertrand, D, et al. Steroids inhibit nicotinic acetylcholine receptors. *Neuroreport* 1991; 2: 277–80.
141. Barbiturates bind to an allosteric regulatory site on nicotinic acetylcholine receptor-rich membranes. *Mol Pharmacol* 1987; 32: 119–26.

142. Cicinelli, E, et al. Twice-weekly transdermal estradiol and vaginal progesterone as continuous combined hormone replacement therapy in postmenopausal women: a 1-year prospective study. *Am J Obstet Gynecol* 2002 Sep; 187 (3): 556–60.
143. Murphy, DD, et al. Brain-derived neurotrophic factor mediates estradiol-induced dendritic spine formation in hippocampal neurons. *Proc Natl Acad Sci* (USA) 1998 Sep 15; 95 (19): 11412–7.
144. Warren, SG, et al. LTP varies across the estrogen cycle; enhanced synthetic plasticity in procedure rats. *Brain Res* 1995; 703: 26–30.
145. Burakat-Walter, I, et al. Thyroid hormone stimulate expression and modification of cytoskeletal protein during rat sciatic nerve regeneration. *Brain Res* 2002 Dec 13; 957 (2): 259–70.
146. Magnaghi, V, et al. Neuroactive steroids and peripheral myelin proteins. *Brain Res Brain Res Rev* 2001; 37: 360–71.
147. Aminof, D, et al. Coordinate regulation of transcription and splicing by progesterone receptor configuration. *Science* 2002; 298: 11–18.
148. Asarian, L, et al. Cyclic estradiol treatment normalizes body weight and restores physiological patterns of spontaneous feeding and sexual receptivity in ovariectomized rats. *Horm Behav* 2002; 42: 461–71.
149. Jung-Testas, I, et al. Progesterone as a neurosteroid: synthesis and actions in rat glial cells. *J Steroid Biochem Mol Biol* 1999; 69: 97–107.
150. Magnaghi, V, et al. Neuroactive steroids and peripheral myelin proteins. *Brain Res Brain Res Rev* 2001; 37: 360–71.
151. Dhall, U, et al. Effect of estrogen and progesterone on noradrenergic nerves and on nerves serving sertonin-like immunoreactivity in basilar arthery. *Brain Res* 1988; 442: 335–9.
152. Ferrari, M. Biochemistry of Migraine. *Pathol Biol* 1992; 40: 287–92.
153. Sekiguchi, M, et al. Nerve vascular changes induced by serotonin under chronic cauda equina suppression. *Spine* 2002; 27: 1634–9.
154. Magnaghi, V, et al. Neuroactive steroids and peripheral myelin proteins. *Brain Res Brain Res Rev* 2001; 37: 360–71.
155. Sawada, D, et al. Estrogen protects dopaminergic neurons from oxidative-stress induced neuronal death. *J Neurosci* 1998; 54: 707–19.
156. Obeta, S, et al. Role of free radicals in neurotoxicity as revealed by free radical trapping steroid receptors. *Toxicology lett* 2002; 132: 87–93.
157. Smith, Y, et al. Neuroimaging of aging and steroid effects on central nervous system physiology. Role of functional plasticity in aging brains. *Fertil Steril* 2001; 76: 651–9.
158. Graeber, M, et al. Reanalysis of the first case of Alzheimer's disease. *Eur Arch Psychiatry Clin Neurosci* 1999; suppl 3: 10–13.
159. Alzheimer, A. Uber eine eigenartige erkrakrung der hirn-flissde. *Alg Zeitschr Psychiatr* 1907; 64: 146–88.
160. National Institute on Aging. Forgetfulness: it's not always what you think. *Health information* 2002; 1–4.
161. Garber, K. An end to Alzheimer's? *Technology Review* 2001 March; 70–78.
162. National Vital Statistics Report 2002; vol50 #15.

163. Halpern, S. *Heart and Darkness. The New York Review of Books* 2002; 49: 16–22.
164. Shenk, D. *The forgetting: Alzheimer's portrait of an epidemic*. Doubleday, 2002.
165. Alzheimer's Disease International. Estimated number of patrients with dementia, 2002; April factsheet.
166. Jorm, AF. The prevalence of dementia: a quantitative integration of the literature. *Acta Psychiatr Scand* 1987; 76: 465–79.
167. Jorm, AF. Sex and age differences in depression. A quantitative analysis of published research. *Aust N Z J Psychiatr* 1987; 21: 46–53.
168. Johnson, G, et al. Tau, where are we now? *J Alzheimer Dis* 2002; 4: 375–98.
169. Auld, D, et al. Alzheimer's disease and the basal forebrain cholinegic system relations to beta-amyloid peptides, cognition and treatment strategies. *Prog Neurobiol* 2002; 68: 209–45.
170. Xiao, A, et al. Slight impairment of (Na,K)ATPase synergistically aggrevates beta-amyloid induced apoptosis in cortical neurons. *Brain Res* 2002; 955: 253–59.
171. Citron, M. Beta-secretase as a target for the treatment of Alzheimer's disease. *J Neurosci Res* 2002; 70: 373–9.
172. Check, E. Nerve inflammation halts trials for Alzheimer's drug. *Nature* 2002; 415: 462.
173. Haddad, I, et al. Cytokines and neuro-immune-endocrine interactions: a role for the hypothalamic-pituitary-adrenal revolving axis. *J Neuroimmunol* 2002; 133: 1–19.
174. Schenk, D. Plaques are diagnostic for Alzheimer's disease. *Nature* 1999; 400: 173–177.
175. Garber, K. An end to Alzheimer's? *Technology Review* 2001 March; 70–7.
176. Ibid.
177. Check, E. Nerve inflammation halts trial for Altheimer's drug. *Nature* 2002; 415: 462.
178. Lemonick, M. The nun study. *Time* magazine. Science and health 2001 May 05; 1–4.
179. Weiner, M, et al. Aging and alzheimers disease: lessons from the nun study. *Gerontologist* 1998; 38: 1–5.
180. Snowdon, D. Aging and Alzheimer's disease. The NUN study. *Gerontologist* 1997; 37: 150–6.
181. Snowdon, D, et al. Brain infarction and the clinical expression of Alzheimer's disease. The nun study. *JAMA* 1997; 277: 813–7.
182. Lemonick, M, et al. The nun study. How one scientist and 678 sisters are helping unlock the secrets of Alzheimer's. *Time* 2001; 157: 54–64.
183. Snowdon, D, et al. Linguistic ability in early life and the neuropathology of Alzheimer's disease and cerebrovascular disease. *Ann N Y Acad Sci* 2000; 903: 34–8.
184. Snowdon, D, et al. Serum folate, homocysteine and the severety of atrophy of the neocortex in Alzhermer's disease. Findings from the nun study. *Am J Clin Nutr* 2000; 71: 993–8.
185. Riley, K, et al. Alzheimer's neurofibrillary pathology and the spectrum of cognitive function: findings from the nun study. *Ann Neurol* 2002; 51: 567–77.
186. Gosche, K, et al. Hippocampal volume as an index of Alzheimer neuropathology: findings from the nun study. *Neurology* 2002; 58: 1476–82.
187. Xu, H, et al. Estrogen reduces neuronal generation of Alzheimer beta-amyloid peptides. *Nature Medicine* 1998; 4: 447–54.
188. Kawahara, M, et al. Intracellular calcium changes in neuronal cells induced by

Alzheimer's beta-amyloid protein are blocked by estradiol and cholesterol. *Cell Mol Neurobiol* 2001; 21: 1–13.

189. Jaffe, A, et al. Estrogen regulates metabolism of Alzheimer amyloid beta precursor protein. *J Biol Chem* 1994; 269: 13065–68.
190. Greenfield, J, et al. Estrogen lowers Alzheimer beta-amyloid generation by stimulating trans-Golgi network vesicle biogenesis. *J Biol Chem* 2002; 277: 12128–36.
191. Jung-Testas, I, et al. Progesterone as a neurosteroid: synthesis and actions in rat glial cells. *J Steroid Biochem Mol Biol* 1999; 69: 97–107.
192. Kawas, C, et al. A prospective study of estrogen replacement therapy and the risk of developing Alzheimer's disease: The Baltimore longitudial study of aging. *Neurology* 2001; 58: 435–440.
193. Schulkin, J. Corticotropin-releasing hormone signals adversity in both the placenta and the brain: regulation by glucocorticoids and allostatic overload. *J Endocrinol* 1999; 161: 349–56.
194. Barbaccia, M, et al. Plasma 5alpha-androstane-3alpha, 17-beta estradiol, and endogeneous steroid that positively modulates GABA receptor function, and anxiety: a study in menopausal women. *Phychoneuroendocrinol* 2000; 25: 659–75.
195. Hogervorst, E, et al. Hormone replacement therapy for cognitive function in postmenopausal women. *Cochrane Database Syst Rev* 2002; (3): CD3122.
196. *http://www.alz.co.uk/help/associations.html*
197. Gridley, KE, et al. Low concentrations of estradiol reduce beta-amyloid (25–35)-induced toxicity, lipid peroxidation and glucose utilization in human SK-N-SH neuroblastoma cells. *Brain Res* 1997 Dec 5; 778 (1): 158–65.
197. Xu, H, et al. Estrogen reduces neuronal generation of Alzheimer beta-amyloid peptides. *Nat Med* 1998 Apr; 4 (4): 447–51.
198. Seshadri, S, et al. Plasma homocysteine as a risk factor for dementia and Alzheimer's disease. *New Engl J Med* 2002; 346: 476–83.
198. Greenfield, JP, et al. Estrogen lowers Alzheimer beta-amyloid generation by stimulating trans-Golgi network vesicle biogenesis. *J Biol Chem* 2002 Apr 5; 277 (14): 12128–36.
199. Modena, M, et al. Effects of hormone replacement therapy on C-reactive protein levels in healthy postmenopausal women: comparison between oral and transdermal administration of estrogen. *Am J Med* 2002; 113: 331–4.
199. Jaffe, AB, et al. Estrogen regulates metabolism of Alzheimer amyloid beta precursor protein. *J Biol Chem* 1994 May 6; 249 (18): 13065–8. cells induced by Alzheimer's beta-amyloid protein are blocked by estradiol 2001 Feb; 21 (1): 1–13.
200. Garber, K. An end to Alzheimer's? *Technology review* 2001 March; 70–8.
201. *http://www.webmd.com*
202. Mariott, I, et al. Long-term estrogen therapy worsens the behavioral and neuropathological consequences of chronic brain inflammation. *Behav Neurosci* 2002; 116: 902–11.

203–7. Ibid.

208. Korth, C. A co-evolutionary theory of sleep. *Med Hypotheses* 1995 Sep; 45(3): 304–10.
209. Marriott, L, et al. Long-term estrogen therapy worsens the behavioral and neuropathological consequences of chronic brain inflammation. *Behav Neurosci* 2002; 116: 901–11.

CHAPTER NINE

1. Orenstein, F. What's killing the women of Marin county? *Elle* special report 2001; 158.
2. Fortin, JM, et al. Identifying patient preferences for communicating risk estimates: A descriptive pilotstudy. *BMC Med Inform.*
3. Breast cancer. Fifty years ago, a women's risk of developing cancer was about 1 in 22, today it's 1 in 8. *Elle* special report 2001; 290.
4. Yaffe, K, et al. Cognitive decline in women in relation to non-protein bound oestradiol concentrations. *Lancet* 2000; 356: 708–12.
5. Lieman, H, et al. Effects of aging and estradiol supplementation on GH Axis dynamics in women. *J Clin Endocrinometab* 2001; 86: 3918–23.
6. Bruning, P, et al. Insulin resistance and breast cancer risk. *Int J Cancer* 1992; 52: 511–16.
7. Hankinson, S, et al. Plasma prolactin levels and subsequent risk of breast cancer in postmenopausal women. *J Natl Cancer Inst* 1999; 91: 629–34.
8. Hoffmeyer, J. The swarming cyberspace of the body. *Cybernetics and human knowing* 1995; 3: 1–10.
9. Baebrecke, E. How death shapes life during development. *Nat Rev Mol Cell Biol* 2002; 3: 779–87.
10. Von Muhlen, D, et al. Postmenopausal estrogen and increased risk of clinical osteoarthritis at the hip, hand, and knee in older women. *J Womens Health Gend Based Med* 2002; 11: 511–8.
11. Brunelli, R, et al. Hormone replacement therapy effects various immune cell subsets and natural cytotoxicity. *Gynecol Obstet Invest* 1996; 41: 128–31.
12. Albrecht, A, et al. Effect of estrogen replacement therapy on natural killer cell activity in postmenopausal women. *Maturitas* 1996; 25: 217–22.
13. Brooks-Asplund, E, et al. Hormonal modulation of interleukin-6, tumor necrosis factor as associated receptor secretion in postmenopausal women. *Cytokine* 2002; 19: 193.
14. Cushman, M, et al. Effect of postmenopausal hormones on inflammation-sensitive proteins. *Circulation* 1999; 100: 717–22.
15. Koh, K, et al. Effects of continuous combined hormone replacement therapy on inflammation in hypertensive overweight postmenopausal women. *Artheriol Thromb vas Biol* 2002; 221: 459–64.
16. Nezhat, F, et al. Comparative immunohistochemical studies of bcl-2 and p53 proteins in benign and malignant ovarian endometriotic cysts. *Cancer* 2002; 94: 2935–40.
17. Yang, X, et al. Synergistic activation of functional estrogen receptor (ER)-alpha by DNA methyltransferase and histone deacetylase inhibition in human ER-alpha negative breast cancer cells. *Cancer Res* 2001; 61: 7025–29.
18. Starkov, A, et al. Regulation of the energy coupling in mitochondria by some steroid and thyroid hormones. *Biochim Biophys Acta* 1997; 1318: 173–183.
19. *http://www.americanheart.org*
20. Bhavnani, B. Pharmacokinetrics and pharmacodynamics of conjugated equine estrogens: chemistry and metabolism. *Proc Soc Exp Biol* 1998; 217: 6–16.
21. Zhang, F, et al. The major metabolite of equilin, 4-hydroxyequilin, autoxidizes to an o-

quinone which isomerizes to the potent cytotoxin 4-hydroxequilenin-o-quinine. *Chem Res Toxicol* 1999 Feb; 12 (2): 204–13.

22. Chen, Y, et al. The equine estrogen metabolite 4-hydroxyequilenin causes DNA single-strand breaks and oxidation of DNA bases in vitro. *Chem Res Toxicol* 1998; 11: 1105–11.
23. Pisha, E, et al. Evidence that a metabolite of equine estrogens, 4-hydroxyequilenin, induces cellular transformation in vitro. *Chem Res Toxicol* 2001; 14: 82–90.
24. Zhang, F, et al. Synthesis and reactivity of the catechol metabolites from the equine estrogen, 8, 9-dehydroestrone. *Chem Res Toxicol* 2001; 14: 754–63.
25. Ansbacher, R. The pharmacokinetics and efficacy of different estrogens are not equivalent. *Am J Obstet Gynecol* 2001 Feb; 184 (3): 255–63. Review.
26. Yildirir, A, et al. Effects of hormone replacement therapy on plasma homocysteine and C-reactive protein levels. *Gynecol Obstet Invest* 2002; 53: 54–8.
27. Post, MS, et al. Effects of transdermal and oral estrogen replacement therapy on C-reactive protein levels in postmenopausal women: a randomised, placebo-controlled trial. *Thromb Haemost*. 2002 Oct; 88 (4): 605–10.
28. Decensi, A, et al. Effect of transdermal estradiol and oral conjugated estrogen on C-reactive protein in retinoid-placebo trial in healthy women. *Circulation* 2002; 106: 1224–8.
29. Modena, MG, et al. Effects of hormone replacement on C-reactive protein levels in healthy postmenopausal women: comparison between oral and transdermal administration of estrogen. *Am J Med* 2002; 113: 331–4.
30. Vehkavaara, S, et al. Effects or oral and transdermal estrogen replacement therapy markers of coagulation, fibronolysis, inflammation and serum lipids and lipoproteins in postmenopausal women. *Thromb Haemost* 2001; 85: 619–25.
31. Rabbani, L, et al. Oral conjugated equine estrogen increases plasma von Willebrands factor in postmenopausal women. *J Am Coll Cardiol* 2002; 40: 1991–9.
32. Boschetti, C, et al. Short-and long-term effects of hormone replacement therapy transdermal estradiol vs oral conjugated equine estrogens, combined with medroxyprogestereone acetate on blood coagulation factors in postmenopausal women. *Thromb Res* 1991; 62: 1–8.
33. Vidal, A, et al. Estrogen replacement therapy induces telomerase RNA expression. *Fertil and Steril* 2002; 77: 611–8.
34. De Meeus, JB, et al. C-reactive protein levels at the onset of labor and at day 3 post partum in normal pregnancy. *Clin Exp Obstet Gynecol* 1998; 25: 9–11.
35. Jerne, N. The generative grammar of the immune system. Nobel lecture, 1984 December 8.
36. Behl, C. Estrogen as a neuroprotective hormone. *Nature Rev* 2002; 3: 433–40.
37. Song, RX, et al. Apoptotic action of estrogen. *Apoptosis* 2003; 8: 55–60.
38. Hoffman, G, et al. Divergent effects of ovarian steroids on neuronal survival during experimental allergic encephalitis in lewis rats. *Exp Neurol* 2001;171: 272–84.
39. Vegeto, E, et al. Estrogen and progesterone induction of survival of monoblast cells undergoing TNF-alpha-induced apoptosis. *FASEB J* 1999; 13: 793–803.
40. Hou, I, et al. Effect of sex hormones on NK and ADCC activity of mice. *Int J Immunopharmacol* 1988; 10: 15–22.

41. Nielsson, N, et al. Estrogen induces suppression of natural killer cell cytotoxicity and augmentation of polyclonal B cell activation. *Cell Immunol* 1994; 158: 131–9.
42. Mor, G, et al. Interaction of estrogen receptors with the FAS ligand in human monocytes. *J Immunol* 2003; 170: 114–22.
43. Mor, G, et al. Role of the fas/fas ligand system in female reproductive organs survival and apoptosis. *Biochem Pharmacol* 2002; 64: 1305–15.
44. Salmaso, C, et al. Regulation of apoptosis in endocrine autoimmunity. *Ann N Y Acad Sci* 2002; 966: 496–501.
45. Chikanza, J. Mechanisms of corticosteroid resistance in rheumatoid arthritis. *Ann N Y Acad sci* 2002; 9676: 39–48.
46. Castagnetta, L, et al. A role for sex steroids in autoimmune diseases. *Ann NY Acad Sci* 2002; 966: 193–203.
47. Formby, B. Immunologic response in pregnancy. *Endocrinol Metab Clin North Am* 1995; 24: 187–208.
48. Ranson, M, et al. Perspectives on anti-HER monoclonal antibodies. *Oncology* 2002; 63 Suppl 1: 17–24. Review.
49. Arteaga, CL. Overview of epidermal growth factor receptor biology and its role as a therapeutic target in human neoplasia. *Semin Oncol* 2002 Oct; 29 (5 Suppl 14): 3–9. Review.
50. Mentlein, R, et al. The brain and thymus have much in common: a functional analysis of their microenvironments. *Immunol Today* 2000; 21: 133–40.
51. Levin, M, et al. Autoimmunity due to molecular mimicry as a cause of neurological disease. *Nat Med* 2002; 8: 509–13.
52. Klenerman, P, et al. Tracking T cells with tetramers: new tales from new tools. *Nat Rev Immuno* 2002 Apr; 2 (4): 263–72. Review.
53. Yao, V, et al. Dendritic cells. *ANZ J Surg* 2002 Jul; 72 (7): 501–6. Review.
54. Nelson, R, et al. Photoperiodic effects on tumor development and immune function. *J Biol Rhythm* 1994; 9: 233–49.
55. Neeck, G, et al. Involvement of the glucocorticoid receptor in the pathogenesis of rheumatoid arthritis. *Ann N Y Acad Sci* 2002; 966: 491–95.
56. Nakamura, H, et al. Expression of CD40/CD40 ligand and bcl-2 family proteins in labial salvary glands of patients with Sjogren's syndrome. *Lab Invest* 1999; 79: 261–9.
57. Pfeilschifter, J, et al. Changes in proinflammatory cytokine activity after menopause. *Endocrine Rev* 2002; 23: 90–119.
58. Neidhart, M. Prolactin in autoimmune diseases. *Proc Soc Exp Biol Med* 1998; 217: 408–14.
59. Eguchi, K. Apoptosis in autoimmune diseases. *Intern Med* 2001; 40: 275–84.
60. Brenner, A, et al. History of allergies and autoimmune diseases and risk of brain tumor in adults. *Int J Cancer* 2002; 99: 252.
61. Tanaseanu, C, et al. The antiphospholipid antibodies. *Haematologia* 2002; 31: 287–302.
62. Hoel, A, et al. Analysis of peripheral blood lymphocyte subsets, NK cells and delayed type hypersensitivity skin test in patients with premature ovarian failure. *Am J Reprod Immunol* 1995; 33: 495–502.

63. Wiemels, J, et al. History of allergies among adults with glioma and controls. *Int J Cancer* 2002; 98: 609–15.
64. Wrensch, M, et al. Prevalence of antibodies to four herpes viruses among adults with glioma and controls. *Am J Epidemiol* 2001; 154: 161–5.
65. Straub, R, et al. Involvement of the hypothalamic-pituitary-adrenal/gonadal axis and the peripheral nervous system. *Arthritis Rheum* 2001; 44: 493–501.
66. Symmons, D. Neoplasms of the immune system in rheumatoid arthritis. *Am J Med* 1985; 78: 22–8.
67. Plater-Zyberg, C, et al. Phenotypic and functional features of CD5 B lymphocytes in rheumatoid athhritis.
68. Zoli, A, et al. Prolactin/cortisol ratio in rheumatoid arthritis. *Ann N Y Acad Sci* 2002; 966: 508–12.
69. Kumagai, S, et al. Possible different mechanisms of B cell activation in systemic lupus erythromatosis and rheumatoid arthritis: opposite expression of low-affininity receptors for IgE (CD23) on their peripheral B cells. *Clin Exp Immunol* 1989; 7848–53.
70. Baecklund, D. Rheumatoid arthritis ups lymphoma risk. *Brit Med J* 1998; 317: 180–1.
71. Ibid.
72. Huisman, A, et al. Glucocorticoid receptor down regulation in early diagnosed rheumatoid arthritis. *Ann N Y Acad Sci* 2002; 966: 64–67.
73. Ibid.
74. Cardarelli, R, et al. Binding to CD20 by anti-B1 antibody or F(ab')(2) is sufficient induction of apoptosis in B-cell lines. *Cancer Immunol Immunother* 2002; 51: 15–24.
75. Souza, SS, et al. Influence of menstrual cycle on NK activity. *J Reprod Immunol* 2001; 50: 51–9.
76. Deans, J, et al. CD20-mediated apoptosis: signaling through lipid rafts. *Immunology* 2002; 107: 176–82.
77. Huisman, A. Glucocortoid receptor down regulation in early diagnosed rheumatoid arthritis. *Ann N Y Acad Sci* 2002; 966: 64–67.
78. Cardarelli, P, et al. Binding to CD20 by anti-B1 antibody or F(ab')(2) is sufficient indiction of apoptos B-cell lines. *Cancer Immunol Immunother* 2002; 51: 15–24.
79. Souza, S, et al. Influence of menstrual cycle on NK activity. *J Reprod Immunol* 2001; 50: 151–9.
80. Kennedy, GA, et al. Incidence and nature of CD20-negative relapses following retuximab therapy aggressive B-cell non-Hodgkin's lymphoma: a retrospective review. *Br J Haematol* 2002 Nov; 11: 6.
81. Incidence of nature of CD20-negative relapses following retuxin therapy in aggressive B-cell non-Hodgkin's lymphoma:a retrospective review. *Brit J Haematol* 2002; 119: 412–6.
82. Niels, Jerne. The generative grammar of the immune system. Nobel lecture, 1984 December 8.
83. Niels, Jerne. The generative grammar of the immune system. Nobel Lecture, 1984 December 8.
84. Sternberg, E, et al. *The mind-body interaction in disease. Mysteries of the mind.* McGill University Press, 1996.

85. Born, J, et al. Effects of sleep and circadian rhythm on human circulating immune cells. *J Immunol* 1997; 158: 4454–64.
86. Physician Desk Reference. *www.pdr.net*.
87. Hoffmeyer, J. Biosemiotics: Towards a new synthesis in biology. *Eur J Semiotic Studies* 1997; 9: 355–76.
88. Alzheimer's facts and statistics. *Healingwithnutrition.com*

CHAPTER TEN

1. Friedan, Betty. *The fountain of age*. Simon & Schuster, New York, NY, 1993. Page 15.
2. Greer, Germaine. *The change: women, aging and the menopause*. Random House, New York, NY, 1991. Page 7.
3. Bachmann, GA. The changes before 'the change'. Strategies for the transition to the menopause. *Postgrad Med* 1994 Mar; 95 (4): 113–5, 119–21, 124. Review.
4. Sheehy, Gail. *The silent passage*. Pocket Books, New York, NY, 1993. Page 14.
5. Mead, Margaret, et al. *Blackberry winter: My earlier years.* (Kodansha Globe), Kodansha International, Reprint edition, June 1995.
6. Coutinho, Elsimar M, et al. *Is menstruation obsolete?* Oxford University Press, New York, NY, 1999. Page 5.
7. Strassmann, BI, et al. Life-history theory, fertility and reproductive success in humans. *Proc R Soc Lond B Biol Sci* 2002 Mar 22; 269 (1491): 553–62.
8. Strassmann, BI. Menstrual cycling and breast cancer: an evolutionary perspective. *J Women's Health* 1999 Mar; 8 (2): 193–202. Review.
9. Strassmann, BI, et al. Predictors of fecundability and conception waits among the Dogon of Mali. *Am J Phys Anthropol* 1998 Feb; 105 (2): 167–84.
10. Grant, EC. Dangers of suppressing menstruation. *Lancet* 2000 Aug 5; 356 (9228): 513–4.
11. Thomas, Sarah L, et al. Nuisance or natural and healthy: should monthly menstruation be optional for women? *Lancet* 2000 March 11; 355: 408–12.
12. Pike, MC, et al. Breast cancer prevention through modulation of endogenous hormones. *Breast Cancer Res Treat* 1993 Nov; 28 (2): 179–93. Review.
13. Pike, MC, et al. The prevention of breast cancer through reduced ovarian steroid exposure. *Acta Oncol* 1992; 31 (2): 167–74. Review.
14. Pike, MC, et al. Do regular ovulatory cycles increase breast cancer risk? *Cancer* 1985 Sep 1; 56 (5): 1206–8.
15. Pike, MC, et al. "Incessant ovulation" and ovarian cancer. *Lancet* 1979 Jul 28; 2 (8135): 170–3.
16. Coutinho, Elsimar M, et al. *Is menstruation obsolete?* Oxford University Press, New York, NY, 1999.
17. Ganong, William F. *Review of medical physiology*. Simon & Schuster, New York, NY, 1995. Page 406.
18. Henderson, K, et al. Comparison of the merits of measuring equine chorionic gonadotrophin (eCG) and blood and faecal concentrations of estrone sulphate for determining the pregnancy status of miniature horses. *Reprod Fertil Dev* 1998; 10 (5): 441–4.
19. Ginsburg, ES, et al. Half-life of estradiol in postmenopausal women. *Gynecol Obstet Invest* 1998; 45 (1): 45–8.

20. Reiss, Uzzi. *Natural hormone balance for women*. Pocket Books, New York, NY, 2001. Pages 38–40.
21. Starkov, AA, et al. Regulation of the energy coupling in mitochondria by some steroid and thyroid hormones. *Biochim Biophys Acta* 1997 Jan 16; 1318 (1–2): 173–83.
22. Nevretdinova, Z, et al. Some aspects of lipid metabolism and thyroid function in arctic ground squirrel, Citellus parryi during hibernation. *Arctic Med Res* 1992 Oct; 51 (4): 196–204.
23. Vasudevan, N, et al. Estrogen and thyroid hormone receptor interactions: physiological flexibility by molecular specificity. *Physiol Rev* 2002 Oct; 82 (4): 923–44. Review.
24. Wang, SH, et al. 2-Methoxyestradiol, an endogenous estrogen metabolite, induces thyroid cell apoptosis. *Mol Cell Endocrinol* 2000 Jul 25; 165 (1–2): 163–72.
25. Cecconi, S, et al. Thyroid hormone effects on mouse oocyte maturation and granulosa cell aromatase activity. *Endocrinology* 1999 Apr; 140 (4): 1783–8.
26. Carter-Su, C, et al. Molecular mechanism of growth hormone action. *Annu Rev Physiol* 1996; 58: 187–207. Review.
27. Gonzalez-Sancho, JM, et al. Inhibition of proliferation and expression of T1 and cyclin D1 genes by thyroid hormone in mammary epithelial cells. *Mol Carcinog* 2002 May; 34 (1): 25–34.
28. Tazebay, Uygar H, et al. The mammary gland iodide transporter is expressed during lactation and in breast cancer. *Nat Med* 2000 Aug; 6 (8): 871–8.
29. Prasad, R, et al. Thyroid hormones modulate zinc transport activity of rat intestinal and renal brush-border membrane. *Am J Physiol* 1999 Apr; 276 (4 Pt 1): E774–82.
30. Pringle, T. The relationship between thyroxine, oestradiol, and postnatal alopecia, with relevance to women's health in general. *Med Hypotheses* 2000 Nov; 55 (5): 445–9.
31. Huopio, H, et al. Acute insulin response tests for the differential diagnosis of congenital hyperinsulinism. *J Clin Endocrinol Metab* 2002 Oct; 87 (10): 4502–7.
32. Ganong, William F. *Review of medical physiology*. Simon & Schuster, New York, NY, 1995. Page 308.
33. Schwartz, MW, et al. Model for the regulation of energy balance and adiposity by the central nervous system. *Am J Clin Nutr* 1999 Apr; 69 (4): 584–96. Review.
34. Heilbronn, LK, et al. Effect of energy restriction, weight loss, and diet composition on plasma lipids and glucose in patients with type 2 diabetes. *Diabetes Care* 1999 Jun; 22 (6): 889–95.
35. Taubes, G. Nutrition: The soft science of dietary fat. *Science* 2001 Mar 30; 291 (5513): 2536–45.
36. Heitmann, Berit L, et al. Genetic effects on weight change and food intake in Swedish adult twins. Am *J Clin Nutr* 1999 Apr; 69 (4): 597–602.
37. Mukherjea, R, et al. Elevated leptin concentrations in pregnancy and lactation: possible role as a modulator of substrate utilization. *Life Sci* 1999; 65 (11): 1183–93.
38. Sites, CK, et al. Relation of regional fat distribution to insulin sensitivity in postmenopausal women. *Fertil Steril* 2000 Jan; 73 (1): 61–5.
39. Kristensen, K, et al. Regulation of leptin by steroid hormones in rat adipose tissue. *Biochem Biophys Res Commun* 1999 Jun 16; 259 (3): 624–30.

40. Kaye, SA, et al. Associations of body mass and fat distribution with sex hormone concentrations in postmenopausal women. *Int J Epidemiol* 1991 Mar; 20 (1): 151–6.
41. Tchernof, A, et al. Sex hormone-binding globulin levels in middle-aged premenopausal women. Associations with visceral obesity and metabolic profile. *Diabetes Care* 1999 Nov; 22 (11): 1875–81.
42. Perrone, G, et al. Evaluation of the body composition and fat distribution in long-term users of hormone replacement therapy. *Gynecol Obstet Invest* 1999; 48 (1): 52–5.
43. Posaci, C, et al. Effects of HRT on serum levels of IGF-I in postmenopausal women. *Maturitas* 2001 Oct 31; 40 (1): 69–74.
44. Cecconi, S, et al. Thyroid hormone effects on mouse oocyte maturation and granulosa cell aromatase activity. *Endocrinology* 1999 Apr; 140 (4): 1783–8.
45. Carter-Su, C, et al. Molecular mechanism of growth hormone action. *Annu Rev Physiol* 1996; 58: 187–207. Review.
46. Gonzalez-Sancho, JM, et al. Inhibition of proliferation and expression of T1 and cyclin D1 genes by thyroid hormone in mammary epithelial cells. *Mol Carcinog* 2002 May; 34 (1): 25–34.
47. Bagis, T, et al. The effects of short-term medroxyprogesterone acetate and micronized progesterone on glucose metabolism and lipid profiles in patients with polycystic ovary syndrome: a prospective randomized study. *J Clin Endocrinol Metab* 2002 Oct; 87 (10): 4536–40.
48. Mueck, AO, et al. Urinary excretion of insulin after estradiol treatment of postmenopausal women. *Clin Exp Obstet Gynecol* 1997; 24 (1): 11–3.
49. Brann, DW, et al. Regulation of leptin gene expression and secretion by steroid hormones. *Steroids* 1999 Sep; 64 (9): 659–63.
50. Nieuwenhuizen, AG, et al. Progesterone stimulates pancreatic cell proliferation in vivo. *Eur J Endocrinol* 1999 Mar; 140 (3): 256–63.
51. Geary, N. Estradiol and appetite. *Appetite* 2000 Dec; 35 (3): 273–4.
52. Rocha, M, et al. The anorectic effect of oestradiol does not involve changes in plasma and cerebrospinal fluid leptin concentrations in the rat. *J Endocrinol* 2001 Nov; 171 (2): 349–54.
53. Davis, SN, et al. Brain of the conscious dog is sensitive to physiological changes in circulating insulin. *Am J Physiol* 1997 Apr; 272 (4 Pt 1): E567–75.
54. Michener, W, et al. The role of low progesterone and tension as triggers of perimenstrual chocolate and sweets craving: some negative experimental evidence. *Physiol Behav* 1999 Sep; 67 (3): 417–20.
55. Tempel, DL, et al. Adrenal steroid receptors: interactions with brain neuropeptide systems in relation to nutrient intake and metabolism. *J Neuroendocrinol* 1994 Oct; 6 (5): 479–501. Review.
56. Willner, P, et al. "Depression" increases "craving" for sweet rewards in animal and human models of depression and craving. *Psychopharmacology (Berl)* 1998 Apr; 136 (3): 272–83.
57. Melzig, ME, et al. In vitro pharmacological activity of the tetrahydroisoquinoline salsolinol present in products from Theobroma cacao L. like cocoa and chocolate. *J Ethnopharmacol* 2000 Nov; 73 (1–2): 153–9.

58. Vassen, L, et al. Human insulin receptor substrate-2 (IRS-2) is a primary progesterone response gene. *Mol Endocrinol* 1999 Mar; 13 (3): 485–94.
59. Tchernof, A, et al. Weight loss reduces C-reactive protein levels in obese postmenopausal women. *Circulation* 2002 Feb 5; 105 (5): 564–9.
60. No author. Healthy living. *New Scientist* 2002 November 2; 25.
61. Zinman, B, et al. Circulating tumor necrosis factor-alpha concentrations in a native Canadian population with high rates of type 2 diabetes mellitus. *J Clin Endocrinol Metab* 1999 Jan; 84 (1): 272–8.
62. Eizirik, DL, et al. Identification of genes and proteins involved in B-cell damage and repair in Type 1 diabetes mellitus. *Diabetes* 1998; 19: 9–11.
63. Sowers, ME, et al. Testosterone concentrations in women aged 25–50 years: associations with lifestyle, body composition, and ovarian status. *Am J Epidemiol* 2001 Feb 1; 153 (3): 256–64.
64. Marsden, P, et al. Severe impairment of insulin action in adipocytes from amenorrheic subjects with polycystic ovary syndrome. *Metabolism* 1994 Dec; 43 (12): 1536–42.
65. Rose, DP, et al. Adverse effects of obesity on breast cancer prognosis, and the biological actions of leptin (Review). *Int J Oncol* 2002 Dec; 21 (6): 1285–92.
66. Wilett, WC. Dietary fat intake and cancer risk: a controversial and instructive story *Semin Cancer Biol* 1998 Aug; 8 (4): 245–53.
67. Holmes, MD, et al. Dietary factors and the survival of women with breast carcinoma. *Cancer* 1999 Sep 1; 86 (5): 826–35.
68. Mokdad, AH, et al. The continuing epidemic of obesity in the United States. *JAMA* 2000 Oct 4; 284 (13): 1650–1.
69. Matkovic, V, et al. Leptin is inversely related to age at menarche in human females. *J Clin Endocrinol Metab* 1997 Oct; 82 (10): 3239–45.
70. O'Sullivan, AJ, et al. The route of estrogen replacement therapy confers divergent effects on substrate oxidation and body composition in postmenopausal women. *J Clin Invest* 1998 Sep 1; 102 (5): 1035–40.
71. Barr, SI. Vegetarianism and menstrual cycle disturbances: is there an association? *Am J Clin Nutr* 1999 Sep; (3 Suppl): 549S–54S. Review.
72. Barnard, ND. Vegetarianism and women's health. *Alternative Therapies in Women's Health* 2000 June; 2 (6): 41–8.
73. MohanKumar, PS, et al. Effects of chronic hyperprolactinemia on tuberoinfundibular dopaminergic neurons. *Proc Soc Exp Biol Med* 1998 Apr; 217 (4): 461–5.
74. Peeva, E, et al. Bromocriptine restores tolerance in estrogen-treated mice. *J Clin Invest* 2000 Dec; 106 (11): 1373–9.
75. Hu, ZZ, et al. Prolactin Receptor Gene Diversity: Stucture and Regulation. *Trends in Endocrinology and Metabolism* 1998; 9 (3): 94–102.
76. Freemark, M, et al. Ontogenesis of prolactin receptors in the human fetus in early gestation. Implications for tissue differentiation and development. *J Clin Invest* 1997 Mar 1; 99 (5): 1107–17.
77. Brosens, JJ, et al. Progesterone receptor regulates decidual prolactin expression in differentiating human endometrial stromal cells. *Endocrinology* 1999 Oct; 140 (10): 4809–20.

78. Nishikawa, S, et al. Progesterone and EGF inhibit mouse mammary gland prolactin receptor and betacasein gene expression. *Am J Physiol* 1994 Nov; 267 (5 Pt 1): C1467–72.
79. Mizoguchi, Y, et al. The regulation of the prolactin receptor gene expression in the mammary gland of early pregnant mouse. *Endocr J* 1997 Feb; 44 (1): 53–8.
80. Rensing, L, et al. Biological timing and the clock metaphor: oscillatory and hourglass mechanisms. *Chronobiol Int* 2001 May; 18 (3): 329–69. Review.
81. DeRijk, R, et al. Exercise and circadian rhythm-induced variations in plasma cortisol differentially regulate interleukin-1 beta (IL-1 beta), IL-6, and tumor necrosis factor-alpha (TNF alpha) production in humans: high sensitivity of TNF alpha and resistance of IL-6. *J Clin Endocrinol Metab* 1997 Jul; 82 (7): 2182–91.
82. Barash, I. Prolactin and insulin synergize to regulate the translation modulator PHAS-I via mitogen-activated protein kinase-independent but wortmannin- and rapamycin-sensitive pathway. *Mol Cell Endocrinol* 1999 Sep 10; 155 (1–2): 37–49.
83. Scavone, JM, et al. Acetaminophen pharmacokinetics in women receiving conjugated estrogen. *Eur J Clin Pharmacol* 1990; 38 (1): 97–8.
84. Nolen, TM. Sedative effects of antihistamines: safety, performance, learning, and quality of life. *Clin Ther* 1997 Jan–Feb; 19 (1): 39–55; discussion 2–3. Review.
85. Walsh, GM, et al. New insights into the second generation antihistamines. *Drugs* 2001; 61 (2): 207–36. Review.
86. Welch, MJ, et al. H1-antihistamines and the central nervous system. *Clin Allergy Immunol* 2002; 17: 337–88. Review.
87. Graeff, FG, et al. Modulation of the brain aversive system by GABAergic and serotonergic mechanisms. *Behav Brain Res* 1986 Jul; 21 (1): 65–72.
88. Kulig, E, et al. The effects of estrogen on prolactin gene methylation in normal and neoplastic rat pituitary tissues. *Am J Pathol* 1992 Jan; 140 (1): 207–14.
89. Vakkuri, O, et al. Decrease in melatonin precedes follicle-stimulating hormone increase during perimenopause. *Eur J Endocrinol* 1996 Aug; 135 (2): 188–92.
90. Rohr, UD, et al. Melatonin deficiencies in women. *Maturitas* 2002 Apr 15; 41 Suppl 1: S85–104. Review.
91. Cos, S, et al. Effects of melatonin on the cell cycle kinetics and "estrogen-rescue" of MCF-7 human breast cancer cells in culture. *J Pineal Res* 1991 Jan; 10 (1): 36–42.
92. Cohen, M, et al. Hypotheses: melatonin/steroid combination contraceptives will prevent breast cancer. *Breast Cancer Res Treat* 1995 Mar; 33 (3): 257–64.
93. Nelson, RJ, et al. Photoperiodic effects on tumor development and immune function. *J Biol Rhythms* 1994 Winter; 9 (3–4): 233–49.
94. Karbownik, M, et al. Anticarcinogenic actions of melatonin which involve antioxidative processes: comparison with other antioxidants. *Int J Biochem Cell Biol* 2001 Aug; 33 (8): 735–53. Review.
95. Stevens, RG, et al. Light in the built environment: potential role of circadian disruption in endocrine disruption and breast cancer. *Cancer Causes Control* 2001 Apr; 12 (3): 279–87. Review.
96. Karbownik, M, et al. Melatonin attenuates estradiol-induced oxidative damage to DNA: relevance for cancer prevention. *Exp Biol Med (Maywood)* 2001 Jul; 226 (7): 707–12.

97. San Martin, M, et al. Progesterone inhibits, on a circadian basis, the release of melatonin by rat pineal perifusion. *Steroids* 2000 Apr; 65 (4): 206–9.
98. Luboshitzky, R, et al. Increased 6-sulfatoxymelatonin excretion in women with polycystic ovary syndrome. *Fertil Steril* 2001 Sep; 76 (3): 506–10.
99. Rimler, A, et al. Melatonin elicits nuclear exclusion of the human androgen receptor and attenuates its activity. *Prostate* 2001 Oct 1; 49 (2): 145–54.
100. Eppler, E, et al. IGF-I in human breast cancer: low differentiation stage is associated with decreased IGF-I content. *Eur J Endocrinol* 2002 Jun; 146 (6): 813–21.
101. Anderson, SM, et al. E2 supplementation selectively relieves GH's autonegative feedback on GH-releasing peptide-2-stimulated GH secretion. *J Clin Endocrinol Metab* 2001 Dec; 86 (12): 5904–11.
102. Ishido, M, et al. Magnetic fields (MF) of 50 Hz at 1.2 microT as well as 100 microT cause uncoupling of inhibitory pathways of adenylyl cyclase mediated by melatonin 1a receptor in MF-sensitive MCF-7 cells. *Carcinogenesis* 2001 Jul; 22 (7): 1043–8.
103. Rose, J, et al. Melatonin-induced downregulation of uterine prolactin receptors in mink (Mustela vison). *Gen Comp Endocrinol* 1996 Jul; 103 (1): 101–6.
104. Akerstedt, T, et al. A 50-Hz electromagnetic field impairs sleep. *J Sleep Res* 1999 Mar; 8 (1): 77–81.
105. Davis, S, et al. Residential magnetic fields, light-at-night, and nocturnal urinary 6-sulfatoxymelatonin concentration in women. *Am J Epidemiol* 2001 Oct 1; 154 (7): 591–600.
106. Davis, S, et al. Night shift work, light at night, and risk of breast cancer. *J Natl Cancer Inst* 2001 Oct 17; 93 (20): 1557–62.
107. Schernhammer, ES, et al. Rotating night shifts and risk of breast cancer in women participating in the nurses' health study. *J Natl Cancer Inst* 2001 Oct 17; 93 (20): 1563–8.
108. Midwinter, MJ, et al. Adaptation of the melatonin rhythm in human subjects following night-shift work in Antarctica. *Neurosci Lett* 1991 Jan 28; 122 (2): 195–8.
109. Rohr, UD, et al. Melatonin deficiencies in women. *Maturitas* 2002 Apr 15; 41 Suppl 1: S85–104. Review.
110. Rato, A, Pedrero, J, Martinez, M, et al. Melatonin blocks the activation of estrogen receptor for DNA binding. *FASEB J* 1999; 13: 857–68.
111. Baldwin, WS, et al. Melatonin: receptor-mediated events that may affect breast and other steroid hormone-dependent cancers. *Mol Carcinog* 1998 Mar; 21 (3): 149–55. Review.
112. Greendale, GA, et al. Bone mass response to discontinuation of long-term hormone replacement therapy: results from the Postmenopausal Estrogen/Progestin Interventions (PEPI) Safety Follow-up Study. *Arch Intern Med* 2002 Mar 25; 162 (6): 665–72.
113. Grady, D, et al. Postmenopausal hormone therapy for prevention of fractures: how good is the evidence? *JAMA* 2001 Jun 13; 285 (22): 2909–10.
114. Ducy, P, et al. Leptin inhibits bone formation through a hypothalamic relay: a central control of bone mass. *Cell* 2000 Jan 21; 100 (2): 197–207.
115. Otsuka, F, et al. A negative feedback system between oocyte bone morphogenetic protein 15 and granulosa cell kit ligand: its role in regulating granulosa cell mitosis. *Proc Natl Acad Sci* (USA) 2002 Jun 11; 99 (12): 8060–5.

116. Ishida, Y, et al. Pharmacologic doses of medroxyprogesterone may cause bone loss through glucocorticoid activity: an hypothesis. *Osteoporos Int* 2002 Aug; 13 (8): 601–5. Review.
117. Torgerson, DJ, et al. Hormone replacement therapy and prevention of nonvertebral fractures: a meta-analysis of randomized trials. *JAMA* 2001 Jun 13; 285 (22): 2891–7. Review.
118. Prasad, R, et al. Osteoporosis with underlying connective tissue disease: an unusual case. *Ann N Y Acad Sci* 2002 Jun; 966: 474–7.
119. Cooper, LF, et al. Estrogen-induced resistance to osteoblast apoptosis is associated with increased hsp27 expression. *J Cell Physiol* 2000 Dec; 185 (3): 401–7.
120. Beral, V, et al. Evidence from randomised trials on the long-term effects of hormone replacement therapy. *Lancet* 2002 Sep 21; 360 (9337): 942–4. Review.
121. Oleksik, AM, et al. Effects of the selective estrogen receptor modulator, raloxifene, on the somatotropic axis and insulin-glucose homeostasis. *J Clin Endocrinol Metab* 2001 Jun; 86 (6): 2763–8.
122. Lufkin, EG, et al. Treatment of postmenopausal osteoporosis with transdermal estrogen. *Ann Intern Med* 1992 Jul 1; 117 (1): 1–9.
123. Weiss, SR, et al. A randomized controlled trial of four doses of transdermal estradiol for preventing postmenopausal bone loss. Transdermal Estradiol Investigator Group. *Obstet Gynecol* 1999 Sep; 94 (3): 330–6.
124. Heiss, CJ, et al. Associations of body fat distribution, circulating sex hormones, and bone density in postmenopausal women. *J Clin Endocrinol Metab* 1995 May; 80 (5): 1591–6.
125. O'Meara, E, et al. Hormone replacement therapy after a diagnosis of breast cancer in relation to recurrence and mortality. *J Natl Cancer Inst* 2001; 93: 754–5.
126. Sivaraman, L, et al. Hormone-induced protection against breast cancer. *J Mammary Gland Biol Neoplasia* 2002; 7: 77–92.
127. Wiley, TS, et al. *Sex, lies & menopause: The shocking truth about hormone replacement.* William Morrow Publishing. New York, NY, 2003 Pages 1–390.
128. Martorano, JT, et al. Differentiating between natural progesterone and synthetic progestins: clinical implications for premenstrual syndrome and perimenopause management. *Compr Ther* 1998 Jun–Jul; 24 (6–7): 336–9. Review.
129. Rebar, RW. Progestogens not effective for PMS. *Journal Watch* 2001 Nov 15; 179.
130. Wyatt, K, et al. Efficacy of progesterone and progestrogens in management of premenstrual syndrome: systematic review. *BMJ* 2001 Oct 6; 323 (7316): 776–80.
131. Jordan, VC, et al. The estrogenic activity of synthetic progestins used in oral contraceptives. *Cancer* 1993 Feb 15; 71 (4 Suppl): 1501–5. Review.
132. *http://www.aafp.org/afp/20000301/1391.html.* Managing Menopause.
133. Tarkan, L. Natural remedies for menopause gain popularity. *The New York Times*, Health & Fitness, 2000 June 20. Page D7.
134. *http://www.lotushcf.org.tw/paper/paper03e.htm.* Traditional chinese dietary for health and nutrition.
135. *http://www.families-first.com/hotflash/faq/soy.htm.* What is Red Clover?
136. *http://www.webhealth.co.uk/Research=_Articles=_Relating=_to=_/About=_Soya=_Research/about=_soya=_research.html.* About Soya Research.

137. Woodman, R. More evidence soy guards against breast cancer. Yahoo! News. Health. 2002 Jul 8.
138. Grady, D. Breast Cancer Study on Alternative Therapy. *New York Times*, National Section, 1999 June 3. Page A16.
139. MacKenzie, D. Swallow it whole: Herbalists say their extracts are more potent than purified drugs. Now science is backing them up. *New Scientist* 2001 May 26; 38–40.
140. Matthews, R. TV homeopathy trial was 'flawed'. *New Scientist* 2002 Dec; 7: 10.
141. Hooley, R, et al. A higher plant seven-transmembrane receptor that influences sensitivity to cytokinins. *Curr Biol* 1998 Mar 12; 8 (6): 315–24.
142. Tomita, N. Risk factors for circulatory disease in patients on antihypertensive drug treatment. *Nippon Koshu Eisei Zasshi* 1998 Feb; 45 (2): 112–20. Japanese.
143. Mehra, MR, et al. Ethnic disparity in clinical outcome after heart transplantation is abrogated using tacrolimus and mycophenolate mofetil-based immunosuppression. *Transplantation* 2002 Dec 15; 74 (11): 1568–73.
144. Dev, AT, et al. Southeast Asian patients with chronic hepatitis C: the impact of novel genotypes and race on treatment outcome. *Hepatology* 2002 Nov; 36 (5): 1259–65.
145. Jensen-Fangel, S, et al. The effect of race/ethnicity on the outcome of highly active antiretroviral therapy for human immunodeficiency virus type 1-infected patients. *Clin Infect Dis* 2002 Dec 15; 35 (12): 1541–8.
146. Kalus, JS, et al. Role of race in the pharmacotherapy of heart failure. *Ann Pharmacother* 2002 Mar; 36 (3): 471–8. Review.
147. Wilson, JF, et al. Population genetic structure of variable drug response. *Nat Genet* 2001 Nov; 29 (3): 265–9.
148. Klinge, CM. Estrogen receptor interaction with co-activators and co-repressors. *Steroids* 2000 May; 65 (5): 227–51. Review.
149. Formby, B, Wiley, TS. Insulin Modulates Expression of the Estrogen-Induced Genes bcl-2, c-fos and LuCa-2 in MCF-7 Breast Tumor Cells: Evidence for an Association between Cancer Risk and Type 2 Diabetes? 58th Annual Meeting & Scientific Sessions, American Diabetes Association 1997 June 13–16.
150. Panet-Raymond, V, et al. Interactions between androgen and estrogen receptors and the effects on their transactivational properties. *Mol Cell Endocrinol* 2000 Sep 25; 167 (1–2): 139–50.
151. Clottes, J. *The shamans of prehistory.* Harry N. Abrams, New York, NY, 1998. Page 120.
152. MacKenzie, D. Swallow it whole: Herbalists say their extracts are more potent than purified drugs. Now science is backing them up. *New Scientist* 2001 May 26; 38–40.
153. Temburni, MK, et al. Receptor targeting and heterogeneity at interneuronal nicotinic cholinergic synapses *in vivo. Journal of Physiology* 2000; 525.1:21–29.
154. *http://www.fcmsdocs.org/Conference/10th/10herbaltherapyforwomen.html.* Herbal Therapy for Women.
155. Ibid.
156. Ibid.
157. Hooley, R, et al. A higher plant seven-transmembrane receptor that influences sensitivity to cytokinins. *Curr Biol* 1998 Mar 12; 8 (6): 315–24.

158. Coughlan, A. Shared roots: Hormones took control long before plants and animals went their separate ways. *New Scientist* 1998 Feb; 28:6.
159. Darwin, Charles, LLD, FRS. The power of movement in plants. John Murray & Sons, London, England, 1880. Page 461.
160. Phillips, H. They may be green, but plants ain't stupid: Not just a pretty face. *New Scientist* 2002 July 27; 40–43.
161. *http://www.bierengezondheid.be/index=_eng.jsp?Page=Dos215&Doc=hop*. Medicinal properties of the hop.
162. Milligan, SR, et al. The endocrine activities of 8-prenylnaringenin and related hop (Humulus lupulus L.) flavonoids. *J Clin Endocrinol Metab* 2000 Dec; 85 (12): 4912–5.
163. Riddle, JM. *Eve's herbs: A history of contraception and abortion in the west*. Harvard University Press, Cambridge, MA, 1997. Pages 25, 26, 222–224.
164. Fraser, Robert, et al. *Golden Bough*. Palgrave Macmillan Publishing. New York, NY, 2002. Pages 103–127, 772.
165. *http://usa.weleda.com/medicines/mistletoe.asp*. Cancer treatments. Introducing an unusual plant. What is Mistletoe?
166. *http://www.weleda.co.nz/Prod08=_Iscador.html*.
167. *http://www.fcmsdocs.org/Conference/10th/10herbaltherapyforwomen.html*. Herbal Therapy for Women.
168. Eluere, C. *The celts: first masters of Europe*. Thames and Hudson, New Horizons, 1992.
169. Fraser, Robert, et al. *Golden bough*. Palgrave Macmillan Publishing, New York, NY, 2002. Page 764.
170. Ibid.
171. Ibid.
172. *http://iscador.com/*. Homepage.
173. *http://www.weleda.co.nz/Prod08=_Iscador.html*.
174. *http://www.paam.net/media.htm*. Iscador in the Media.
175. Lavelle, EC, et al. Mistletoe lectins enhance immune responses to intranasally co-administered herpes simplex virus glycoprotein D2. *Immunology* 2002 Oct; 107 (2): 268–74.
176. Tabiasco, J, et al. Mistletoe viscotoxins increase natural killer cell-mediated cytotoxicity. *Eur J Biochem* 2002 May; 269 (10): 2591–600.
177. *http://www.westonaprice.org/askdoctor/ask=_cancer.html*. Ask the Doctor About a Treatment for Cancer.
178. Kruzel, TA. The role of lectins in the formation of disease and their potential use in treatment. Southwest College of Naturopathic Medicine & Health Sciences.
179. Siegle, I, et al. Combined cytotoxic action of Viscum album agglutinin-1 and anticancer agents against human A549 lung cancer cells. *Anticancer Res* 2001 Jul–Aug; 21 (4A): 2687–91.
180. *http://www3.cancer.gov/legis/testimony/camtestimony.html*. Integrative Oncology: Cancer care for the next millenium.
181. Lewin, J, et al. Progesterone: a novel adjunct to intravesical chemotherapy. *BJU Int* 2002 Nov; 90 (7): 736–41.

182. Maggiolini, M, et al. Estrogen receptor alpha mediates the proliferative but not the cytotoxic dose-dependent effects of two major phytoestrogens on human breast cancer cells. *Mol Pharmacol* 2001 Sep; 60 (3): 595–602.
183. *http://www.sbherbals.com/NutritionTip15.html.* Nutrition tip #15: Soy-Pros & Cons.
184. Schellenberg R, et al. Treatment for the premenstrual syndrome with agnus castus fruit extract: prospective, randomized, placebo controlled study. *British Medical Journal* 2001; 322: 134–137.
185. Bergmann, J, et al. The efficacy of the complex medication Phyto-Hypophyson L in female, hormone-related sterility. A randomized, placebo-controlled clinical double-blind study. *Forsch Komplementarmed Klass Naturheilkd* 2000 Aug; 7 (4): 190–9. German.
186. Wu, LS, et al. Ginseng flowers stimulate progesterone production from bovine luteal cells. *Am J Chin Med* 2000; 28 (3–4): 371–7.
187. Freedman, RR, et al. Estrogen raises the sweating threshold in postmenopausal women with hot flashes. *Fertil Steril* 2002 Mar; 77 (3): 487–90.
188. Stachenfeld, NS, et al. Estrogen and progesterone effects on transcapillary fluid dynamics. *Am J Physiol Regul Integr Comp Physiol* 2001 Oct; 281 (4): R1319–29.
189. Loprinzi, CL, et al. Tamoxifen-induced hot flashes. *Clin Breast Cancer* 2000 Apr; 1 (1): 52–6.
190. Saitz, R. Alternative Therapies for menopausal symptoms: evidence is limited. *Journal Watch* 2003 Jan 15; 15.
191. *http://nerdatabank.nic.in/csirmedicine.htm.* North East India: Medicinal Plants.
192. *http://www.motherearthherbs.com/phytosterols.html.* Hormonally active plants.
193. Davis, SR. Phytoestrogen therapy for menopausal symptoms? *BMJ* 2001 Aug 18; 323 (7309): 354–5.
194. *http://www.j-t-s.org/Other/HRT/faq.htm.* Transition into the Light. HRT-Hormone Replacement Therapy.
195. *http://www.eatright.org/erm/erm030800.html.* Phytochemicals: The Power of Produce.
196. *http://www.fcmsdocs.org/Conference/10th/10herbaltherapyforwomen.html.* Herbal Therapy for Women.
197. Schneeman, BO. Building scientific consensus: the importance of dietary fiber. *Am J Clin Nutr* 1999 Jan; 69 (1): 1.
198. Katdare, M, et al. Inhibition of aberrant proliferation and induction of apoptosis in preneoplastic human mammary epithelial cells by natural phytochemicals. *Oncol Rep* 1998 Mar–Apr; 5 (2): 311–5.
199. Ganong, William F. *Review of medical physiology*. Simon & Schuster, New York, NY, 1995. Page 333.
200. Chan, AF, et al. Persistence of premenstrual syndrome during low-dose administration of the progesterone antagonist RU 486. *Obstet Gynecol* 1994 Dec; 84 (6): 1001–5.
201. Wyatt, K, et al. Efficacy of progesterone and progestogens in management of premenstrual syndrome: systematic review. *BMJ* 2001 Oct 6; 323 (7316): 776–80.
202. Miyagawa, K, et al. Medroxyprogesterone interferes with ovarian steroid protection against coronary vasospasm. *Nat Med* 1997 Mar; 3 (3): 324–7.
203. Apgar, BS, et al. Using Progestins in Clinical Practice. *American Family Physician* 2000 Oct: 15.

204. Dalton, K. Progesterone or progestogens? *Br Med J* 1976 Nov 20; 2 (6046): 1257.
205. Jordan, VC, et al. The estrogenic activity of synthetic progestins used in oral contraceptives. *Cancer* 1993 Feb 15; 71 (4 Suppl): 1501–5. Review.
206. Ganong, William F. Review of Medical Physiology. Simon & Schuster, New York, NY, 1995. Page 414.
207. *http://www.neurosci.pharm.utoledo.edu/MBC3320/estrogens.htm*
208. Chen, CL, et al. Hormone replacement therapy in relation to breast cancer. *JAMA* 2002 Feb 13; 287 (6): 734–41.
209. Dupont, WD, et al. Menopausal estrogen replacement therapy and breast cancer. *Arch Intern Med* 1991 Jan; 151 (1): 67–72.
210. Xie, B, et al. Sex hormone-induced mammary carcinogenesis in female noble rats: the role of androgens. *Carcinogenesis* 1999 Aug; 20 (8): 1597–606.
211. Fuller, PJ. The steroid receptor superfamily: mechanisms of diversity. *FASEB J* 1991 Dec; 5 (15): 3092–9. Review.
212. *http://www.earlymenopause.com/hrt=_triest.htm*. Different Forms of HRT: Tri-Est.
213. *http://www.families-first.com/hotflash/faq/cenestin.htm*. When will Cenestin be available?
214. *http://www.equineadvocates.com/*. Promoting the humane and responsible treatment of horses.
215. Whittaker, PG, et al. Serum equilin, estrone, and estradiol levels in postmenopausal women receiving conjugated equine oestrogens ('Premarin'). *Lancet* 1980 Jan 5; 1 (8158): 14–6.
216. Nelson, HD, et al. Postmenopausal hormone replacement therapy: scientific review. *JAMA* 2002 Aug 21; 288 (7): 872–81. Review.
217. Ross, D, et al. Randomized, double-blind, dose-ranging study of the endometrial effects of a vaginal progesterone gel in estrogen-treated postmenopausal women. *Am J Obstet Gynecol* 1997 Oct; 177 (4): 937–41.
218. Warren, MP, et al. A new clinical option for hormone replacement therapy in women with secondary amenorrhea: effects of cyclic administration of progesterone from the sustained-release vaginal gel Crinone (4% and 8%) on endometrial morphologic features and withdrawal bleeding. *Am J Obstet Gynecol* 1999 Jan; 180 (1 Pt 1): 42–8.
219. Asthana, S, et al. Cognitive and neuroendocrine response to transdermal estrogen in postmenopausal women with Alzheimer's disease: results of a placebo-controlled, double-blind, pilot study. *Psychoneuroendocrinology* 1999 Aug; 24 (6): 657–77.
220. Garnero, P, et al. Effects of intranasal 17beta-estradiol on bone turnover and serum insulin-like growth factor I in postmenopausal women. *J Clin Endocrinol Metab* 1999 Jul; 84 (7): 2390–7.
221. Suvanto-Luukkonen, E, et al. Percutaneous estradiol gel with an intrauterine Ievonorgestrel releasing device or natural progesterone in hormone replacement therapy. *Maturitas* 1997 Apr; 26 (3): 211–7.
222. Pasquale, SA, et al. Peripheral progesterone (P) levels and endometrial response to various dosages of vaginally administered P in estrogen-primed women. *Fertil Steril* 1997 Nov; 68 (5): 810–5.

223. De Lignieres, B. Oral micronized progesterone. *Clin Ther* 1999 Jan; 21 (1): 41–60; discussion 1–2. Review.
224. Stanczyk, EZ. Pharmacokinetics of progesterone administered by the oral and parenteral routes. *J Reprod Med* 1999 Feb; 44 (2 Suppl): 141–7. Review.
225. De Lignieres, B. Oral micronized progesterone. *Clin Ther* 1999 Jan; 21 (1): 41–60; discussion 1–2. Review.
226. Arafat, ES, et al. Sedative and hypnotic effects of oral administration of micronized progesterone may be mediated through its metabolites. *Am J Obstet Gynecol* 1988 Nov; 159 (5): 1203–9.
227. Rapkin, AJ, et al. Progesterone metabolite allopregnanolone in women with premenstrual syndrome. *Obstet Gynecol* 1997 Nov; 90 (5): 709–14.
228. Cavailles, V, et al. Comparative activity of pulsed or continuous estradiol exposure on gene expression and proliferation of normal and tumoral human breast cells. *J Mol Endocrinol* 2002 Jun; 28 (3): 165–75.
229. Timiras, Paola S, et al. *Hormones and aging*. CRC Press, New York, NY, 1995. Page 78.
230. Burry, KA, et al. Percutaneous absorption of progesterone in postmenopausal women treated with transdermal estrogen. *Am J Obstet Gynecol* 1999 Jun; 180 (6 Pt 1): 1504–11.
231. Leonetti, HB, et al. Transdermal progesterone cream for vasomotor symptoms and postmenopausal bone loss. *Obstet Gynecol* 1999 Aug; 94 (2): 225–8.
232. Wiley, TS, et al. Pharmacokinetics and clinical effects of percutaneousely administered progesterone to breast cancer patients. A preliminary study. The Rasmus Institute for Medical Research.
233. Bhattacharjee, Y. More Than the Patch: New Ways to Take Medicine Via Skin. *New York Times*, Health & Fitness 2002 July 2; Section F: Page 5.
234. Moser, K, et al. Passive skin penetration enhancement and its quantification in vitro. *Eur J Pharm Biopharm* 2001 Sep; 52 (2): 103–12. Review.
235. Cicinelli, E, et al. Twice-weekly transdermal estradiol and vaginal progesterone as continuous combined hormone replacement therapy in postmenopausal women: a 1-year prospective study. *Am J Obstet Gynecol* 2002 Sep; 187 (3): 556–60.
236. Wren, BG, et al. Effect of sequential transdermal progesterone cream on endometrium, bleeding pattern, and plasma progesterone and salivary progesterone levels in postmenopausal women. *Climacteric* 2000 Sep; 3 (3): 155–60.
237. *http://www.endo101.com/getprog.htm*. Sources of progesterone for endometriosis.
238. Ghen, MJ, et al. *The Ghen and Rains Physicians' guide to pharmaceutical compounding*. IMPAKT Communications Inc., Green Bay, WI, 2000. Page 1.
239. Ibid.
240. Ibid.
241. Hagen, C, et al. Effects of two years' estrogen-gestagen replacement on climacteric symptoms and gonadotropins in the early postmenopausal period. *Acta Obstet Gynecol Scand* 1982; 61 (3): 237–41.
242. Medina, D, et al. Mechanisms of hormonal prevention of breast cancer. *Ann N Y Acad Sci* 2001 Dec; 952: 23–35. Review.

243. Ginger, MR, et al. Persistent changes in gene expression induced by estrogen and progesterone in the rat mammary gland. *Mol Endocrinol* 2001 Nov; 15 (11): 1993–2009.
244. Wray, S. Development of luteinizing hormone releasing hormone neurones. *J Neuroendocrinol* 2001 Jan; 13 (1): 3–11. Review.
245. *http://www.ourstolenfuture.org/NewScience/phytoestrogens/phyto1.htm.* Our stolen future: Phytoestrogens vs. synthetic compounds.
246. Ganong, William F. *Review of medical physiology.* Simon & Schuster, New York, NY, 1995. Page 413.
247. Medina, D, et al. Mechanisms of hormonal prevention of breast cancer. *Ann N Y Acad Sci* 2001 Dec; 952: 23–35. Review.
248. Ganong, William F. *Review of medical physiology.* Simon & Schuster, New York, NY, 1995. Page 404.
249. Eskin, BA. *The menopause comprehensive management.* The Parthenon Publishing Group, New York, NY, 2000. Page 248.
250. Ibid.
251. Medina, D, et al. Mechanisms of hormonal prevention of breast cancer. *Ann N Y Acad Sci* 2001 Dec; 952: 23–35. Review.
252. Ganong, William F. *Review of medical physiology.* Simon & Schuster, New York, NY, 1995. Page 404.
253. Amsterdam, A, et al. Steroid regulation during apoptosis of ovarian follicular cells. *Steroids* 1998 May–Jun; 63 (5–6):314–8. Review.
254. Evans, RW, et al. Progesterone inhibition of uterine nuclear estrogen receptor: dependence on RNA and protein synthesis. *Proc Natl Acad Sci* (USA) 1980 Oct; 77 (10): 5856–60.
255. Bush, DE, et al. Estrogen replacement reverses endothelial dysfunction in postmenopausal women. *Am J Med* 1998 Jun; 104 (6): 552–8.
256. Tesarik, J, et al. Nongenomic effects of 17 beta-estradiol on maturing human oocytes: relationship to oocyte developmental potential. *J Clin Endocrinol Metab* 1995 Apr; 80 (4): 1438–43.
257. Lindheim, SR, et al. Serum progesterone before and after human chorionic gonadotropin injection depends on the estradiol response to ovarian hyperstimulation during in-vitro fertilization-embryo transfer cycles. *J Assist Reprod Genet* 1999 May; 16 (5): 242–6.
258. Requena, A, et al. Endocrinological and ultrasonographic variations after immature oocyte retrieval in a natural cycle. *Hum Reprod* 2001 Sep; 16 (9): 1833–7.
259. Child, TJ, et al. Basal serum levels of FSH and estradiol in ovulatory and anovulatory women undergoing treatment by in-vitro maturation of immature oocytes. *Hum Reprod* 2002 Aug; 17 (8): 1997–2002.
260. Cano, F, et al. Effect of aging on the female reproductive system: evidence for a role of uterine senescence in the decline in female fecundity. *Fertil Steril* 1995 Sep; 64 (3): 584–9.
261. Trounson, A, et al. In vitro maturation and the fertilization and developmental competence of oocytes recovered from untreated polycystic ovarian patients. *Fertil Steril* 1994 Aug; 62 (2): 353–62.

262. Sauer, MV, et al. Three hundred cycles of oocyte donation at the University of Southern California: assessing the effect of age and infertility diagnosis on pregnancy and implantation rates. *J Assist Reprod Genet* 1994 Feb; 11 (2): 92–6.
263. Zheng, T, et al. Lactation and breast cancer risk: a case-control study in Connecticut. *Br J Cancer* 2001 Jun 1; 84 (11): 1472–6.
264. Swanson, SM, et al. Hormone levels and mammary epithelial cell proliferation in rats treated with a regimen of estradiol and progesterone that mimics the preventive effect of pregnancy against mammary cancer. *Anticancer Res* 1997 Nov–Dec; 17 (6D): 4639–45.
265. Wiley, TS, et al. *Sex, lies & menopause: The shocking truth about hormone replacement.* William Morrow Publishing, New York, NY, 2003. Acknowledgements.

CONCLUSION

1. *http://www.cancer.org/docroot/STT/stt=_0=_2002.asp?sitearea=STT&level=1.* Cancer Facts & Figures 2002.
2. Lobo R. Medscape Women's Health, Clinical Management. Menopause management for the millennium. October 17, 2000. *http://www.medscape.com/Medscape/WomensHealth/ClinicalMgmt.*
3. Leung, G, et al. No effect of a high-fat diet on promotion of sex hormone-induced prostate and mammary carcinogenesis in the Noble rat model. *Br J Nutr* 2002 Oct; 88(4): 399–409.
4. Leyenaar, J, et al. Self-reported physical and emotional health of women in a low-fat, high-carbohydrate dietary trial (Canada). *Cancer Causes Control* 1998 Dec; 9(6): 601–10.
5. Morimoto, LM, et al. Obesity, body size, and risk of postmenopausal breast cancer: the Women's Health Initiative (United States). *Cancer Causes Control* 2002 Oct; 13(8): 741–51.
6. Moradi, T, et al. Physical activity and risk for breast cancer a prospective cohort study among Swedish twins. *Int J Cancer* 2002 Jul 1; 100(1): 76–81.
7. Dubnov, G, et al. Weight control and the management of obesity after menopause: the role of physical activity. *Maturitas* 2003 Feb 25; 44(2): 89–101.
8. *http://www.ananoya.com/news/story/sm 682525.html.* Breast Cancer Deaths unaffected by Self-Checks—Report.
9. Josefson, D. Mammography is no better than physical examination, study shows. *BMJ* 2000 Sep 30; 321(7264): 785.
10. Moss, Ralph W. *Questioning chemotherapy*. Equinox Press, Brooklyn, NY, 1995. Page 44.
11. Josefson, D. Mammography is no better than physical examination, study shows. *BMJ* 2000 Sep 30; 321(7264): 785.
12. *http://www.ananova.com/news/story/sm=_682525.html.* Breast Cancer Deaths unaffected by Self-Checks—Report.
13. Villanueva, P, et al. Accuracy of pharmaceutical advertisements in medical journals. *Lancet* 2003 Jan 4; 361(9351): 27–32.
14. Pear, R. Investigators Find Repeated Deception in Ads for Drugs. *New York Times*, National, 2002 Dec 4. Page A22.
15. Ibid.
16. Abelson, R. Drug Sales Bring Huge Profits, and Scrutiny, to Cancer Doctors. *New York Times*, 2003 Jan 26.

17. Ibid.
18. Ibid.
19. Ibid.
20. Ibid.
21. *http://cbc.ca/cgi-bin/templates/view.cgi?category=Regional&story=/news/2000/05/04/mb=_stonewallcondom050400.* Teen Sex Debate Continues in Stonewall.
22. U.S. Bureau of the Census, "U.S. Population Estimates by Age, Sex, Race, and Hispanic Origin, 2001.
23. *http://cbc.ca/cgi-bin/templates/view.cgi?category=Consumers&story=/news/2000/07/20/career=_pill00720.* New Birth Control Pill Could Delay Menopause.
24. *http://www.cancer.org/docroot/STT/stt=_0=_2002.asp? sitearea=STT&level=1.* Cancer Facts & Figures 2002.
25. *http://www.nih.gov/.*
26. Collaborative Group on Hormonal Factors in Breast Cancer. Breast cancer and breastfeeding: collaborative reanalysis of individual data from 47 epidemiological studies in 30 countries, including 50,302 women with breast cancer and 96,973 women without the disease. *Lancet* 2002 Jul 20; 360 (9328): 187–95.
27. Ibid.
28. Greaves, Mel. *Cancer: The evolutionary legacy.* Oxford University Press Inc., New York, NY, 2000. Page 149.
29. Ibid.
30. Gould, Nigel. Drastic cure for cancer. *The Belfast Telegraph*, 2002 Sep 27.
31. Abadjieva, TI. Treatment of androgenetic alopecia in females in reproductive age with topical estradiolbenzoate, prednisolon and salicylic acid. *Folia Med (Plovdiv)* 2000; 42(3): 26–9.
32. Varma, M, et al. Effect of estradiol and progesterone on daily rhythm in food intake and feeding patterns in Fischer rats. *Physiol Behav* 1999 Dec 1–15; 68 (1–2): 99–107.
33. Geisler, JG, et al. Estrogen can prevent or reverse obesity and diabetes in mice expressing human islet amyloid polypeptide. *Diabetes* 2002 Jul; 51 (7): 2158–69.
34. Anderson, EJ, et al. Body composition and energy balance: lack of effect of short-term hormone replacement in postmenopausal women. *Metabolism* 2001 Mar; 50 (3): 265–9.
35. Frohlich, J, et al. Hormones, genes and the structure of sexual arousal. *Behav Brain Res* 1999 Nov 1; 105 (1): 5–27. Review.
36. Read, J. ABC of sexual health: sexual problems associated with infertility, pregnancy, and aging. *BMJ* 1999 Feb 27; 318 (7183): 587–9. Review.
37. Shah, MG, et al. Estrogen and skin. An overview. *Am J Clin Dermatol* 2001; 2 (3): 143–50. Review.
38. Thornton, MJ. The biological actions of estrogens on skin. *Exp Dermatol* 2002 Dec; 11 (6): 487–502.
39. Balog, JA, et al. 17beta-Estradiol increases, aging decreases, c-Fos expression in the rat accessory olfactory bulb. *Neuroreport* 2001 Dec 4; 12 (17): 3787–90.
40. O'Meara, ES, et al. Hormone replacement therapy after a diagnosis of breast cancer in

relation to recurrence and mortality. *J Natl Cancer Inst* 2001 May 16; 93 (10): 754–62.

41. O'Meara, ES, et al. Hormone replacement therapy after a diagnosis of breast cancer in relation to recurrence and mortality. *J Natl Cancer Inst* 2001 May 16; 93 (10): 754–62.
42. Song, RX, et al. Effect of long-term estrogen deprivation on apoptotic responses of breast cancer cells to 17beta-estradiol. *J Natl Cancer Inst* 2001 Nov 21; 93 (22): 1714–23.
43. Song, RX, et al. Effect of long-term estrogen deprivation on apoptotic responses of breast cancer cells to 17beta-estradiol. *J Natl Cancer Inst* 2001 Nov 21; 93 (22): 1714–23.
44. Song, RX, et al. Effect of long-term estrogen deprivation on apoptotic responses of breast cancer cells to 17beta-estradiol. *J Natl Cancer Inst* 2001 Nov 21; 93 (22): 1714–23.
45. *http://www.desaction.ie/*. DES Action Ireland.
46. Harris, Jay R, et al. *Diseases of the breast*. Lippincott-Raven Publishers, New York, NY, 1996. Page 355.
47. Swanson, SM, et al. Hormone levels and mammary epithelial cell proliferation in rats treated with a regimen of estradiol and progesterone that mimics the preventive effect of pregnancy against mammary cancer. *Anticancer Res* 1997 Nov–Dec; 17 (6D): 4639–45.
48. Collaborative Group on Hormonal Factors in Breast Cancer. Breast cancer and breast-feeding: collaborative reanalysis of individual data from 47 epidemiological studies in 30 countries, including 50,302 women with breast cancer and 96,973 women without the disease. *Lancet* 2002 Jul 20; 360 (9328): 187–95.
49. *http://www.ilo.org/public/english/employment/gems/eeo/law/sweden/1=_plas.htm*. Parental Leave Act: Sweden: Equal Employment Opportunities.
50. *http://www.hreoc/gov.au/sex=_discrimination/pml/*. Valuing Parenthood: Options for Paid Parental Leave: Interim Paper 2002.

Glossary

Acetylcholine: a neurotransmitter released and hydrolyzed in certain synaptic transmissions of the nervous system and in the initiation of muscle contraction.

Activational effects of hormones: transient actions of hormones.

Active immunity: type of immunity produced by the body when stimulated by a vaccine or by exposure to a pathogen.

Adaptation: in evolutionary biology, any structure, physiological process, or behavioral trait that makes an animal better able to survive and reproduce compared to other similar species. Also used to describe the process of evolutionary change leading to the formation of such a trait.

Adaptive behavior: behavior patterns that make an organism more fit to survive and reproduce in comparison with other members of the same species.

Adenocarcinoma: type of cancer of the glandular epithelium or lining (i.e., lung, breast, colon).

Adenosine triphosphate (ATP): a ubiquitous small molecule involved in many biological energy exchange reactions, consisting of the nitrogenous base adenine, the sugar ribose, and three phosphate residues.

Adhesion: tissues that stick together; occurs in response to bleeding or inflammation caused by disease or surgery.

Adipose tissue: fat cells.

Adjuvant chemotherapy: additional drug or radiation treatment after the primary or first treatment (i.e., surgery first, then "adjuvant" chemotherapy after).

Adrenalcorticotropic hormone (ACTH): pituitary hormone that stimulates the adrenal gland to produce cortisone.

Adrenal gland: pyramid-shaped endocrine gland located on top of each kidney that secretes hormones such as adrenaline, noradrenaline, cortisol, and other corticosteroids and androgens.

Adrenalectomy: surgical removal of part or all of an adrenal gland (near each kidney).

Adrenaline (epinephrine): neurotransmitter produced by the adrenal gland that is released in response to fear, heightened emotion, or physiological stress.

Agonist/Antagonist: these are terms from pharmacology that refer to two opposing actions associated with the binding of a ligand or compound to its receptor. In the case of a ligand that is an *agonist*, the fit between ligand and receptor is perfect, and binding is followed by transmission of a signal to the cell. *Antagonists*, while considerably rarer, are of tremendous interest from the point of view of drug design and therapeutics. Tamoxifen is one such hormone antagonist, which was developed to block the action of estrogen in women who have had breast cancer, but it also has agonist action.

AIDS: acquired immune deficiency syndrome; a condition in which certain cells of the immune system are killed by infection with HIV.

Allele: one of a number of different forms of the same gene for a specific trait. For example, there are both blue and brown alleles of the eyecolor gene.

Allergy: reaction of the immune system that results when the body is stimulated by antigens or specific immune cells.

Allopatric speciation: the production of new species through the branching or splitting of existing ones. The process begins with the geographic isolation of one or more populations from the bulk of the parent species.

Altruism: behavior that is directly beneficial to others at some cost or risk to the altruistic individual.

Alzheimer's disease/senile dementia: a middle- to late-life degenerative neurologic disease of unknown etiology that results in the progressive death of multiple brain neuronal populations with profound cognitive impairment. The early degeneration of basal forebrain cholinergic neurons is thought to contribute to prominent memory deficits.

Amenorrhea or amenorrheic: absence of menstruating.

Amino acids: a group of organic compounds that act as building blocks for proteins.

Amniotic sac: fluid-filled structure that cushions and protects the developing fetus in placental mammals such as humans.

Amplitude: the maximum height of a wave peak or the maximum depth of a wave trough.

Amygdala: group of neuronal nuclei in the dorsomedial temporal lobe bilaterally that subserve informational learning in conjunction with the hippocampus.

Analgesic: a drug that relieves pain.

Androgenic: a substance or hormone that produces male or masculine characteristics.

Androgens: hormones secreted in small amounts by the adrenal glands that produce male or masculine characteristics (e.g., testosterone).

Angiogenesis: the formation of new blood vessels.

Angiotensin: a hormone substance in the blood that causes blood vessels to narrow or constrict, thereby raising blood pressure.

Annual rhythms (type I): annual rhythms that are dependent to some degree upon the environment for their repression; Type I rhythms do not persist in constant environmental conditions.

Anovulation: failure to ovulate.

Anoxia: deficiency or absence of oxygen.

ANP: see **Atrial naturetic peptide.**

Antagonism: the condition of being an opposing principle, force, or factor, as when two hormones have opposite effects on target tissues.

Antagonist: see **Agonist.**

Anthropic principle: doctrine that one explanation for why the universe has the properties we observe is that were the properties different, it is likely that life would not have formed and therefore we would not be here to observe the changes.

Anthropology: the science of humankind; the systematic study of human evolution, human variability, and human behavior, past and present.

Antibiotic: any of a large number of substances, produced by various microorganisms and fungi, capable of inhibiting or killing bacteria and usually not harmful to higher organisms (e.g., penicillin, streptomycin).

Antibody: a protein produced as a defense mechanism to attack a foreign substance invading the body.

Antigen-binding site: area on a molecule that allows it to bind to an antigen.

Antigens: any organic substances recognized by the body as foreign that stimulate the immune system.

Antioxidants: substances that stop oxidation when a substance is exposed to oxygen. Oxygen is essential for our bodies to function. Unfortunately, when oxidation takes place, this can create highly reactive chemical fragments called *free radicals*. It is these free radicals that have been linked to cancer, coronary heart disease, rheumatoid arthritis, and premature aging. Environmental pollutants, smoking, and ultraviolet light can also increase production of free radicals. Antioxidants prevent this oxidation from taking place. They include beta-carotene, vitamin E, vitamin C, and selenium.

Aorta: large artery in mammals that carries oxygen-rich blood from the left ventricle of the heart to all parts of the body except the lungs.

Aortic body: sensory structures in the aorta that respond to changes in blood CO_2 and pH levels by sending neural impulses to the respiratory control center.

Apoptosis: process of suicidal cell death.

Appetitive behavior: the flexible introductory phase of a behavior sequence during which the organism is searching to obtain something to meet a need, as in seeking food, a mate, stimulation of a specific type, etc.

Arimidex: anastrozole tablets. A first-line treatment of breast cancer in postmenopausal women. It slows the growth of advanced cancer within the breast and cancer that has spread to other parts of the body. It is also used to treat advanced breast cancer in postmenopausal women whose disease has spread to other parts of the body following treatment with tamoxifen (Nolvadex), another anticancer drug. Arimidex combats the kind of breast cancer that thrives on estrogen. One of the hormones produced by the adrenal gland is converted to a form of estrogen by an enzyme called *aromatase*. Arimidex suppresses this enzyme and thereby reduces the level of estrogen circulating in the body; it is manufactured by AstraZeneca Pharmaceuticals LP.

Aromatase: an enzyme that catalyzes the conversion of testosterone into estradiol.

Arteriosclerosis: narrowing of the arteries due to age or high blood pressure.

Artery: tough, flexible blood vessel covered with smooth muscle that carries blood away from the heart to the tissues of the body.

Arthritis: inflammation of a joint.

Artificial selection: technique in which the intervention of humans allows only selected organisms to produce offspring. For example, animal husbandry.

Assay: a tool used to examine, evaluate, and research; a test.

Asthma: allergic reaction in which smooth muscles contract around the passages leading to the lungs.

Atherosclerosis: "hardening of the arteries"; disease of the arteries caused by fatty plaques deposited on the inner walls, making the arteries narrower, eventually constricting blood flow.

Atom: the smallest indivisible unit of an element still retaining the element's characteristics.

ATP: see **Adenosine triphosphate**.

Atrial naturetic peptide: referring to a peptide or substance secreted from the atrium of the heart that conveys information immediately from the heart to various organs of the body, including the endocrine organs and the brain.

Atrophic vaginitis: vaginal dryness due to depletion or absence of estrogen.

Atypical hyperplasia: precancerous changes.

Autoimmune: immune responses directed against the body's own tissue.

Autoimmune disease: a disease in which the organism's immune system attacks and destroys one or more of the organism's own tissues, as in the case of arthritis.

Autoimmunity: a condition characterized by a specific humoral or cell-mediated immune response against the constituents of the body's own tissues. It may result in hypersensitivity reactions or, if severe, in autoimmune disease.

Autologous stem cell transplant: a more sophisticated descendant of the bone marrow transplant. This procedure is used in combination with high-dose chemotherapy with or without radiation. After taking potentially toxic doses of chemotherapy drugs, one receives a life-saving infusion of one's own stem cells—young bone marrow cells, harvested from the bloodstream before treatment—that have been enhanced with a synthetic growth hormone.

Autonomic nervous system: the two main branches of the autonomic nervous system, emanating from the spinal cord, that control involuntary, unconscious actions of smooth and cardiac muscle and glands, and act in opposition to each other. One branch is known as the sympathetic system, and the nerves controlling it are found in the thoracic and lumbar segments of the spinal cord. The sympathetic system primarily uses the neurotransmitters adrenaline and noradrenaline to mobilize the organism in a fight-or-flight reaction in emergencies. The parasympathetic system, located in the cranial and sacral segments of the spinal cord, uses the transmitter acetylcholine to relax the body.

Axilla: The armpit.

Axon: the usually long extension of a nerve fiber that generally conducts impulses away from the body of the nerve cell.

Axonal transport: the processes through which molecules and particulate matter are carried to different regions of the neuron. Orthograde transport, for example, carries molecules from the cell body to nerve terminals in targets, whereas retrograde transport carries molecules from terminals to the cell body.

B-cell (B-lymphocyte): a type of white cell or lymphocyte that matures in the lymph glands and later circulates in the blood; involved in the immune response, especially in the production of free antibodies.

Basal forebrain cholinergic neurons: an extended group of neuronal nuclei at the base of the brain that innervate multiple cerebrocortical areas and utilize acetylcholine as a neurotransmitter. The neurons have been implicated in memory function.

Basal metabolic rate (BMR): the rate at which energy is released within the body under conditions of minimal activity.

Base pair: an association between two of the five fundamental chemical groups (A, T, C, U) that make up all DNA and RNA molecules. Base pairs are the smallest structures that form units of meaning in the genetic code. The more base pairs, the larger the molecule.

Behavioral ecology: a subdiscipline within animal behavior that deals with the ways in which animals interact with their environment and the survival value of behavior, as well as its contribution to reproductive success.

Behavior genetics: the study of the role that genes play in controlling behavior.

Benign: nonmalignant.

Beta cells: cells that make insulin. These cells are found in the islets of Langerhans in the pancreas.

Beta-endorphins: a natural painkiller produced in the body; beta-endorphins also have a calming effect and enhance feelings of well-being.

Bilateral symmetry: arrangement of an organism's body parts so that if an imaginary line were drawn down the length of the body, the body's parts would mirror on either side of the line.

Bioflavonoids: substances found in fruits such as blackberries, black currants, lemons, and plums. They help to increase the function of vitamin C. They also help to keep the connective tissues such as the skin healthy and strengthen capillary function and hence the circulation.

Biological clock: an internal timing mechanism that involves both an internal self-sustaining pacemaker and cyclic environmental synchronizers.

Biological cycles: changes in the activities of living things in an ebb-and-flow pattern. Such changes occur in almost all physical aspects, including sleep–wakefulness, hormone levels, and numbers of white cells in the blood. The predominant pattern is approximately twenty-four hours and usually follows the solar day closely.

Biological rhythm: a cyclical pattern of behavior, occurring at some regular period.

Biological species: groups of actually or potentially interbreeding natural populations that are reproductively isolated from other such groups.

Biomass: the total weight of living material of a species or population.

Biopsy: removal of a sample of tissue for laboratory examination.

Biosphere: the entire part of the Earth's land, soil, waters, and atmosphere in which living organisms are found.

Biphasic effects of progesterone: the ability of progesterone at different levels or doses to at first stimulate and later inhibit cell growth or sexual behavior.

Blood–brain barrier: in the brain, a state of highly selective permeability to many substances that readily move into or out of other tissues, attributed in part to lack of the usual looseness of capillary structure.

Blood glucose meter: a handheld machine that tests blood glucose levels. A drop of blood (obtained by pricking a finger) is placed on a small strip that is inserted in the meter. The meter calculates and displays the blood glucose level.

Blood pressure: measure of the force that blood exerts against a vessel wall.

Bone marrow: soft tissue in the cavities of bones where blood cells are formed.

Bottleneck: population bottleneck, a relatively short period of time during which the size of a population becomes unusually small, resulting in a random change in gene frequencies because of the decrease in genetic diversity due to the limited number of individuals left to reproduce.

Brain nucleus: aggregation of neuron cell bodies within the central nervous system.

Brain stem: the portion of the brain, composed of the medulla oblongata, the pons, and the midbrain, that governs a variety of vegetative functions and contains sensory and motor fibers of passage.

BRCA-1: a gene for heritable breast cancer, located by Dr. Mark Skolnick's research team in September 1994. BRCA-1 has since been shown to also play a role in sporadic breast cancer—disease in women who do not have a family history of breast cancer.

BRCA-1, 2: breast (and other) cancer associated genes 1 and 2. Considerable increase in risk of cancer when inherited in mutant form.

Breakthrough bleeding: non-menstrual unscheduled uterine bleeding not associated with trauma of miscarriage.

CA-125: a protein used as a tumor marker; found in the blood. Used primarily to monitor ovarian cancer.

Calcium: one of the mineral nutrients needed to maintain bone strength.

Calorie: the amount of heat (or equivalent chemical energy) needed to raise the temperature of 1 gram of water by 1°C.

Cancer: uncontrolled or unregulated growth of malignant cells. There are more than one hundred different types of cancer.

Capillary: the smallest blood vessels; the fine channel between the arteriole (one of the small terminal branches of an artery) and the venule (a small vein).

Capillary action: the tendency of a liquid to rise in a small tube due to adhesion to its inner surfaces and cohesion among water molecules.

Carbohydrate: organic compound containing carbon, hydrogen, and oxygen; human body's main source of energy; sugars, starches, cellulose, and chitin.

Carbon cycle: movement of carbon between organic compounds that make up living tissues and carbon dioxide in the air.

Carcinogen: an identified substance or process that damages DNA and induces cancer.

Carcinoma: cancer found in epithelial tissue, which includes the skin, glands, and the lining of internal organs.

Carcinoma in situ: malignant cells confined to original site of origin; not invasive.

Cardiac: pertaining to the heart; near or toward the heart.

Cardiac conduction system: cardiology's name for the complex bundle of fibers relaying info-energy within and from the heart; the electrical system of the heart.

Cardiac muscle: tissue made up of striated cells not under voluntary control; and found only in the heart.

Cartilage: a firm, elastic, flexible, translucent type of connective tissue; in development, a precursor of bone formation.

Casodex: bicalutamide tablets. For use in combination therapy with luteinizing hormone-releasing hormone (LHRH) analogue for the treatment of Stage D-2 metastatic carcinoma of the prostate, stops adrenal testosterone; manufactured by AstraZeneca Pharmaceuticals LP.

Castration: removal of the ovaries or testes. Also see **Oopherectomy.**

Catecholamines: a family of neurotransmitters used by the sympathetic nervous system peripherally and by a number of brain systems, including the locus ceruleus (arousal and attention), the substantia nigra (which degenerates in Parkinson's disease), and the mesocortical/subcortical (deranged in schizophrenia) systems. The amines are also hormones produced by the adrenal medulla. Catecholamines are defined chemically as 3,4-dihydroxy derivatives of phenylethylamines. Prominent members include dopamine, norepinephrine, and epinephrine.

Celebrex: celecoxib tablets. Prescribed for acute pain, menstrual cramps, and the pain and inflammation of osteoarthritis and rheumatoid arthritis; manufactured by Pfizer, Inc.

Cell: the smallest structural unit of an organism that is capable of independent functioning.

Cell adhesion molecules: specific molecules expressed on the cell surface that mediate cell-cell interactions, such as selective adhesivity. Also known as I-CAMS.

Cell cycle: period from the beginning of one replication of DNA to the beginning of the next, subdivided into the phases G1, S, G2, and M.

Cell division: process by which a single cell divides into two daughter cells.

Cell-mediated immunity: one of the immune processes in which killer T-cells cause the cells of pathogenic organisms to rupture and die.

Cell-mediated response: the response of activated cytotoxic T-cells, which includes the identification of, binding to, and lysis of cancerous and virus-infected cells.

Cell membrane: a cell structure that surrounds the cell and regulates the passage of materials between the cell and its environment; aids in the protection and support of the cell.

Cell nucleus: central, membrane-bound zone of cell containing chromosomes.

Cell respiration: the energy-yielding metabolism of foods in which oxygen is used.

Cell theory: the universally accepted proposal that cells are the functional units of organization in living organisms and that all cells today come from preexisting cells.

Cell wall: cell structure that surrounds the cell membrane for protection and support in plants, algae, and some bacteria.

Central nervous system (CNS): that part of the nervous system that is condensed and centrally located; consists of the brain and spinal cord in humans.

Cerebral cortex: the outermost region of the cerebrum, the "gray matter," consisting of several dense layers of neural cell bodies and including numerous conscious centers, as well as regions specialized in voluntary movement and sensory reception.

Cerebrum: the anterior, dorsal portion of the vertebrate brain, the largest portion in humans, consisting of two cerebral hemispheres and controlling many localized functions, among them voluntary movement, perception, speech, memory, and thought.

Cervical dysplasia: abnormal cell changes on the cervix that may progress to cancer if unchecked. Also called *cervical intraepithelial neoplasia* (CIN).

Cervix: the necklike base and opening of the uterus.

Chakra: from the Sanskrit meaning "wheel," chakras, according to Indian yogic teachings, are the body's energy centers, resembling whirling vortices of subtle ("L") energy. There are seven chakras, the fourth being the central or "heart" chakra. These energy centers relate to the levels of flowing Qui (pronounced "chee"), referred to in the two-thousand-year-old system of Chinese medicine.

Chemical synapse: space between neurons across which neurotransmitters must pass for neural impulse to begin in the second neuron.

Chemotaxis: attraction to or repulsion of cells by specific molecules.

Chemotherapy: treatment of cancer with certain chemicals that interfere with cell division and affect not only the cancer cells but all young and dividing cells of the body, such as blood cells. Chemotherapy alone may destroy immunity if given too long and too intensely. It is not usually curative except in rare instances.

Cholesterol: a lipid molecule that is needed for making parts of the cell fabric as well as steroid hormones, made in the liver, but which, if deposited in artery walls, leads to atherosclerosis.

Choline acetyltransferase: the enzyme that catalyzes the synthesis of acetylcholine from choline and acetyl CoA.

Choriocarcinoma: cancer derived from embryonic (placental) tissue.

Chromatin: the substance of chromosomes, a molecular complex consisting of DNA, histones, nonhistone chromosomal proteins, and usually some RNA of unknown function.

Chromosomal mutation: a massive change in DNA, generally breakage involving a whole chromosome that has not been repaired or has been repaired improperly.

Chromosomes: coiled, threadlike structures of DNA, bearing the genes and found in the nucleus of all plant and animal cells; twenty-three pairs of each in every human cell.

Circadian clock: mechanism(s) generating a master circadian rhythm; located in the suprachiasmatic nucleus in mammals.

Circadian rhythm: a biological rhythm of about a day in length or period.

Circadian time 12: the time is relative to a circadian "day" consisting of twenty-four circadian hours, each of which may be longer or shorter than sixty minutes depending upon whether the free-running "day" is longer or shorter than twenty-four hours.

Circannual rhythm: a biological rhythm of about a year in length or period.

Claritin: loratadine tablets. An antihistamine that relieves the sneezing, runny nose, stuffiness, itching, and tearing eyes caused by hay fever. It is also prescribed for relief of the swollen, red, itchy patches of skin labeled chronic hives; manufactured by Schering Corporation.

Climacteric: the transition from reproductive to nonreproductive status among women; begins about ten years before menopause.

Clinical trials: study of new treatments or procedures, in a research setting, to determine toxicity levels, proper dosage, and efficacy compared to existing treatments.

Clone: group of cells (or individuals) derived from a single ancestor. Term also applied, as a verb, to the synthetic production of multiple copies of a gene (or individual cells or organisms) by genetic and cellular engineering methods.

Closed circulatory system: a system in which blood is enclosed within arteries, veins, and capillaries throughout and is not in direct contact with cells other than those lining these vessels.

Codon: a nucleotide triplet in the genetic program (genome), designating a particular amino acid.

Coenzyme: a small organic molecule required for an enzymatic reaction.

Coevolution: the change in gene frequencies resulting from two species acting as strong selective forces on one another.

Cognition: the processes in the minds of animals of their general mental functions, including perception, representation, and memory.

Cohesion: the attraction between the molecules of a single substance, which holds it together as a whole.

Coincidence hypothesis: a hypothesis concerning the regulation of a seasonal event in which occurrence of the event depends upon the "coincidence" (simultaneous occurrence) of specific elements or phases of two or more rhythms.

Collagen: a fibrous protein that forms a connective tissue supporting the skin, bone, tendons, and cartilage; injections of collagen are sometimes used to fill in wrinkles, burns, and scars.

Combinatorial strategy: use of a limited series of elements to generate a large number of unique aggregates, or combinations.

Common descent: descent of two or more species (or individuals) from a common ancestor (e.g., the similarity in blood chemistry of apes and humans is due to common descent).

Competitive exclusion principle: two species cannot exist at the same locality if they have identical ecological requirements.

Competitive inhibition: enzyme inhibition involving molecules of similar compounds that compete for the active site.

Complement: a substance in blood serum and plasma that in combination with antibodies destroys bacteria, foreign cells, and other antigens. Part of the immune response.

Conception: the fertilization of an egg by sperm, resulting in pregnancy.

Conditioning, instrumental: process of association between the response of an organism and a reinforcing stimulus.

Conformation, molecular: the structure of a molecule in three-dimensional space; tertiary structure of a molecule. The conformation of a protein is dictated by the primary structure, the sequence of amino acids that comprise the molecule.

Congenital: present at birth.

Congenital adrenal hyperplasia (CAH): an inherited adrenal enzyme deficiency that results in overproduction of androgens, beginning in the prenatal period.

Conjugated estrogen: a mixture of estrogens, either natural or artificial, that can be prescribed to relieve symptoms of menopause and to treat infertility.

Connective tissue: a principal type of vertebrate-supporting tissue, often with an extracellular matrix of collagen. Included are bone, cartilage, ligaments, and blood.

Contraceptive: an agent or device used to prevent conception.

Contraindication: any factor in your medical history that would mean that it would be unwise to take a particular medication or follow a certain line of treatment.

Cooperative oncology groups: four groups comprised of a network of doctors conducting clinical trials research, including the East Coast Oncology Group (ECOG), New Hope, Cancer and Leukemia Group B (CALGB), and the National Surgical Adjuvant Breast and Bowel Project (NSABP).

Copulation: the act of sexual intercourse.

Coronary heart disease: narrowing of the arteries that supply blood to the heart.

Corpus callosum: a broad white neural tract in the mammalian brain that connects the cerebral hemispheres and correlates their activities.

Corpus luteum: a temporary structure forming from a collapsed follicle after ovulation that produces progesterone in the second half of the menstrual cycle.

Cortex: the outer layer or rind of an organ, such as adrenal cortex, kidney cortex; the portion of stem between the epidermis and the vascular tissue.

Corticosteroid: steroid hormones produced by adrenal glands that are instrumental in the proper metabolism of carbohydrates and proteins and many other functions (i.e., the function of the heart, lungs, muscles, kidneys, and other major organs).

Corticosteroid binding globulin: a protein that binds and transports most glucocorticoids in the bloodstream.

Corticotropin-releasing factor (CRF): hormone released by the hypothalamus that stimulates the pituitary to secrete adrenocorticotropic hormone (ACTH).

Cortisol: steroid hormone produced and released by the adrenal gland; helps to regulate such things as blood sugar, blood pressure, and bone growth.

Counterregulatory (stress) hormones: hormones released during stressful situations. The hormones include glucagon, epinephrine (adrenaline), norepinephrine, cortisol, and growth hormone. They cause the liver to release glucose and the cells to release fatty acids for extra energy. If there's not enough insulin present in the body, these extra fuels can lead to hyperglycemia and ketoacidosis.

Crepuscular: daily cycles with peak activity around dusk and/or dawn.

Cultural evolution: changes in human culture resulting from the accumulated experience of humankind. Cultural evolution can produce adaptations to the environment faster than organic evolution can.

Culture: (1) a purposeful growth of microorganisms for scientific study; (2) humans' systems of learned behavior, symbols, customs, beliefs, institutions, artifacts, and technology, characteristic of a group and transmitted by its members to their offspring.

Cycle: repeating units that make up a pattern of biological rhythms.

Cyclic AMP (cAMP): adenosine monophosphate in which the phosphate is linked between the 3' and 5' carbons of the ribose group; serves as an intracellular gene regulator under a variety of circumstances and precursor to ATP—body's energy.

Cyst: a fluid-filled sac.

Cyto-: pertaining to the cell.

Cytokine: a generic term for nonantibody proteins released by one cell population on contact with specific antigens, which act as intercellular mediators, as in the generation of an immune response.

DCIS: ductal carcinoma in situ. a noninvasive cancer, limited to the breast's ductal system, sometimes referred to as "precancer." Improved detection technology has enabled doctors to detect microcalcifications as tiny dots on a mammogram, which sometimes signal the presence of DCIS.

Death rate: in human populations, the number of deaths per thousand population per year.

Dedifferentiation: the process in which a mature, specialized cell returns to its original, embryonic, unspecialized state, as in cancer.

Deletion: loss of part or whole gene or chromosome.

Dendrites: prolongations of a nerve cell that carries a message, or stimulus, toward the body. For example, sensory nerve cell bodies receive stimuli from receptors in the skin via their dendrites.

Depolarized: the reduction in the difference in charge (potential) between the outside and inside of a membrane.

Developmental cell death: the normal ontogenetic process in which 50 to 80 percent of cells die in virtually all organ systems, including the nervous system.

Diabetes mellitus: a genetic disease of carbohydrate metabolism characterized by abnormally high levels of glucose in the blood and urine, and the inadequate secretion or utilization of insulin.

Diapause phase: a period of dormancy, common in insect species, which occurs during the more rigorous portions of the annual climatic cycle.

Diethylstilbestrol (DES): a synthetic estrogen agonist. DES was formerly administered clinically to prevent miscarriage, which may have had masculinizing or defeminizing effects on the brains of female children born to these mothers.

Differentiation: in development, the process whereby a cell or cell line becomes morphogically, developmentally, or physiologically specialized. Differentiation involves restricting, or repressing, all genes for other cell types.

Dihydroepiandrosterone (DHEA): a precursor of androgens, the male sex hormones.

Dihydrotestosterone (DHT): a derivative of testosterone that is more potent, molecule for molecule, but does not act equally on all androgen-sensitive tissues.

Dilation and curettage (D&C): minor surgery during which the endometrium is scraped with a spoon-shaped instrument called a curette.

Dimorphic: having more than one form, size, or appearance; usually referring to the difference between males and females of a species.

Diploid: possessing a double set of chromosomes, one set derived from the mother, the other from the father.

Direct fitness: a measure of an individual's potential to contribute genes to future generations via personal reproduction.

Dirty margins: malignant cells at the edge of a pathology slide from a surgical biopsy, which means that not all the cancerous tissue have been removed.

Disease: any change, other than an injury, that interferes with the normal functioning of the body.

Diuretic: any substance that increases the volume of urine by forcing the release of stored water from the tissues.

Diurnal: an animal with an activity period during the light portion of the daily cycle.

Diversity: variety; variability; the range of types in a major taxon; plant diversity. In ecology, a measure of the number of species coexisting in a community.

DNA (deoxyribonucleic acid): the chemical that comprises an individual's genetic code. Two pairs of interlocked bases match up in specific patterns; in a damaged gene those pairs are altered, either by heredity or the environment.

DNA replication: the semiconservative synthesis of DNA in which the chromosome opens, the two strands separate, and each is used as a template for producing a new opposing strand.

DOD: Department of Defense, which undertook a $210 million breast cancer research program in fiscal year 1993.

Dominant: describes a trait that is expressed in the phenotype even when the organism is carrying only one copy of the underlying hereditary material (one copy of the responsible gene).

Dopamine: the catecholamine transmitter used by substantia nigra neurons in the midbrain that regulate aspects of motor function. Dopaminergic deficits result in Parkinsonian signs and symptoms.

Dormacy: period during which an organism's growth and activity decrease or stop temporarily, usually during unfavorable environmental conditions.

Double-blind study: a clinical trial in which neither the patients nor the medical personnel know who is receiving an experimental treatment and who is receiving standard therapy or a placebo.

Double helix: the configuration of the native DNA molecule, which consists of two parallel strands wound helically around each other.

Dual, duality, duality symmetries: situation in which two or more theories appear to be completely different yet actually give rise to identical physical consequences.

Dysfunctional uterine bleeding: (breakthrough bleeding) uterine or vaginal bleeding that takes place in the absence of ovulation; usually attributed to abnormal or irregular production of hormones by the ovary.

Dysmenorrhea: painful menstrual cramps.

Dyspareunia: painful intercourse.

Ecological niche: the range of ecological variables (e.g., temperature, moisture, etc.) in which a species can exist and reproduce.

Ecology: study of the interactions of organisms with one another and with their physical surroundings.

Ecosystem: ecological system; the interacting community of all the organisms in an area and their physical environment, together with the flow of energy among its components.

Effector: a tissue or organ that responds to an action potential or a hormone.

Electrical synapse: contact between neurons formed by gap junctions, in which an action potential passes directly from one neuron to the next.

Electrochemical coding: release of different and unique combinations of neurotransmitters by neurons in response to different frequencies and patterns of electrical impulse activity.

Electromagnetic field: force field of the electromagnetic force, consisting of electric and magnetic lines of force at each point in space.

Electromagnetic force: one of the four fundamental forces, a union of the electric and magnetic forces.

Electromagnetic wave: a wavelink disturbance in an electromagnetic field; all such waves travel at the speed of light. Visible light, X rays, microwaves, and infrared radiation are examples.

Electroreceptor: sensory receptors that detect electric fields.

Element: a substance that cannot be separated into simpler substances by purely chemical means. For example carbon, helium, etc.

Embryogenesis: the growth of a new individual from a fertilized egg to the moment of hatching at birth.

Encoding: basic function of genes; to carry coded instructions.

Endocrine glands: a series of ductless glands that release hormones into the body through the blood or lymph.

Endocrine hormone: a hormone that acts at some distance from its source (usually transported in the blood), as opposed to paracrine hormones, which act on neighboring cells, and autocrine hormones, which remain within the producing cell.

Endocrine system: the endocrine glands taken together, and their hormonal actions and interactions.

Endocrinology: the science of hormone production, action, and control; the study of hormones.

Endogenous: originating or produced within an organism, a tissue, or a cell. The opposite of exogenous.

Endogenous clock mechanism: any internal processes that are genetically based and play a role in setting or regulating biological rhythms.

Endometriosis: a condition in which the tissue that normally lines the uterus (endometrium) grows in other areas of the body, causing pain, irregular bleeding, and frequently infertility. The tissue growth typically occurs in the pelvic area, outside of the uterus, on the ovaries, bowel, rectum, bladder, and the delicate lining of the pelvis, but it can occur in other areas of the body as well.

Endometrium: lining of the inside of the uterus.

Endorphins: neuropeptides, synthesized in the central nervous system of vertebrates, that produce morphinelike effects.

Endothelium: cells that form the inner lining of blood and lymph vessels.

Enkephalin: The brain's own morphine (from the Greek "in the head"), a five-amino-acid peptide that binds to the opiate receptor, causing, among other things, analgesia or the euphoria associated with exercise, the "runner's high."

Entrainment: the process by which a biological clock is set or reset by synchronizing with the period of some external, environmental stimulus. Entrainment can be observed in the physical as well as the organic world. Fireflies have a tendency toward entrainment, which can be observed as they blink in unison. Electronic oscillators will, if their frequencies are close enough, entrain with the fastest frequency, while pendulum clocks running side by side will entrain if the pendula are the same length. Most people are familiar with the high school experiment in which two tuning forks of the same size will set each other's frequency—that's entrainment. William Condon settled on this term to describe a process that makes syncing possible, wherein one central nervous system drives another, or two central nervous systems drive each other.

Entropy: in thermodynamics, the amount of energy in a closed system that is not available for doing work; also defined as a measure of the randomness or disorder of such a system. Negative entropy is free energy in the form of organization.

Environment: the surrounding conditions, influences, or forces that influence or modify an organism, population, or community.

Enzyme: a protein that converts a molecule to a different product rapidly and with high specificity. They do not get used up themselves in the reaction.

Enzyme activation: increased (catalytic) activity of an enzyme due to stimulation of preexisting enzyme molecules, in contrast to an increase in molecule number.

Enzyme induction: increased enzyme molecule number, generally due to an increase in the rate of synthesis of the enzyme, commonly associated with a consequent rise in activity. In a formal sense, steady-state number may also increase due to a decrease in the rate of breakdown or decay.

Epigenesis: the integrated, interactive process of behavior development involving the genetics of the organism and its environment, including all of its experiences.

Epigenetic: pertaining to extragenomic factors. Epigenetic influences refer to signals originating outside the gene(s) of the subject cell or cells.

Epilepsy: a group of cerebrocortical disorders characterized by the convulsive, synchronous electrical discharge of cortical neurons that may result in overt seizures and loss of consciousness.

Epinephrine (adrenaline): the predominant catecholamine elaborated by the adrenal medulla, mediating the stress response and mobilization for emergency. Epinephrine also is a transmitter used by a number of brain stem neuronal populations that regulate cardiovascular function.

Epithelium: a tissue consisting of tightly adjoining cells that cover a surface or line a canal or cavity, and that serves to enclose and protect.

Equilibrium: state in which no net change occurs.

Erythrocyte: a hemoglobin-filled, oxygen-carrying, circulating red blood cell.

Essential amino acid: one of the amino acids that the body cannot synthesize and thus must be provided by the diet.

Essential fatty acid: one of the fatty acids that the body cannot synthesize and thus must be provided by the diet.

Estradiol: the strongest form of estrogen, a form of natural human estrogen secreted mostly by the ovarian follicle; responsible for the development of secondary sex characteristics in teenage girls and promoting growth of the endometrium during the first part of the menstrual cycle.

Estrogen: the female steroid sex hormone, which is mainly produced by ovaries.

Estrogen receptor: a protein on some cells to which an estrogen molecule can attach. Estrogen-receptor-positive tumors are often more responsive to hormone treatment than are receptor-negative cancers.

Estrogen replacement therapy (ERT): the use of estrogen alone to treat menopause.

Estrone: a form of estrogen; less potent and abundant than estradiol.

Estrous cycle: the period of behavioral and physiological changes from one ovulatory event to another.

Estrus: the period of sexual receptivity in females.

Etiology: the causative agent of a disease.

Evista: see **Raloxifene.**

Evolution: the gradual process by which the living world has been developing following the origin of life; a change in the frequency of alleles in a population over generations. The change is caused by natural selection and/or genetic drift.

Evolutionarily stable strategy (ESS): a strategy that when employed by most individuals in a population cannot be outcompeted by some alternative strategy.

Excitatory synapse: a space between neurons in which the secretion of a neurotransmitter stimulates neural impulses in the receiving neuron.

Excretion: the removal of metabolic wastes, particularly nitrogenous wastes, from the body.

Exocrine gland: gland that releases secretions through tubelike structures called *ducts*.

Exogenous: derived or developed outside the body; originating externally or, in medical usage, having a cause external to the body.

Exon: a segment of an interrupted gene that is encoded in the processed messenger RNA product.

Expresses sequence: the portion of mRNA remaining after the introns or unexpressed sequences have been removed.

Extinction: the loss of a species due to the death of all its members.

Extracellular: outside, between, or among cells.

Fallopian tubes: the tubes running from the uterus to the ovaries through which eggs travel after ovulation.

Faslodex: for treatment of hormone receptor-positive metastatic breast cancer in postmenopausal women with disease progression following antiestrogen therapy; manufactured by AstraZeneca Pharmaceuticals.

Fats: the most concentrated source of calories in the diet. Saturated fats are found primarily in animal products. Unsaturated fats mainly come from plants and can be monounsaturated (olive or canola oil) or polyunsaturated (corn and other oils).

Fatty acid: organic acids important for precursors to build other fatty acids; not water-soluble; regulate cholesterol metabolism; used in digestion.

Femara: letrozole tablets. Aromatase inhibitor (substance that blocks the action of aromatase); manufactured by Novartis Pharmaceuticals for the treatment of advanced breast cancer in postmenopausal women with disease progression following antiestrogen therapy.

Fermentation: anaerobic breakdown of glucose to form alcohol and carbon dioxide or lactate.

Fertility rate: the number of births per thousand women from fifteen to forty-four years of age; a clearer indicator of reproductive activity in a population than the birth rate.

Fertilization: fusion between the male gamete (spermatozoon) and the female gamete (ovum). It results in the joining of a haploid set of maternal chromosomes with a haploid set of paternal chromosomes in the newly formed zygote, which thereby becomes diploid.

Fever: human body's response to an infection that results in increased body temperature in an effort to kill pathogens with heat.

Fiber: the parts of plants that the body can't digest, such as fruit and vegetable skins. Fiber aids in the normal functioning of the digestive system, specifically the intestinal tract.

Fibrinogen: a globular blood protein that is converted into fibrin by the action of thrombin as part of the normal blood clotting process.

Fibroadenoma: a hard, benign growth usually seen in the breasts of young women.

Fibrocystic breast disease: a common benign breast condition in which an abundance of cysts arises from the glands within the breast tissue.

Fibroids: benign tumors that grow in the uterus, made up of smooth muscle cells; common after the age of thirty-five. Also called *leiomyoma* or *myoma*.

Fine-needle aspiration: removal of fluid or cells to determine whether a lump is benign or malignant, using a hypodermic needle.

Fitness: the potential for an individual to contribute genes to future generations as a function of its adaptive traits.

Folic acid: a B vitamin; deficiencies are associated with the development of cervical dysplasia. Also see **Cervical dysplasia.**

Follicle: a tiny cyst or sac in which each egg in the ovary develops.

Follicle stimulating hormone (FSH): hormone secreted from the pituitary gland in the brain that stimulates the ripening of the follicles in the ovary. This begins the process of ovulation by stimulating the ovaries to produce the estrogen hormones. At menopause the FSH level rises dramatically as the body tries unsuccessfully to induce ovulation.

Follicular cyst: an ovarian cyst that develops from a follicle that never matured.

Forebrain: the anterior of the three primary divisions of the brain; the parts of the brain developed from the embryonic forebrain.

Formication: relatively rare menopausal symptom in which a woman feels a tingling sensation, as if insects are crawling on her skin.

Fosamax: alendronate sodium tablets. For the treatment and prevention of osteoporosis in postmenopausal women. It is also used to increase bone mass in men with osteoporosis, and is prescribed for both men and women who have developed a form of osteoporosis sometimes caused by steroid medications such as prednisone. This drug can also be used to relieve Paget's disease of bone, a painful condition that weakens and deforms the bones; manufactured by Merck and Company.

Frame shift mutation: a small insertion or deletion in a structural gene such that all mRNA codons downstream are misread in translation.

Free radical: an often highly reactive agent that can damage the cell fabric and other molecules.

Free-running rhythm: the activity cycle that an animal exhibits when placed in a constant environment; its period is different from any known cyclic environmental variable.

Frontal lobe: an anterior division of the cerebral hemisphere, believed to be a site of higher cognition. It subserves motor function and synthetic reasoning and plays a major role in affective behavior.

Functional neuroanatomy: the study of the size, structure, and arrangement of cells within the nervous system, particularly the brain.

G proteins: nearly ubiquitous guanosine triphosphate binding proteins that transduce the activation of multiple receptor subtypes into cellular information.

Galactorrhea: abnormal milk production by mammary gland due to prolactin.

Gallbladder: a sac located on the underside of the liver that stores the bile helpful in the digestion of fats.

Gap junction: dense structures that physically connect plasma membranes of adjacent cells along with channels for cell-to-cell transport.

Gastrointestinal tract: the entire digestive tube from the mouth to the anus.

Gene: a unit of DNA, which carries the instructions to make a protein. Genetic material is contained in the nucleus of a cell. A damaged gene can send faulty instructions, which can result in malignant growth. Controls the coding and inheritance of phenotypic traits; some genes also occur in a closed loop in the mitochondria.

Gene family: a closely related group of genes that encode proteins exhibiting amino acid sequence similarities. A gene family may arise evolutionarily through duplication of a primordial gene.

Gene flow: transmission of genes between populations through cross-breeding between groups which increases the variety of genes available to each and creates or maintains the genetic makeup of the population.

Gene mutation: change involving the nucleotides of DNA.

Gene pool: all the genes of a population at a given time (summing genes within a species yields the species' gene pool).

Gene product: in generic terms, the protein or messenger RNA encoded by a gene.

Gene sequencing: determining the specific sequence of nucleotides in a gene.

Gene splicing: the use of recombinant DNA techniques to form covalent bonds between DNA of different sources.

Genetic: inherited or inborn.

Genetic code: the chemical code based on four nucleotides, carried by DNA and RNA, which specifies amino acids in sequence for protein synthesis.

Genetic drift: genetic changes in populations caused by random phenomena rather than by natural selection.

Genetic engineering: the manipulation of genes through recombinant DNA techniques.

Genetic equilibrium: the state of a population wherein the frequency of certain alleles remains constant generation after generation.

Genetic load: recessive genes in a population that are harmful when expressed in the rare homozygous condition.

Genetic program: the information coded in an organism's DNA.

Genetic variability: a broad term indicating the presence of different genetic constitutions in a population or populations.

Genome: the totality of DNA unique to a particular organism or species.

Genotype: the entire set of genes an individual possesses, including those not expressed.

Genus: group of closely related species.

Germ cell: the egg or sperm cell.

Germ theory of infectious disease: idea that infectious diseases are caused by microorganisms.

Gestation: the period from fertilization of the ovum until delivery of the young.

Gland: any organ that produces and secretes a chemical substance used by another part of the body.

Glia: nonneuronal cells in the nervous system that provide support, elaborate growth cues, terminate the actions of some transmitters, and serve multiple functions that are still being defined. Glia comprise several cell types, including astrocytes, oligodendroglia, and microglia.

Glial cell: any of the nonneuronal constituent cells of the brain or the peripheral nervous system; some 90 percent, of the brain's cells are glia, not neurons.

Glucocorticoids: steroid hormones that are elaborated by the adrenal cortex and that participate in normal metabolism and in stress responses. The hormones appear to act directly on neuronal populations, including those in areas of the cerebral cortex.

Glucose: the end product of carbohydrate metabolism, the chief source of energy, its utilization is controlled by insulin. Excess glucose is converted to glycogen and stored in the liver and muscles for use as needed, and beyond that is converted to fat and stored as adipose tissue.

Glycogen: a highly branched polysaccharide consisting of alpha glucose subunits; a carbohydrate storage material in the liver, muscle, and other animal tissues.

Glycohemoglobin: a test that reflects average blood glucose control for about three months before the test. One such test is the hemoglobin A1c.

Glycolysis: a biochemical pathway including the enzymatic, anaerobic breakdown of glucose in cells, yielding ATP, pyruvate, and NADH.

Gonadotropin-releasing hormone (GNRH): peptide hormone released by the hypothalamus that instructs the pituitary gonadotropins (LH and FSH) to be released in order to set the menstrual cycle in motion each month. It is also called *LHRH*.

Gonadotropins: pituitary hormones that stimulate the gonad.

Gonads: glands responsible for the production of gametes and where certain gonadal hormones are produced. These consist of ovaries in females and the testes in males.

Graves' disease: autoimmune disease; due to the presence of an abnormal chemical stimulator of thyroid hormone production. Some symptoms might be bulging eyes, enlarged thyroid gland, rapid heartbeat, tremors, alteration of menstruation and fertility. It is more common in women than men.

Group selection, theory of: the theory that a social group can be the object of selection if the cooperative interaction among the members of the group enhances the fitness of the group.

Growth curve: a graph of population numbers per unit of time, especially in a period of rapid initial growth leading into population size stabilization or to a population crash.

Growth factor: a molecule that regulates cell division (mitosis), whether derived from distant (endocrine), proximate (paracrine), or the same (autocrine) cells.

Growth hormone: (GH): a pituitary hormone whose actions promote normal growth in developing organisms, tissue, repair, and energy metabolism in adults.

Habituation: decreased efficacy of synaptic conduction consequent to repeated exposure to a stimulus.

Hair follicle: tubelike pocket of epidermal cells that extends into the dermis and produces hair.

Half-life: length of time required for half of a drug to be excreted or metabolized.

Hashimoto's thyroiditis (chronic thyroiditis): autoimmune disease in which an inflammation of the thyroid gland frequently results in hypothyroidism (lowered thyroid function).

Heart: hollow muscular organ that contracts at regular intervals, forcing blood through the circulatory system.

Heart disease: a description of several disease states. Coronary artery disease is the most common form of heart disease. It occurs when the arteries that nourish the heart muscle narrow or become blocked.

Helper T-cell: a white cell and lymphocyte of the immune system that helps other lymphocytes respond to the early stages of an infection.

Hemorrhage: uncontrolled bleeding.

Her-2 breast cancer: c-erb2 gene-driven breast cancer.

Herceptin: trastuzumab tablets. For the treatment of patients with metastatic breast cancer whose tumors overexpress the HER-2 protein and who have received one or more chemotherapy regimens for their metastatic disease; manufactured by Genentech, Inc.

Heredity: passing of genetic traits from parents to their young.

Heritability: a property of phenotypic traits; the proportion of a trait's interindividual variance that is due to genetic variance.

Hermaphrodite: individual who has both male and female reproductive organs.

Hertz (Hz): cycles per second, the unit for measuring the vibratory rate of electromagnetic radiation; a measure of impulse frequency; 1 Hz = 1/1 cycle per second.

Heterozygous: a condition in which an individual has two different alleles at a particular locus.

Hibernation: a condition of deep sleep and reduced metabolic activity observed in some animals, particularly during the winter months.

High-density lipoprotein (HDL): "good" cholesterol. HDL transports cholesterol away from the cells. The HDL level should be above 0.9 mmol (millimole) per liter of blood.

Hindbrain: the parts of the brain derived from the embryonic hindbrain, including the cerebellum, pons, and medulla oblongata.

Hippocampal formation: cortical part of the olfactory system, located on the medial aspect of the temporal lobe, and consisting most prominently of the fimbria, hippocampus proper, dentate gyrus, subiculum, and hippocampal gyrus. The formation has been implicated in memory function and has been employed extensively to study long-term potentiation.

Hippocampus: an area of the brain involved in learning and memory.

Histamine: chemical released from mast cells and other cells when allergy-causing antigens attach themselves to mast cells; responsible for producing allergy symptoms.

Histocompatibility locus antigens (HLA): cell surface proteins that differ between individuals and initiate rejection reactions in transplants. Normal function is to facilitate recognition of foreign antigens (e.g., microbial) by the immune system.

Hodgkin's lymphoma (disease): a malignancy (cancer) of lymphoid tissue found in the lymph nodes, spleen, liver, and bone marrow.

Homeobox: a region within homeotic or control genes, consisting of some one hundred nucleotides, whose base sequence is very similar in a variety of organisms. Homeoboxes are thought to play a key role in the activation of control genes.

Homeostasis: the ability of living organisms to maintain a constant internal environment. For example, the human body maintains a constant amount of dissolved oxygen in the blood at all times by means of various mechanisms that sense the oxygen level and increase or decrease the breathing rate.

Homeostasis, genetic: the capacity of the genotype to compensate for disturbing environmental influences.

Homologous chromosomes (homologue): Chromosomes that exist in pairs; each homologue possesses the same genes or loci, but the homologues may have different alleles at the same locus; one member of each pair comes from each parent.

Homology: a similarity between two structures that is due to inheritance from a common ancestor.

Homozygous: a condition in which an individual has the same two alleles at a particular locus.

Hormone: a substance, usually a peptide or steroid, produced by one tissue and conveyed by the bloodstream to another to effect a change in physiological activity, such as growth or metabolism. The same problems of nomenclature that limit the applicability of terms like neuropeptide or cytokine apply here.

Hormone replacement therapy (HRT): a chemical formulation of estrogen or estrogen and progesterone for treating postmenopausal women.

Hot flashes: waves of heat due to erratic vasodilation of blood vessels that occur during menopause in response to estrogen depletion or during treatment with drugs that block estrogen production.

Human chorionic gonadotropin (HCG): the placental hormone of pregnancy.

Human immunodeficiency virus (HIV): the retrovirus that causes AIDS (acquired immune deficiency syndrome).

Hydrophilic: "water-loving," a characteristic of charged molecules in which they readily interact with water molecules.

Hydrophobic: with regard to a molecule or side group, tending to dissolve readily in organic solvents but not in water; resisting wetting; not containing polar groups or subgroups.

Hyperglycemia: a condition in which blood glucose levels are too high (.250 mg/dl). Symptoms include frequent urination, increased thirst, and weight loss.

Hyperphagia: a condition in which an animal does not stop eating when it normally would.

Hyperplasia: literally, "too many cells." The two stages that precede DCIS are intraductal hyperplasia, where more than the normal number of cells are crowded into the breast duct, and intraductal hyperplasia with atypia, where some of those cells have an abnormal appearance.

Hyperpolarized: a description for a membrane whose polarity is greater than its typical resting potential.

Hyperprolactinemia: increased or excessive release of prolactin.

Hypertension: a disorder characterized by high blood pressure.

Hyperthyroidism: a condition caused by an excess of circulating thyroid hormone; symptoms in humans include nervousness, sleeplessness, hyperactivity, weight loss, and, if prolonged, a bulging of the eyeballs.

Hypoglycemia (or insulin reaction): a condition in which blood glucose levels drop too low (generally, below 70 mg/dl). Symptoms include moodiness, numbness in the arms and hands, confusion, and shakiness or dizziness. When left untreated, this condition can become severe and lead to unconsciousness and coma.

Hypophysectomy: removal of the pituitary, or master endocrine gland, usually surgically.

Hypothalamus: a gland in the brain that produces hormones that initiate the reproductive cycle. The dense aggregation of neuronal subpopulations at the base of the brain, in the wall of the third ventricle extending from optic chiasm to mammillary bodies, that governs autonomic and visceral functions, including endocrine secretion, water balance, intermediary metabolism, temperature regulation, sexuality, appetite, and emotional behavior.

Hypothesis: a proposition set forth as an explanation for a specified group of phenomena, either asserted merely as a provisional conjecture to guide investigation or accepted as highly probable in the light of established facts.

Hypothyroidism: a condition caused by abnormally low levels of circulating thyroid hormone; symptoms include physical and mental sluggishness, weight gain, hair loss, and infertility.

Hypoxia: oxygen deprivation.

Hysterectomy: surgical removal of the uterus.

Immune: condition in which a body is able to permanently fight a disease using B-cells and T-cells produced the first time the body was exposed to the disease.

Immune response: the entire array of physiological and development responses involving specific protective actions against a foreign substance; including phagocytosis, the production of antibodies, complement fixation, lysis, agglutination, and inflammation.

Immune system: the body's complicated primary defense against disease-causing microorganisms.

Immunosuppression: suppression of any or all parts of the immune system; may happen to people who take immunosuppressive drugs to prevent the immune system from rejecting the new organ.

Imprinting: a process that occurs when an animal learns to make a particular response to only one type of animal or object. The sensory modes used for establishing such a connection can be visual, auditory, olfactory, or some combination of these, depending upon the animal.

Impulse: neural impulse; a wave of excitement transmitted through a neuron.

In vitro: the test tube or other artificial environment.

Inbreeding: crossing individuals with similar characteristics who are often closely related.

Incontinence: inability to control elimination of urine or feces.

Induced ovulation: ovulation in response to stimulation by a male.

Infection: condition that results when the body is invaded by a pathogen.

Infertility: inability to conceive.

Inflammation: natural tissue reaction to injury or infection. Involves infiltrating white blood cells and vascular (blood capillary) responses.

Inflammatory response: a nonspecific immune reaction brought on by the release of kinins, histamine, and other agents that increases permeability in nearby capillaries and causes redness and swelling of tissue.

Inhibiting hormone: any of several hypothalamic neurosecretions targeted for the adenohypophysis, that responds by slowing the release of one of its hormones.

Inhibitory block: according to the classical definition of instinct, the neurological inhibitors of behavior that are selectively removed by the perception of the appropriate releaser.

Inhibitory synapse: a synapse in which the secretion of neurotransmitter increases the threshold voltage requirement of the receiving neuron, thereby inhibiting it.

Innate: behavior that has either a fixed genetic basis or a high degree of genetic preprogramming.

Instinct: innate behavior involving appetitive and consummatory phases.

Insulin: a large peptide secretion of the pancreas whose primary function is to control blood glucose levels. Insulin and related peptides are also well known for their growth-factor actions, that is, they induce and support the division of numerous cell types.

Insulin resistance: a condition in which the body does not respond to insulin properly. This is the most common cause of Type 2 Diabetes.

Interleukin-1 or -2: chemical messengers released by antigen-presenting cells and helper T-cells that stimulate cell division in aroused T- and B-lymphocytes.

Interneuron: a neuron that connects two or more neurons.

Interstitial cells: cells of the testis that have an endocrine function.

Intracellular: within cells.

Intraductal papilloma: a benign tumor in the lining of the breast duct.

Intron: a region of DNA separating two parts of a structural gene; transcribed but later removed from mRNA during post-transcriptional modification.

Invasive carcinoma: also known as infiltrating carcinoma. Cancer that can spread beyond its site of origin. Metastatic.

Ion: any electrostatically charged atom or molecule.

Ion channel: in the neural membrane, sodium and potassium channels that, through the opening and closing of gates, selectively admit or reject ions.

Ionizing: property of conferring charge (by electron transfer) on "recipient" molecules (e.g., by many, but not all, forms of radiation).

Irritability: the ability of a cell to undergo a change in membrane potential.

Irritable bowel syndrome: characterized by a combination of abdominal pain and altered bowel function. There are many possible causes. For instance, there may be a disturbance in the muscle movement of the intestine or a lower tolerance for stretching and movement of the intestine. There is no abnormality in the structure of the intestine.

Islets of Langerhans: the islets, beta, alpha, and delta endocrine cells within the pancreas that secrete the hormones insulin, glucagon, and somatostatin, respectively.

Isoflavones: these chemicals form the bulk of soya protein. In the human gut, bacteria convert isoflavones into compounds that can have an estrogenic action, although they are not actually hormones.

Ketoacidosis (or diabetic coma): a severe condition caused by a lack of insulin or an elevation in stress hormones. It is marked by high blood glucose levels and ketones in the urine, and occurs almost exclusively in those with Type 1 Diabetes.

Ketones: acids produced when the body breaks down fat for fuel. This occurs when there is not enough insulin to permit glucose to enter the cells and fuel them or when there are too many stress hormones.

Kidneys: organs that filter waste from your blood.

Killer T-cell: special type of immune cell that transfers proteins into the cell membrane of a pathogen, causing the pathogen to rupture and die.

Kinase: an enzyme that catalyzes the transfer of a phosphate group to specific proteins, thereby altering structure and function.

Knockout gene: a genetically engineered mutant gene that is introduced into an embryo to study the specific effects of that gene.

Labor: series of rhythmic contractions that cause the opening of the cervix to expand so that it will be large enough to allow the baby to pass through.

Lactation: milk production and its release during suckling of young.

Laws of thermodynamics: in physics, laws governing the interconversions of energy.

Lesion: a general term used to describe an abnormal physical finding on exam or X-ray.

Leukemia: group of cancers derived from white blood cells.

Leukocyte: a vertebrate white blood cell, including eosinophils, neutrophils, basophils, monocytes, and lymphocytes.

Libido: sex drive.

Ligament: a tough, flexible, but inelastic band of connective tissue that connects bones or that supports an organ in place.

Ligand: from the Latin *ligare,* "that which binds" (same root as religion). Any of a variety of small molecules that specifically bind to a cellular receptor and in so doing convey an informational message to the cell.

Light reaction: that part of photosynthesis directly dependent on the capture of photons; specifically, the photolysis of water, the thylakoid electron transport system, and the chemiosmotic synthesis of ATP and NADPH.

Limbic system: the emotional brain; a group of structures in the brain important in regulating such behavior as eating, drinking, aggression, sexual activity, and expressions of emotion. Proportionately smaller in humans than in other primates, it operates below the level of consciousness. In fact, the base of limbic, *lim,* comes from the Latin meaning "bottom threshold," as in subliminal, and is the origin of the name.

Lipase: any fat-digesting enzyme.

Lipid: fat molecule.

Lipitor: atorvastatin calcium tablets. A cholesterol-lowering drug and HMG-CoA reductase blocker; manufactured by Pfizer, Inc.

Lipolysis: the physiological process that breaks down stored triglycerides from adipose tissue into glycerol and fatty acids; opposite of lipogenesis.

Liposome: a spherical bilayer of phospholipids that forms spontaneously in water.

Locus: specific place on a chromosome where a gene is located.

Longevity: maximum life span recorded for the species.

Long-term memory: learning that persists more than a few hours, the memory trace of which is physically located in a different part of the brain than short-term memory.

Long-term potentiation: Persistent strengthening of synaptic efficacy elicited by coincident electrical activation of different incoming neural pathways to the same nerve process.

Low-density lipoprotein (LDL) cholesterol: one type of cholesterol that deposits lipids/fat in the blood vessels; the "bad cholesterol."

Lumpectomy: also called a *wide excision.* Breast-conserving surgery in which the doctor attempts to remove malignant tissue and a small rim of healthy tissue.

Lupron Depot: leuprolide acetate. Lupron is a synthetic version of naturally occurring gonadotropin releasing hormone (GnRH). Lupron suppresses shedding of the endometrium during menstruation and is used to treat endometriosis. Some doctors also prescribe Lupron for infertility and for early puberty; it is manufactured by TAP Pharmaceuticals, Inc.

Lupus: any of a group of skin diseases in which the lesions are characteristically eroded.

Luteinizing hormone (LH): the hormone secreted by the pituitary that is responsible for triggering ovulation; a pituitary gonadotrophin that causes follicles to ovulate, corpora lutea to secrete progesterone, and Leydig cells to secrete testosterone.

Luteinizing hormone-releasing hormone (LHRH): one of the general class of gonadotrophin hormones, luteinizing hormone-releasing hormone promotes ovulation and egg maturation. When released in the brain, LHRH causes mating behaviors (lordosis) in small animals and probably in humans as well. It is related to the alpha-mating factor, which promotes sexual reproduction in the primitive organisms known as yeasts. This hints at an evolutionary conservation of function (behavior) uniting the simplest and the most complex of organisms.

Lymph: fluid that bathes all the tissues. The lymphatic system plays an important part in immune function by getting rid of toxins from the body.

Lymph node: a rounded, encapsulated mass of lymphoid tissue through which lymph ducts drain, consisting of a fibrous mesh containing numerous lymphocytes and phagocytes.

Lymphatic system: the system of lymphatic vessels, lymph nodes, lymphocytes, the thoracic duct, and the thymus, which together serve to drain body tissues of excess fluids and to combat infections.

Lymphocyte: any of several varieties of similar-appearing leukocytes involved in the production of antibodies and in other aspects of the immune response.

Lymphoid tissue: tissue in which lymphocytes are activated and aggregate.

Lymphoma: group of cancers which affect lymphoid tissue (e.g., lymph nodes).

Lysosome: a small membrane-bounded cytoplasmic organelle, generally containing strong digestive enzymes or other cytotoxic materials.

Macrophage: a large phagocyte that forms from a monocyte.

Macular degeneration: the deterioration of the macula (the central part of therctina of the eye); leads to blurring of central vision, while peripheral vision remains intact. May be caused by atherosclerosis.

Magnetic resonance imaging (MRI): a diagnostic test during which tissues are studied with the aid of a high-powered magnet and a computer.

Major histocompatibility complex (MHC): genes that code for cell surface proteins and glycoproteins that make individuals biochemically unique; part of the HLA system. See also **Histocampatibility locus antigens (HLA)**.

Malignant: clinical term for life-threatening cancer. Cells that have lost the regulatory mechanism and now grow unchecked.

Mammary gland: breast gland in female mammals that produces milk to nourish the young for some time after they are born.

Mammogram: an X-ray of the breasts to screen for breast cancer.

Mass extinction: the extermination of a large proportion of the plant and animal life on Earth by a climatic, geological, cosmic, or other environmental event.

Mastectomy: according to Dr. Susan Love, "the ultimate wide excision." The current procedure involves removing all the breast tissue and a wedge of skin that includes the nipple, as well as some lymph nodes. The radical mastectomy, introduced in the United States in the 1890s by Dr. William Halsted, involved removing pectoral muscles and lymph nodes above the breast as well.

Meiosis: "reduction-division," the specialized division of cells that will form sperm or eggs and reduce the chromosome number by half.

Melanin: the characteristic animal surface pigmentation; also found in plants.

Melanoma: type of aggressive cancer derived from melanin pigment-producing skin cells.

Melatonin: a hormone produced by the pineal gland during the hours of darkness that affects diurnal body rhythms.

Meme: a small mental representation of cultural information, such as a commercial jingle, car design, clothing fashion, dance step, or simple phrase. The "science" of memetics studies the ways in which memes can act as "brain viruses" and "infect" our consciousness by becoming annoying, dominating, distracting memories.

Menarche: a woman's first menstruation, at puberty.

Menopause: cessation of estrogen production; the end of a woman's ability to reproduce. The cessation of menstruation because of the depletion of eggs in the ovary; the whole group of physical, physiological, and behavioral occurrences and changes associated with the cessation of menstruation.

Menses: the period of shedding of the lining (endometrium) of the uterus and associated fluids if an ovum is not fertilized, most notably in primates.

Menstrual cycle: the period from the end of one ovulatory cycle, as demarcated by the beginning of menstrual flow, to the end of the next cycle in female primates.

Menstruation: monthly bleeding during which the endometrial lining is shed. The periodic discharge of blood, secretion, and tissue debris resulting from the normal, temporary breakdown of the uterine mucosa in the absence of implantation following ovulation.

Messenger RNA (mRNA): (1) in prokaryotes, RNA directly transcribed from an operation or structural gene, containing one or more contiguous regions specifying a polypeptide sequence; (2) in eukaryotes, RNA transcribed from a structural gene, tailored and usually capped and polyadenylated in the nucleus and transported to the cytoplasm, containing a single contiguous region specifying a polypeptide sequence as well as leader and follower sequences.

Metabolic pathway: an orderly series or progression of enzyme-mediated chemical reactions leading to a final product, each step catalyzed by its own specific enzyme.

Metabolism: all the physical and chemical processes that take place in the body in order for it to grow and function.

Metabolite: (1) a metabolic waste, especially one that is toxic; (2) an intermediate in a biochemical pathway.

Metastasis, metastasize: usually refers to the movement of two malignant cells from one part of the body to another.

Mg/dl: milligrams per deciliter. This is the unit of measure used when referring to blood glucose levels.

Microcalcifications: dots of calcium that can show up on a mammogram; benign 80 percent of the time, but, if small and clustered together, a possible indication of DCIS.

Microorganism: any organism too small to be seen readily without the aid of a microscope; such as bacterium, protist, or yeast.

Midbrain: the middle of the three divisions of the vertebrate embryonic brain; the adult structures derived from the embryonic midbrain.

Midluteal phase: a portion of the menstrual cycle characterized by high concentrations of estradiol and progesterone, occurring about midway between ovulation and onset of menstruation.

Mitochondria: granular or rod-shaped bodies in the cytoplasm of cells that function in the metabolism of fat and proteins, probably of bacterial origin; the energy source of the cell.

Mitosis: the process of cell division that results in two identical daughter cells.

Molecular biology: a branch of biology concerned with the ultimate physicochemical organization of living matter; the study of biological systems using biochemical methods.

Molecular clock: the clocklike regularity of the change of a molecule (gene) or a whole genotype over geological time.

Molecule: the smallest particle into which an element or a compound can be divided without changing its chemical and physical properties. A molecule is composed of several, perhaps many, atoms.

Monoclonal: derived from a single cell line or same cell type.

Monocyte/macrophage: an immune system cell formed from a bone marrow precursor that circulates in the blood for several days before migrating into tissues throughout the body that respond rapidly (in hours or days, rather than weeks) to trauma, injury, and infections. They play prominent roles in wound repair and healing and ingesting and digesting debris (dead cells).

Monogamy: a mating system in which a male and female bond for some period of time and share in the rearing of offspring.

Monosaccharide: a sugar not composed of smaller sugar subunits (e.g., glucose, fructose).

Morphology: the form and structure of an organism considered as a whole.

Mortality rate: the number of deaths per unit of time occurring among a specified number of individuals in a given area or population.

Motor neuron: a neuron that synapses with a muscle membrane.

Motor neuron disease: a progressive mid- to late-life degenerative neurologic disease in which primary motor neurons in the spinal cord and their afferents in the cerebral cortex degenerate, leading to paralysis, spasticity, and death due to respiratory compromise. Some forms are known as amyotrophic lateral sclerosis (Lou Gehrig's disease).

Mucosa: the highly glandular mucous membrane lining of an organ; also a type of epithelium.

Mucous membrane: lining tissue that specializes in secreting mucus.

Mucus: a viscid, slippery secretion rich in mucins, which is secreted by mucous membranes and serves to moisten and protect such membranes.

Multicellular: consisting of a number of specialized cells that cooperatively carry out the functions of life.

Multiple sclerosis: nerve disease that results from autoimmune destruction of the myelin sheath that surrounds nerve fibers.

Mutagen: a chemical or physical agent that causes mutations.

Mutate: (1) to alter, cause a change, or cause a mutation or DNA change to occur in, to mutagenize; (2) to change in state or genetic condition, to become altered, to undergo a mutation.

Mutation: any inheritable alteration in the genetic material, most commonly an error of replication during cell division, resulting in the replacement of an allele by a different one. In addition to such gene mutations, there are also chromosomal mutations (i.e., major chromosomal changes, including polyploidy).

Mutation pressure: the constant resupplying of mutations to the gene pool due to a base mutation rate.

Mutation rate: the rate at which new mutations occur, generally in terms of mutations per locus per gamete per generation.

Myelin: substance composed of lipids and protein that forms an insulated sheath around an axon.
Myelin sheath: fatty sheath surrounding the axons of many vertebrate neurons.
Myoma: a benign fibroid tumor in the uterine muscle.
Myometrium: muscle layer of the uterus.

Natural killer (NK) cell: a free-roving lymphocyte that identifies, binds to, and lyses cancerous and virus-infected cells as part of the nonspecific immune response.
Natural selection: the disproportionate survival and reproductive success of organisms that possess certain alleles, a result of the influence of those alleles. The process by which in every generation individuals of lower fitness are removed from the population.
NBCC: National Breast Cancer Coalition, a grass-roots lobbying and advocacy group founded in 1991 by Dr. Susan Love and Susan Hester, with breast cancer survivor Fran Visco as its first president.
NCI: National Cancer Institute, the largest division of the National Institutes of Health, created by a special act of Congress in 1937 and funded separately under a bypass budget.
Negative feedback: an automated control mechanism in which an action, brought about by a chemical or physical stimulus, directly or indirectly reduces the stimulus. Such an inhibiting effect constitutes a negative feedback loop.
Neoblast: an unspecialized embryonic cell retained in the adult bodies of certain primitive animals and called to the site of an injury to take part in regenerative healing.
Neocortex: the nonolfactory cerebral cortex that increases in size from reptiles to mammals and humans and subserves a variety of higher integrative functions.
Neoplasia: the formulation and growth of new tissue; refers to benign or malignant growth.
Nephropathy: kidney damage. This condition can be life-threatening. When the kidneys fail to function, dialysis (filtering blood through a machine) or kidney transplantation becomes necessary.
Nerve: (1) a filamentous band of nerve cell axons and dendrites and protective and supporting tissue that connects parts of the nervous system with other parts of the body; (2) pertaining to the nerve or nervous system (e.g., nerve cell, nerve net, nerve fiber).
Nerve cell body: the largest part of a neuron; typically contains the nucleus.
Nerve growth factor: a trophic protein elaborated by targets and possibly glia that is required for the normal survival and function of peripheral sympathetic and sensory neurons and basal forebrain cholinergic neurons. Effects on other brain populations are under intense investigation.
Nervous system: system that receives and relays information about activities within the body and monitors and responds to internal and external changes.
Neural impulse: a transient membrane depolarization, followed by immediate repolarization, traveling in a wavelike manner along a neuron.
Neurocardiology: the field that studies the heart as a neurohormonal organ.
Neuroepidermal junction: a structure formed from the union of skin and nerve fibers at the site of tissue in animals capable of regeneration. It produces the specific electrical currents that bring about the subsequent regeneration.
Neurohormone: a chemical produced by nerve cells that has effects on other nerve cells or other parts of the body.

Neuroleptic agents: antipsychotic drugs, used to treat psychoses, that exert beneficial effects on mood and disordered thought.

Neuron: any of the impulse-conducting cells that constitute the brain, spinal column, and nerves, consisting of a nucleated cell body with one or more dendrites and a single axon. Also called *nerve cell.* Neurons have usually been associated with the functioning of the brain, but their presence in close association with immune cells is clear evidence that they mediate brain/immune interactions.

Neuropathy: damage to the nerves. Neuropathies are often broken down into two categories. Peripheral neuropathies affect the nerves controlling sensation (and less commonly, muscles) in the feet, hands, and joints. Autonomic neuropathies affect the nerve function of various organs, including those of the digestive system and urinary tract.

Neuropeptides: neurotransmitters made up of amino acids that are active not only in the brain but, like microcosmic keys fitting into tiny keyholes in the cells of the body, act like "bits of brain" that float throughout the body and help unlock a cell's memory.

Neurotransmitter: a chemical released by the presynaptic membrane of a synapse that attaches to receptor molecules on the postsynaptic membrane and causes a change in the permeability of that membrane.

Neurotransmitters: chemical signals that communicate among neurons, and potentially between neurons and glia, resulting in such diverse effects as electrical impulse activity, altered gene expression, growth, and survival.

Neutrophil: the most common and abundant white cell involved with fighting bacterial infections.

Niche: a conglomerate of properties of the environment making it suitable for occupation by a specific species.

Nicotine: poisonous substance in tobacco that enters the bloodstream and causes the release of epinephrine.

NIH: National Institutes of Health, the federal government's center for medical research, founded in 1887 and located in Bethesda, Maryland.

Nocturnal: animals whose primary activity occurs during the dark portion of the daily cycle.

Nolvadex: see **Tamoxifen.**

Nonspecific defense: defense mechanism of the body that guards against all infections rather than a particular pathogen.

Norepinephrine: also called *noradrenaline;* the sympathetic catecholamine in the peripheral nervous system and a transmitter used by the locus ceruleus in the brain.

Normalizing (stabilizing) selection: the elimination by selection of variants beyond the normal range of variation of a population.

Nucleic acid: a high-molecular-weight nucleotide polymer. There are two types, DNA and RNA.

Nucleotide: A compound consisting of a nitrogenous base and a phosphate group linked to the 1' and 5' carbons or ribose, respectively; the repeating subunit of DNA and RNA.

Nucleotide base: essential subunit of genetic code in all genes, consisting of adenine, thymine, cytosine, or guanine (A, T, C, or G).

Nucleus: the sac within each cell that contains the chromosomes.

Nucleus accumbens: a subcortical nucleus of neurons that may play a role in the pathogenesis of schizophrenia when deranged.

Obesity: an abnormal and excessive amount of body fat greater than 20 percent. Obesity also occurs in people who are not overweight but have more body fat than muscle. Obesity is considered a chronic illness. It is on the rise and is a risk factor for Type 2 Diabetes.

Olfactory: having to do with the sense of smell.

Olfactory system: neural structures at the base of the brain that process odorant information and the motor responses thereto and that play a role in memory processing. The system includes the olfactory bulb, olfactory tract and striae, and the structures of the hippocampal formation.

Oncogenes: tumor genes that can, if damaged, encourage uncontrolled malignant cell growth.

Oncologist: a physician specializing in cancer treatment.

Oncology: study of cancer treatment.

Oophorectomy: surgical removal of one or both ovaries.

Opposed HRT: estrogen and progestogen taken together as hormone replacement therapy.

Oral agents: medications taken orally that are designed to lower blood glucose. They are used by some people with Type 2 Diabetes and are not to be confused with insulin.

Oral contraceptive: drug for birth control; usually consists of a combination of progestogen and estrogen.

Orchiectomy: surgical removal of a testicle(s).

Organelle: a functionally and morphologically specialized part of a cell.

Organic molecule: a molecule containing carbon and generally produced by living organisms.

Orgasm: in humans, the climax of sexual excitement, usually accompanied in men by ejaculation and in women by rhythmic contractions of the cervix.

Oscillator: the internal mechanism that is the clock in a biological rhythm.

Osteoblast: a cell that forms bone by producing the specific type of collagen that forms bone's underlying structure.

Osteocyte: cell in compact and spongy bone that is responsible for bone growth and changes in the shape of bones.

Osteogenesis: the formation of new bone, whether in embryogenesis, postnatal development, or fracture healing.

Osteoporosis: the condition in which bones become thin and porous as a result of calcium loss.

Ovarian cyst: a saclike structure in the ovary that causes an enlargement of the ovary.

Ovarian failure: the inability of the ovary to produce estrogen; also known as menopause.

Ovary: female reproductive organ that also houses eggs and produces hormones.

Ovulation: the release of one or more eggs from an ovary.

Ovum: egg produced in an ovary.

Oxidation: the loss of electrons from an element or compound; the loss of hydrogens from a compound.

Oxidation-reduction reaction: a chemical reaction in which one reactant is oxidized and another is reduced.

Oxidative respiration: the breakdown of biochemicals to produce cellular energy, utilizing oxygen as the final electron acceptor.

Oxytocin: a hormone produced by the pituitary gland that causes uterine contractions.

P53: (protein 53). Important protein in protecting cells from stress or DNA damage. Commonly deleted or mutated in cancer. *P53* gene encoding p53 protein (*note:* italicized for gene, roman for protein; similarly for all genes and their protein products) = 53 dalton in molecular weight.

Pancreas: a gland located in the abdomen that produces both digestive enzymes (exocrine pancreas) and hormones (endocrine pancreas). Key hormones produced by the pancreas are insulin and glucagon, which play roles in regulating blood glucose levels.

Pap test: cervical smear sample analyzed microscopically for abnormal, potentially cancerous cells.

Parasite: an organism living in or on another living organism from which it obtains its organic sustenance to the detriment of its host.

Parkinson's disease: a middle- to late-life, progressive, degenerative neurologic disorder in which death of the substantia nigral dopaminergic neurons is accompanied by slowed movement (bradykinesia), muscle rigidity, masklike face, and stooped (festinating) gait.

Passive immunity: type of immunity that results when antibodies produced by other animals against a pathogen are injected into the bloodstream.

Patches: regions of localized concentrations of resources.

Pathogen: an organism that is capable of causing disease in another organism; generally refers to viruses and parasitic bacteria and fungi.

Pathogenesis: the processes through which abnormal physiological mechanisms give rise to specific signs and symptoms.

Pelvic inflammatory disease (PID): an infection of the female pelvic organs, usually due to a sexually transmitted disease.

Peptide: a chain of two or more amino acids; the building blocks of proteins.

Peptide hormone: any hormone consisting of one or more amino acids.

Perimenopause: a time of decreasing fertility leading up to menopause.

Period: the duration of one cycle of a biological rhythm. Menstruation.

Peripheral nervous system: the system of nerves that links the brain and spinal cord—the central nervous system—to the rest of the human body. The peripheral nerves consist of the cranial nerves (twelve pairs), the spinal nerves (thirty-one pairs), and the autonomic nerves (sympathetic and parasympathetic), which are distributed to smooth muscles, cardiac muscle, and glands.

Phagocytosis: incorporation of foreign organisms by defending immune cells.

Phase transition: evolution of a physical system from one phase or cycle to another.

Phenotype: unique physical features of a cell or individual that result from the influence of both the organism's genotype and environmental factors.

Phenotypic expression: a generic term referring to the production of specific gene products, including particular species of messenger RNA and the proteins they encode (i.e., blue versus brown eyes).

Pheromone: a species-specific odor cue released by animals that influences the behavior and/or physiology of other similar species.

Photon: a quantum of electromagnetic radiant energy.

Photoperiodism: the response of an organism to photoperiods, involving sensitivity to the onset of light or darkness and a capacity to measure time.

Photosynthesis: the organized capture of light energy and its transformation into usable chemical energy in the synthesis of organic compounds.

Phylogeny: the evolutionary history of a group of organisms.

Physiology: (1) a branch of biology dealing with the processes, activities, and phenomena of individual living organisms, organs, tissues, and cells; (2) the normal functioning of an organism.

Phytoestrogens: a group of foods that contain substances that have a hormonelike action, such as soya beans, fennel, celery, parsley, clover, and linseed oil.

Pigment: any chemical substance that absorbs light, whether or not its normal function involves light absorption (e.g., chlorophyll, cytochrome *c*, hemoglobin, melanin).

Pineal gland: an endocrine gland located near the midline of the brain that produces melatonin, a hormone involved in biological rhythms, particularly in annual cycles.

Pituitary gland: pea-sized gland located between and behind the eyes in the base of the brain that secretes hormones to control many other important glands in the body, including ovaries, thyroid, and adrenal glands; controlled by the hypothalamus.

Placebo: a substance having no pharmacological effect but administered as a control in testing experimentally or clinically the efficacy of a biologically active preparation.

Placenta: the organ formed by the union of the uterine mucosa with the extraembryonic membranes of the fetus, which provides for the nourishment of the fetus, the elimination of waste products, and the exchange of dissolved gases.

Plasma: liquid portion of the blood that contains water, dissolved fats, salts, sugars, and proteins.

Plasticity, neuronal: a generic term referring to mutability of structure and function, frequently induced by environmental experience.

Platelets: minute blood cells associated with clotting.

Pleiotropic: a description for a gene or set of genes that influences the phenotype of more than one characteristic.

Pleiotropy: the situation where one gene has many effects.

Point mutation: gene mutation that affects a single nucleotide.

Polarized: a description for a membrane that has a potential difference due to an unequal distribution of ions across the membrane.

Polycystic ovaries: abnormal condition in the ovaries in which the eggs are not released after they are mature.

Population: usually a local or breeding group; a group in which any two individuals have the potential of mating with each other.

Population genetics: the scientific study of genetic variation within populations, of the genetic correlation between related individuals in a population, and of the genetic basis of evolutionary change.

Positive feedback: a process in which a positive change in one component of a system brings about changes in other components, which in turn bring about further positive changes in the first component.

Posterior pituitary: in humans, the posterior lobe of the pituitary, a stalked extension of neural tissue extending from the hypothalamus.

Potential energy: energy stored in chemical bonds, in nonrandom organization, in elastic bodies, in elevated weight, or any other static form in which it can theoretically be transformed into another form with the capacity to do work.

Premature menopause: ovarian failure that occurs before the age of thirty-five to forty.

Premenopausal: prior to menopause.

Premenstrual syndrome (PMS): a disorder causing a range of symptoms such as nervousness, irritability, bloating, depression, headache, fatigue, tenderness of the breasts, and acne, that occur each month following ovulation and leading up to menstruation; usually five to fourteen days before.

Preovulatory gonadotrophin surge: sudden large increase of luteinizing hormone (LH) that acts as the final hormonal stimulus for the next ovulation.

Preovulatory phase: the portion of the menstrual cycle just prior to ovulation in which estradiol levels reach peak concentrations.

Presynaptic membrane: the membrane of an axon or of the synaptic knob of an axon in the region of a synaptic cleft, into which it secretes neurotransmitters in the course of the transmission of a nerve impulse.

Primary follicle: cluster of cells that surround an ovum and prepare it for release from the ovary.

Primary immune response: the slower, initial response against invasion of the body by organisms or foreign molecules, during which immature, inactive lymphocytes are activated into specialized B- and T-cell lymphocytes.

Primates: an order of placental mammals (i.e., monkeys, apes, humans).

Progesterone: an ovarian hormone that interacts with estrogen to control the menstrual cycle. A type of steroid hormone produced mainly by the ovaries and placenta that is needed to prepare for and maintain pregnancy.

Progestin: a synthetic form of the hormone progesterone.

Prolactin: a pituitary hormone that induces lactation and prevents ovulation.

Prolapse: sagging of the uterus, bladder, and/or vagina due to loss of muscle and ligament support.

Proliferative phase: the first half of the menstrual cycle, when the endometrium is being built up by estrogen.

Promoter: a DNA sequence to which RNA polymerase must bind in order for transcription to begin.

Proopiomelanocortin (POMC): a polyprotein that contains ACTH (adrenocorticotropic hormone), endorphin, and MSHs (melanocyte stimulating hormones), which are released from the pituitary gland in response to environmental stress. POMC is also localized to other brain areas.

Prophylactic: preventive.

Prostaglandin: any of a group of naturally occurring, chemically related hydroxy fatty acids that stimulate contractility of the uterine and other smooth muscle and have the ability to lower blood pressure, regulate acid secretion of the stomach, regulate body temperature and platelet aggregation, and control inflammation and vascular permeability; they also affect the action of certain hormones.

Prostate gland: a gland in the lower abdomen of men that contributes to the formation of seminal fluid.

Protein: a complex organic macromolecule that is composed of one or more chains of amino acids. Proteins are fundamental components of all living cells and include many substances, such as enzymes, hormones, and antibodies, that are necessary for the proper functioning of an organism.

Prozac: fluoxetine hydrochloride, also known as Sarafem, tablets. Prescribed for the treatment of depression, obsessive-compulsive disorder, bulimia, other eating disorders, obesity, premenstrual dysphoric disorder (PMDD, PMS); manufactured by Eli Lilly & Company.

Psoriasis: a chronic, heredity, recurrent dermatosis marked by discrete vivid red macules, papules, or plaques covered with silvery lamellated scales.

Psychobiology: the study of the mechanism and function of the central nervous system from both psychological and biological perspectives.

Psychoneuroimmunology (PNI): the field that studies the interaction between the mind, body, and social systems and how this interaction influences health and healing. A term coined in the early 1980s to emphasize and promote research that is interdisciplinary in focus and attempts to understand how mental (psychological) function affects immunological activities mediated via traditional neuronal connections. *Neuroimmunomodulation* is another variant term in which psyche is subsumed (implied) within "neuro."

Psychopharmacology: the study of the brain's behavior in terms of chemical, physiological, and psychological parameters.

Puberty: the period during which an individual reaches reproductive maturity.

Pulsatile secretion: pattern of hormone secretion that creates bursts instead of a steady flow. It is characteristic of the way GNRH and some pituitary hormones are released.

Punctuated equilibrium: a theory that evolution does not occur gradually but that life exists over long periods of time with little evolutionary change, interrupted periodically by great changes.

Radiation therapy: treatment of cancer by destroying the cells with ionizing radiation. This process destroys not only the cancer but healthy cells as well; it causes long-term deterioration of tissues, such as atrophy, loss of vascularity, poor healing, and skin changes.

Raloxifene: also known as Evista, raloxifene hydrochloride. Prescribed to treat and prevent osteoporosis, manufactured by Eli Lilly & Company.

Randomized control study: a trial in which people are assigned at random either to receive a new treatment or procedure, or to be given a placebo or standard treatment. The control group provides an essential basis for comparison for the treatment group's results.

RAS: gene commonly mutated in many forms of cancer. Encodes a protein involved in intracellular signaling and growth control.

Recapitulation: the appearance of a structure or other attribute of a larval or immature individual of a species that resembles a similar attribute of the adults of an ancestral species; it is interpreted as evidence for descent from that ancestor.

Receptors: molecules that sit on cell surfaces and play a role in chemical "communication." For example, insulin cannot allow glucose into our cells unless the receptors on the cells respond properly to the insulin.

Recessive: describes a trait that is expressed only when the organism is carrying two copies of the underlying hereditary material (two copies of the responsible gene).

Reciprocal altruism: behavior functions to increase the fitness of the individual insofar as it increases the likelihood that the individual will be the recipient of beneficial behavior at another time.

Recombinant DNA: a general term for the laboratory manipulation of DNA in which DNA molecules or fragments from various sources are severed and combined enzymatically and reinserted into living organisms.

Recombination: a reshuffling of the genes in a new zygote as a result of crossing over and reassortment of the chromosomes during meiosis. A new set of genotypes is thus produced in each generation.

Recurrence: the reappearance of a cancer. Local recurrence can occur at the site of a lumpectomy, and is not considered a metastasis. More serious recurrences can show up in lymph nodes, the mastectomy scar or chest wall, the second breast, or distant organs.

Red blood cells (corpuscles): hemoglobinized blood cells that carry oxygen to all parts of the body.

Red Queen hypothesis: the hypothesis that sexual reproduction has evolved because the genetic variation that results is adaptive in the evolutionary "arms race" between hosts and their pathogens and parasites as well as between predators and prey.

Redifferentiation: the process in which a previously mature cell that has dedifferentiated becomes a mature, specialized cell again.

Reductase: 5 alpha-reductase catalyzes the conversion of testosterone into 5 alpha-dihydrotestosterone (DHT).

Refractory state: a brief period when a neuron cannot generate a second impulse.

Releasing factors: hormones or neurosecretions from the hypothalamus that travel either via the hypothalamic-pituitary portal system or along axons between the hypothalamus and the pituitary where they exert their effect in terms of production and release of hormones.

Releasing hormone: a chemical messenger released by the hypothalamus that stimulates hormonal release by the pituitary.

REM sleep: a normal period of sleep during which the muscles are very relaxed but the eyes move rapidly under closed lids; accompanied by high brain electrical activity.

Repair enzyme: any of several different complexes of enzymes that recognize improper base pairing in DNA, excise a region of one of the strands, and rebuild the DNA.

Repressor: special protein that binds to the operator and thus turns off an operon.

Reproductive success: the production of viable offspring that reproduce in turn; levels of reproductive success may differ between individuals.

Resonance: one of the natural states of oscillation of a physical system.

Resting state: a state of seeming inactivity in a neuron, but one in which the membrane activity maintains a polarized state in preparation for conduction.

Restriction enzyme: in bacteria, an enzyme that recognizes and serves a specific, short DNA sequence, thus protecting the cell from all but a few highly adapted, host-specific viruses; such enzymes have proved useful for experimental DNA manipulation.

Rheumatoid arthritis: a chronic inflammatory disease that primarily affects the joints and surrounding tissues, but can also affect other organ systems.
Ribonucleic acid (RNA): a compound found with DNA in cell nuclei and chemically close to DNA; transmits genetic code from DNA to direct the formation of proteins. May take two forms: messenger RNA (mRNA) or transfer RNA (tRNA).
Ritualization: evolutionary process by which behavior patterns become modified to serve as communication signals.
Rituxan: rituximab tablets. For the treatment of patients with relapsed or refractory low-grade of follicular, CD20 positive, B-cell non-Hodgkin's lymphoma; manufactured by Genentech, Inc.

S phase: the phase of the cell cycle during which DNA synthesis occurs.
Saturated fats: a fat is saturated when its molecules hold the maximum amount of hydrogen. The more saturated a fat becomes, the harder it is for the body to use it, so the fat gets deposited and stored. Saturated fats include hard cheese, butter, and palm oil.
Scan: various radiographic tests used as a diagnostic tool for the detection of disease.
Schwann cells: the cells that surround all of the nerves outside of the brain and spinal cord.
Sciatic nerve: the main nerve in the leg. It includes both motor nerve fibers carrying impulses to the leg muscles, and sensory nerve fibers carrying impulses to the brain.
Scientific method: systematic approach to problem-solving that involves observation and experimentation.
Secondary immune response: a rapid response to a second or subsequent invasion of the body by organisms or foreign molecules, during which memory cells quickly produce large numbers of active, specialized B- and T-cell lymphocytes.
Secondary sex characteristic: sex characteristic that appears at puberty (e.g., pubic and axillary hair).
Selective breeding: method of improving a species by choosing animals or plants that have desirable characteristics to produce offspring that have the parents' desirable traits.
Self-propagating: a description of the events occurring during an action potential, with each regional depolarization by sodium voltage-gated channels causing a similar event at an adjacent area downstream.
Semen: combination of sperm and seminal fluid.
Senescence: the biological characteristics of aging.
Sensory neuron: a neuron that is modified to respond to a particular set of stimuli (e.g., touch, temperature).
Serotonin: a naturally produced substance that is involved in nerve signal transmission. A transmitter derived from dietary tryptophan to play a role in sleep, blood clotting, and mood.
Serum (plasma): a clear liquid component of blood that carries the red blood cells, white blood cells, and platelets.
Sex chromosomes: those chromosomes that carry the genes that control gender (maleness or femaleness). Referred to as X or Y.
Sex hormone binding globulin (SHBG): a protein produced in the liver that binds most sex hormones in the bloodstream and tempers their effects on cells.

Sex-influenced: description of a trait that is caused by a gene whose expression differs in males and females.

Sex linkage: the type of linkage produced when a gene is located on the X or the Y chromosome.

Sex-linked trait: an inherited trait coded on the sex chromosomes, and thus having a special distribution related to sex.

Sexual cycle: cycle of ovarian follicular development, ovulation, and corpora lutea formation, including hormone secretion.

Sexual selection: selection for attributes that enhance reproductive success.

Simultaneous reconstruction: in autologous simultaneous reconstruction, the plastic surgeon builds a breast for a mastectomy patient out of her own tissue at the same time as her mastectomy. Two procedures are most common: the tunnel tram-flap, in which a segment from the abdomen is tunneled up to the chest, its blood supply intact; and the free-flap, in which the tissue and skin are severed and attached to a new vein and artery pulled down from the armpit.

Sinoatrial (SA) node: the heart's rhythmic center. It is a tiny patch of tissue in the heart's back wall near the top of its right atrium that is the center of the cardiac conduction system. It functions as the heart's own internal pacemaker and is central to the complex "nervous system" of the heart.

Smooth muscle: the muscle tissue of the glands, viscera, iris, piloerection, and other involuntary functions, usually controlled by the autonomic nervous system.

Society: a group of individuals belonging to the same species and organized in a cooperative manner. Usually assumed to extend beyond sexual behavior and parental care of offspring.

Sociobiology: a study that involves the application of the principles of evolution to the study of the social behavior and social systems of animals.

Sodium ion gate: either of the two gates controlling sodium ion passage through an ion channel, including an activation gate and inactivation gate.

Sodium/potassium ion exchange pump: a poorly understood molecular entity in the plasma membrane, capable of actively transporting sodium out of the cell and potassium in, at a cost of ATP energy.

Software: in neuroscience, by analogy with computer science, the functional program that dictates particular operations in the nervous system.

Somatic: having to do with body cells (i.e., those that do not produce gametes).

Somatic nervous system: division of the peripheral nervous system that regulates activities that are under conscious control.

Species: a group of populations of organisms that are enough alike in structure and behavior so that individuals can interbreed and produce fertile offspring if they have access to one another. Individuals from one species are reproductively isolated from other species.

Spleen: an abdominal organ consisting of lymphoid, reticular, and endothelial tissues with blood supply and red blood cells circulating freely in intercellular spaces; functions include the scavenging of debris and the maintenance of blood volume. Also part of the immune system.

Stabilizing natural selection: natural selection that operates during periods when the environment is stable; maintains the genetic and phenotypic status quo within a population.

Staging: the process of categorizing disease states to help predict outcomes from treatment or natural history. There are four stages of cancer, listed in order of increasing severity.

Stage 1 cancer, the least threatening, means the disease has been caught at an early stage—no positive lymph nodes (cancer) and a tumor less than 2 cm in diameter. Patients in this group usually do not have chemotherapy, since seven will survive without it, two will die in spite of it, and only one will survive because of it.

Stage 2 can mean several things—a small tumor with positive but mobile axillary lymph nodes; a tumor up to 5 cm in diameter with positive mobile nodes or negative nodes; or a tumor over 5 cm in diameter with negative nodes.

Stage 3 is a large tumor, over 5 cm in diameter, with positive nodes, or a small tumor with fixed nodes.

Stage 4 means that a patient's cancer has widely disseminated, or spread to other organs.

Stasis: a period of evolutionary equilibrium or inactivity.

Stem cell: a self-renewing type of cell that also produces differentiated products. Founder cell of specialized cells such as blood, epithelia, epidermis, and liver. Sustains production of such cells or tissues. Major target for many types of cancer.

Stereotactic core biopsy: use of a high-speed needle, guided by computer, to remove tissue samples; an alternative to some surgical biopsies.

Steroid: a family of lipid molecules including cholesterol and the naturally occurring hormones: estrogens, progesterone, and testosterone.

Steroid hormone: a class of hormones consisting of the steroid molecule with carious side group substitutions, believed to freely pass across the cell membrane and, once bound by a specific carrier protein, interact directly with the chromatin in gene control; included are the vertebrate sex hormones.

Stimulant: drug that speeds up the actions of the nervous system.

Stimulus: an aspect of the environment that influences the activity of a living organism or part of an organism, especially through a sense organ.

Stop codon: in mRNA, one or more of the codons UAA, UAG, or UGA, signaling the end of polypeptide translation.

Stress: physical or emotional strain or pressure. The stress response is thought to be mediated by a variety of neurohumoral mechanisms, including the concerted action of the limbic system, the central and peripheral autonomic systems, and the adrenal gland.

Stress incontinence: inability to retain urine during sneezing, coughing, or laughing.

Stroma: one of the cell types of the uterine lining.

Structural protein: protein that is incorporated into cellular or extracellular structures.

Substance P: a putative peptide, excitatory transmitter that is localized to multiple subpopulations, including sensory and sympathetic neurons. The peptide contains eleven amino acids and is synthesized as part of a larger parent molecule, preprotachykinin, which also may contain the peptide transmitter NKA (substance K).

Sugar: a form of carbohydrate that provides calories and raises blood glucose levels. There are a variety of sugars, such as white, brown, confectioner's, invert, and raw. Fructose, lactose, sucrose, maltose, dextrose, glucose, honey, corn syrup, molasses, and sorghum are also sugars.

Sugar substitutes: sweeteners used in place of sugar. Note that some sugar substitutes have calories and will affect blood glucose levels, such as fructose and sugar alcohols like sorbitol and mannitol. Others have very few calories and will not affect blood glucose levels, such as saccharin, acesulfame-K, and aspartame (NutraSweet).

Superoxide dismutase (SOD): an enzyme that combats free radical production.

Suppressor gene: gene that inhibits cancerous transformation in cell. Normally directly restrains proliferative activity or induces alternative activities (e.g., senescence, differentiation, or death). Loss of proper function of such a gene (via deletion or mutation) contributes to collective mutation in cancer cells.

Suppressor T-cell: specific subpopulation of T-cells whose role is to moderate, slow, and stop the specific immune responses.

Suprachiasmtic nucleus (SCN): a brain nucleus involved in the visual pathway that has been clearly identified for its involvement in biological rhythms mediated by photoperiod.

Surface adhesion molecules: molecules localized to the extracellular space that mediate specific interactions with selective cell types, such as selective adhesivity.

Symbiosis: the living together in intimate association of two species.

Sympathetic nervous system: a division of the peripheral autonomic system distributed throughout the body that consists of afferent cholinergic neurons and efferent noradrenergic (norepinephrine-containing) neurons. In general terms, the system regulates multiple vegetative functions, including the cardiorespiratory and gastrointestinal systems, and mediates the so-called fight-or-flight physiologic-behavioral repertoire.

Synapse: the junction between one nerve cell and another, or between a nerve cell and some other cell.

Synaptic cleft: the minute space between the synaptic knob of one neuron and the dendrite or cell body of another, into which neurotransmitters are released in the transmission of nerve impulses between cells.

Syncing or in sync: to synchronize; in recent years, due to the research of men like Condon and Birdwhistell, which demonstrates that human beings synchronize with each other.

Syndrome: a collection of symptoms.

Synergism: the interaction of two or more agents or forces so that their combined effect is greater than the sum of their individual effects, as when two hormones combine to affect target tissues.

T4 receptor (CD4): a surface molecule that typifies certain T lymphocytes that have "helper" functions (helper cells). When the T4 molecule is activated, it signals the cell to execute its program, which consists of secreting a variety of molecules that then act on other cells to "help" them perform the actual tasks of immunity, killing virally infected cells or tumors, for example.

T-cell: white cell or specifically a lymphocyte of a variety that matures in the thymus and interacts with invading cells and other cells of the immune system.

Tamoxifen: also known as Nolvadex; tamoxifen citrate tablets. An estrogen blocker and an anticancer drug, it is given to treat breast cancer. It also has proved effective when cancer has spread to other parts of the body. It is most effective in stopping the kind of breast cancer that thrives on estrogen. It is also prescribed to reduce the risk of invasive breast cancer following surgery and radiation therapy for ductal carcinoma in situ. The drug can also be used to reduce the odds of breast cancer in women at high risk of developing the disease. It is manufactured by AstraZeneca Pharmaceuticals LP.

Taxis (pl. taxes): directed reactions to a stimulus involving an orientation of the long axis of the body in line with the stimulus source.

Taxol: a drug first derived from the Pacific yew tree, now produced synthetically. A common chemotherapy treatment.

Telomere: a cap on the end of chromosomes that does not contain a genetic code for proteins but has a protective function.

Temperature-compensated rhythm: the relative insensitivity of biological rhythms to the effects of temperature; this contrasts with the fact that many chemical reactions double in rate for every 10° C increase in temperature.

Testes: male sex glands enclosed in scrota that produce the male sex hormone testosterone, as well as sperm.

Testosterone: the male steroid sex hormone or androgen, which is mainly produced by testes. Women's ovaries also produce a small amount of testosterone.

Thalamus: a large subdivision of the diencephalon, consisting of a mass of nuclei in each lateral wall of the centrally located third ventricle of the brain.

Theory: a proposed explanation whose status is still conjectural, in contrast to well-established propositions that are often regarded as facts. Theory and hypothesis are terms often used colloquially to mean an untested idea or opinion. A theory properly is a more or less verified explanation accounting for a body of known facts or phenomena, whereas a hypothesis is a conjecture put forth as a possible explanation of a specific phenomenon or relationship that serves as a basis for argument or experimentation.

Thermiogenesis: in endothermic animals, the production of body heat through an increase in the metabolic rate that is, the release of energy from fuels.

Thermodynamics: (1) the branch of physics that deals with the interconversions of energy as heat, potential energy, kinetic energy, radiant energy, entropy, and work; (2) the processes and phenomena of energy interconversions.

Thermoreceptors: sensory cells that are sensitive to changes in temperature.

Thermoregulation: (1) an animal's control over its internal temperature; (2) the physiological mechanisms that maintain a body at a particular temperature in an environment with a fluctuating temperature.

Threshold: the minimum stimulus necessary to initiate an all-or-none response.

Thrombin: in the blood-clotting reactions, a proteolytic enzyme that catalyzes the conversion of fibrinogen to fibrin by the removal of two short peptide segments and, in turn, is produced from prothrombin by the action of thromboplastin.

Thymus: a glandular body above the lungs, involved in T-cell lymphocyte development.

Thyroid gland: large, butterfly-shaped gland located in front of and on each side of the trachea that secretes thyroxin and other hormones responsible for numerous metabolic processes; essential for the regulation of the body's metabolism, including heartbeat, temperature control, and other essential processes.

Tissue: a group of associated cells, identical in structure and function.

Toxic/toxicity: damage to tissue.

Toxin: poison.

Trait: characteristic that a living thing can pass on to its young.

Trans fatty acids: the process of hydrogenation in food manufacturing changes the essential unsaturated fats contained in food into trans fatty acids. These have been linked to an increased rate of heart attack.

Transcription, gene: the complex of processes that comprise synthesis of messenger RNA from the DNA genetic code. In turn, messenger RNA is translated into protein product that functions in the cell.

Transduction: in biological systems, conversion of one form of information into another.

Transfer RNA (tRNA): type of RNA that carries amino acids to the ribosomes, where the amino acids are joined together to form polypeptides.

Transformation: in a bacterium, the direct incorporation of a DNA fragment from its medium into its own chromosome.

Transgenic: description of an organism that contains foreign genes.

Translation: synthesis of protein from specific, encoding messenger RNA.

Translocation: movement or relocation of genetic material from one chromosome to another. Common mutational mechanism observed in blood cell cancers and sarcomas.

Trophic factor: a molecule that supports survival of a cellular population.

Trophic hormones (trophic neurosecretions): hormonal or neurosecretory products from endocrine glands or neurosecretory cells that influence the production and release of other hormone products from endocrine glands.

Trophoblast: the outer layer of placenta cells that communicates with the uterus and regulates nutrition of the fetus.

Tubal ligation: interruption of the fallopian tubes to prevent pregnancy or prevent the backflow of endometrial tissue that leads to endometriosis.

Type 1 diabetes: a form of diabetes that tends to develop before age thirty but may occur at any age. It's caused by an immune system attack on the insulin-producing beta cells, which are destroyed, so the pancreas can no longer produce insulin. People who have Type 1 diabetes must take insulin to survive.

Type 2 diabetes: Type 2 diabetics are insulin-resistant. However, some simply cannot produce enough insulin to meet their bodies' needs, and others have a combination of these problems. Many people with Type 2 diabetes control the disease through diet and exercise, but some must also take oral medications or insulin.

Ultradian rhythm: a cyclical rhythm of less than twenty-four hours.

Ultraviolet light: UV, electromagnetic radiation having a shorter wavelength than visible light and longer than X rays.

Undifferentiated: unspecialized, a term applied to cells that are in a primitive or embryonic state.

Unopposed HRT: Hormone replacement therapy given as estrogen only; no progestogen is added into the regime.

Unsaturated fats: fats that are usually liquid at room temperature, such as vegetable oils. They are essential for health and hence are classed as essential fatty acids.

Urethra: membranous canal that carries urine from the bladder to the exterior of the body; sensitive to estrogen in women.

Uterine: derived from the womb or uterus.

Uterine atrophy: shrinkage of the uterus.

Uterus: hollow muscular female organ in which the fetus develops; consists of the body, cervix, and endometrium; also known as the womb.

Vagina: canal extending from the uterus to the exterior of a woman's body; extremely sensitive to lack of estrogen at menopause.

Vascular system: the circulatory system of an animal.

Vasometer: term used to describe menopausal symptoms characterized by dilation of blood vessels; hot flashes are vasometer symptoms.

Vasopressin: a hormone that has a variety of effects throughout the body. When released from the posterior pituitary, it affects water balance. When released from the hypothalamus, it acts as a secretagogue at the pituitary, stimulating secretion of adrenocorticotropic hormone (ACTH). Hypothalamic vasopression is typically released during stress.

Vein: blood vessel that collects blood from the body and carries it back to the heart.

Velocity: the speed and the direction of an object's motion.

Venous thrombosis: blood clot in any vein.

Ventricle: (1) a cavity or a body part or organ; (2) one of the large muscular chambers of the four-chambered heart; (3) one of the systems of communicating cavities of the brain, consisting of two lateral ventricles and a median third ventricle.

Vibrational pattern: the precise number of peaks and troughs as well as their amplitude as a *string* oscillates.

Vioxx: rofecoxib tablets or oral suspension. A new kind of painkiller used in the treatment of osteoarthritis, painful menstruation (dysmenorrhea), and other types of acute pain; manufactured by Merck & Company.

Virus: a noncellular organism consisting of DNA and RNA enclosed in a protein coat, often together with a few enzymes; replicating only within a host cell, utilizing host ribosomes, enzymes, and energy.

Vitamin: any organic substance that is essential to the nutrition of an organism, usually by supplying part of a coenzyme.

Vulva: woman's external genital organs including the mons pubis, labia majora, labia minora, clitoris, and other structures.

White blood cell: blood cell produced in bone marrow that protects the body against invasion by foreign cells or substances; also controls the immune system.

Withdrawal bleeding: bleeding that occurs as a response to a drop in blood levels of progesterone.

Women's Health Initiative: a fifteen-year, $625 million National Institutes of Health study of breast cancer, osteoporosis, and heart disease, incorporating both randomized clinical and observational trials.

X chromosome: sex chromosome; in humans, females have two X chromosomes and males have only one.

X-linked: the condition, common to many genes of functions unrelated to sex, of being present on the X chromosome; thus males have only one copy rather than the normal diploid two, and recessive X-linked alleles are always expressed in males, thus radically affecting patterns of inheritance.

Y chromosome: male sex chromosome; in humans, XY individuals are male and XX individuals are female.

Bibliography

Abbas, Abul K., et al. *Cellular and Molecular Immunology.* Philadelphia: W. B. Saunders Company, 1994.

———. *A Natural History of the Senses.* New York: Vintage Books, 1990.

Ackerman, Diane. *A Natural History of Love.* New York: Vintage Books, 1994.

Angier, Natalie. *Natural Obsessions.* Boston: Mariner Book, 1999.

Baker, Robin, Ph.D. *Sperm Wars.* New York: Basic Books, 1996.

Balick, Michael J., et al. *Plants, People, and Culture.* New York: Scientific American Library, 1997.

Barbach, Lonnie, Ph.D. *The Pause.* New York: Signet Books, 1994.

Baumslag, N., et al. *Milk, Money and Madness: The Culture and Politics of Breastfeeding.* Westport, Conn.: Bergin and Garvey, 1995.

Bazell, Robert. *Her* 2. New York: Random House, 1998.

Becker, Jill B., et al. *Behavioral Endocrinology.* Cambridge, Mass.: MIT Press, 1992.

Becker, Robert O., et al. *The Body Electric.* New York: William Morrow and Company, 1985.

Beckwith, Bill E., et al. *Neuropeptides in Development and Aging.* New York: New York Academy of Sciences, 1997.

Behe, Michael J. *Darwin's Black Box.* New York: The Free Press, 1996.

Benyus, Janine M. *Biomimicry.* New York: Quill, 1997.

Black, Ira B. *Information in the Brain: A Molecular Perspective.* Cambridge, Mass.: MIT Press, 1991.

Bleier, Ruth. *Feminist Approaches to Science.* New York: Teachers College Press, 1991.

Blum, Deborah. *Sex on the Brain.* New York: Viking, 1997.

Blum, Deborah, et al. *A Field Guide for Science Writers.* New York: Oxford University Press, 1997.

Blum, Richard, et al. *Society and Drugs.* San Francisco: Jossey-Bass Inc., 1970.

Bona, Constantin A., et al. *Book of British Birds.* London, England: Drive Publications Limited, 1969.

———. *Molecular Basis of the Immune Response.* New York: Annals of the New York Academy of Sciences, 1988.

Bradlow, Leon H., et al. *Cancer Prevention: Novel Nutrient and Pharmaceutical Developments.* New York: New York Academy of Sciences, 1999.

Breggin, Peter R., M.D., et al. *Talking Back to Prozac.* New York: St. Martin's Paperbacks, 1994.

Brust, John C. M. *The Practice of Neural Science.* New York: McGraw-Hill, 2000.

Burkholz, Herbert. *The FDA Follies.* New York: Basic Books, 1994.

Buss, David M. *The Evolution of Desire.* New York: Basic Books, 1994.

Cairns-Smith, A. G. *Evolving the Mind.* Cambridge, England: Cambridge University Press, 1996.

Calvin, William H. *How Brains Think.* New York: Basic Books, 1996.

Campbell, Bernard G., et al. *Humankind Emerging.* New York: HarperCollins College Publishers, 1996.

Caporale, Lynn Helena. *Molecular Strategies in Biological Evolution.* New York: Annals of the New York Academy of Sciences, 1999.

Capra, Fritjof. *The Web of Life.* London: HarperCollins Publishers, 1996.

Carr, Bruce R., et al. *Reproductive Medicine*, 2d ed. Stamford, Conn.: Appleton & Lange, 1998.

Cavalli-Sforza, Luigi Luca. *Genes, Peoples, and Languages.* New York: North Point Press, 2000.

Chernin, Kim. *Reinventing Eve.* New York: HarperPerennial, 1987.

Chinen, Allan B., M.D. *Once Upon a Midlife.* New York: Jeremy P. Tarcher/Putnam, 1992.

Chopra, Deepak, M.D. *Quantum Healing.* New York: Bantam Books, 1990.

Clark, William R. *A Means to an End.* New York: Oxford University Press, 1999.

Collier, Peter, et al. *Destructive Generation.* New York: The Free Press, 1996.

Committee on Nutritional Status During Pregnancy and Lactation. *Nutrition During Lactation.* Washington, D.C.: National Academy Press. 1991.

Coney, Sandra. *The Menopause Industry.* New York: Penguin Books, 1994.

Cooper, Jack R., et al. *The Biochemical Basis of Neuropharmacology.* New York: Oxford University Press, 1996.

Coutinho, Elsimar M., et al. *Is Menstruation Obsolete?* New York: Oxford University Press, 1999.

Cowan, George A., et al. *Complexity: Metaphors, Models, and Reality.* Reading, Mass.: Addison-Wesley Publishing Company, 1994.

Creatsas, George, et al. *The Young Woman at the Rise of the 21st Century.* New York: New York Academy of Sciences, 2000.

Crossen, Cynthia. *Tainted Truth.* New York: Simon & Schuster, 1994.

Csermely, Peter. *Stress of Life from Molecules to Man.* New York: New York Academy of Sciences, 1998.

Cummings, Stephen, M.D., et al. *Everybody's Guide to Homeopathic Medicines.* New York: Jeremy P. Tarcher/Perigee Books, 1991.

Darwin, Charles. *The Origin of Species.* New York: Bantam Books, 1999.

Davies-Floyd, Robbie, et al. *Cyborg Babies.* New York: Routledge, 1998.

DeGregorio, Michael W., et al. *Tamoxifen and Breast Cancer.* New Haven, Conn.: Yale University Press, 1994.

Deloache, Judy, et al. *A World of Babies.* Cambridge, Mass.: Cambridge University Press, 2000.

De Moulin, D. *A Short History of Breast Cancer.* Boston: Kluwer Academic Publishers, 1989.

Desmond, Adrian. *Huxley.* Reading, Mass.: Helix Books, 1997.

Desmond, Adrian, et al. *Darwin.* New York: W. W. Norton & Company, 1991.

De Waal, Frans. *Good Natured.* Cambridge: Harvard University Press, 1996.

Diamond, Jared. *The Third Chimpanzee.* New York: HarperPerennial, 1992.

Djerassi, Carl. *The Politics of Contraception.* Stanford, Calif.: Stanford Alumni Association, 1979.

Driver, Jim. *The Mammoth Book of Sex, Drugs & Rock 'N' Roll.* New York: Carroll & Graf Publishers, Inc., 2001.

Eberhard, William G. *Female Control: Sexual Selection by Cryptic Female Choice.* Princeton, N.J.: Princeton University Press, 1996.

Engleman, Edgar G., et al. *Genetic Control of the Human Immune Response.* New York: Rockefeller University Press, 1980.

Eskin, Bernard A. *The Menopause Comprehensive Management.* New York: Parthenon Publishing Group, Inc., 2000.

Fabian, A. C. *Evolution*. Cambridge, England: Cambridge University Press, 1998.

Fabris, N., et al. *Ontogenetic and Phylogenetic Mechanisms of Neuroimmunomodulation*. New York: New York Academy of Sciences, 1992.

Farrington, Benjamin. *What Darwin Really Said*. New York: Schocken Books, 1966.

Flamigni, C., et al. *The Gonadotropins: Basic Science and Clinical Aspects in Females*. New York: Academic Press, 1982.

Formby, B., and T.S. Wiley, "Breast Cancer Cell Growth and Programmed Death by Progesterone." In *Breast Cancer* ed., A. Pasqualini. New York: Marcel Dekker, 2002.

Fox, Matthew. *Mystical Visions*. Santa Fe, N. Mex.: Bear & Company Publishing, 1986.

Fraser, Ian S., et al. *Estrogens and Progestogens in Clinical Practice*. New York: Churchill Livingstone, 1998.

Frazer, Alan, et al. *Biological Bases of Brain Function and Disease*. New York: Raven Press, 1994.

Frazer, James George. *The Golden Bough*. New York: Simon & Schuster, 1922.

Friedewald, Vincent, M.D., et al. *Ask the Doctor: Breast Cancer*. Kansas City, Mo.: Andrews and McMeel, 1997.

Ganong, William F. *Review of Medical Physiology*. New York: Simon & Schuster, 1995.

Gass, George H., et al. *Handbook of Endocrinology*, 2d ed., vol. 1. New York: CRC Press, 1996.

Geene, Brian. *The Elegant Universe*. New York: Vintage Books, 2000.

Gehan, E.A., et al. *Statistics in Medical Research: Development in Clinical Trials*. New York: Plenum, 1994.

Glenville, Marilyn. *Natural Alternatives to HRT*. London: Kyle Cathie Limited, 1997.

Godagama, Shantha. *The Handbook of Ayurveda*. Boston: 1998.

Gosden, Roder. *Cheating Time*. New York: W. H. Freeman and Company, 1996.

Gould, James L., et al. *Sexual Selection: Mate Choice and Courtship in Nature*. New York: Scientific American Library, 1989.

Gratzer, Walter. *A Bedside Nature: Genius and Eccentricity in Science 1869–1953*. New York: W. H. Freeman and Company, 1998.

Greaves, Mel. *Cancer: The Evolutionary Legacy*. New York: Oxford University Press, 2000.

Greene, Brian. *The Elegant Universe*. New York: W. W. Norton & Company, Inc., 1999.

Gribbin, John. *Almost Everyone's Guide to Science*. New Haven, Conn.: Yale University Press, 1999.

Haeger, Knut. *History of Surgery*. New York: Bell Publishing Company, 1988.

Hall, Edward T. *The Dance of Life: The Other Dimension of Time*. New York: Doubleday, 1983.

———. *Hanging Loose* 75. Brooklyn, N.Y.: Hanging Loose Press, 1999.

Haraway, Donna. *Primate Visions*. New York: Routledge, 1989.

———. *Simians, Cyborgs, and Women*. New York: Routledge, Chapman and Hall, Inc., 1991.

Harris, Jay R., et al. *Diseases of the Breast*. Philadelphia: Lippincott-Raven Publishers, 1996.

Hill, D. L. *A Review of Cyclophosphamide*. Springfield, Ill.: Thomas, 1975.

Hiller, Lejaren A. *Surgery Through the Ages*. New York: Hastings House, 1944.

Hope, Sally, et al. *Hormone Replacement Therapy*. New York: Oxford University Press, 1999.

Hornblum, Allen M. *Acres of Skin*. New York: Routledge, 1998.

Hrdy, Sarah Blaffer. *Mother Nature*. New York: Pantheon Books, 1999.

———. *The Woman That Never Evolved*. Cambridge: Harvard University Press, 1981.

Ikenze, Ifeoma, et al. *Menopause & Homeopathy: A Guide for Women in Midlife*. Berkeley, Calif.: North Atlantic Books, 1998.

Janeway, Charles A., et al. *Immunobiology*. New York: Elsevier Science Ltd./Garland Publishing, 1999.

Jankovic, Branislav, et al. *Neuroimmune Interactions: Proceedings of the Second International Workshop on Neuroimmunomodulation*. New York: New York Academy of Sciences, 1987.

Janlovic, Branislav D., et al. *Neuroimmune Interactions*. New York: New York Academy of Sciences, 1987.

Jeanes, Allene, et al. *Physiological Effects of Food Carbohydrates*. Washington, D.C.: American Chemical Society, 1975.

Jennings, Peter, et al. *The Century*. New York: Doubleday Dell Publishing, 1998.

Jovanovic, Lois, M.D., et al. *A Woman Doctor's Guide to Menopause*. New York: Hyperion, 1993.

Kalat, James W. *Biological Psychology*. Pacific Grove, Calif.: Brooks/Cole Publishing Company, 1998.

Kitzinger, S., et al. *Being Born*. New York: Grosset & Dunlap, 1986.

Kosslyn, Stephen M., et al. *Frontiers in Cognitive Neuroscience*. Cambridge, Mass.: MIT Press, 1992.

Kotulak, Ronald. *Inside the Brain*. Kansas City, Mo.: Andrews and McMeel, 1996.

Kramer, Peter D. *Listening to Prozac*. New York: Penguin Books, 1997.

Kuklick, Henrika. *The Savage Within*. New York: Cambridge University Press, 1991.

Kushner, R. *Breast Cancer: A Personal and Investigative Report*. New York: Harcourt Brace Jovanovich, 1975.

Lark, Susan M. *The Estrogen Decision Self-Help Book*. Berkeley, Calif.: Celestial Arts, 1993.

———. *The Menopause Self-Help Book*. Berkeley, Calif.: Celestial Arts, 1990.

Laux, Marcus, M.D., et al. *Natural Woman, Natural Menopause*. New York: HarperCollins Publishers, 1997.

Leavitt, Wendell W., et al. *Steroid Hormone Receptor Systems*. New York: Plenum Press, 1979.

Lee, John. *Natural Progesterone: The Multiple Roles of Remarkable Hormone*. Charlbury, Oxon, Wales: Jon Carpenter Publishing, 1999.

Lee, John R., M.D., et al. *What Your Doctor May Not Tell You About Menopause*. New York: Warner Books, 1996.

Lee, Martin A., et al. *Acid Dreams*. New York: Grove Press, Inc., 1985.

Lerner, Barron H. *The Breast Cancer Wars: Hope, Fear, and the Pursuit of a Cure in Twentieth-Century America*. New York: Oxford University Press, 2001.

Lippman, M.E., et al. *Regulatory Mechanisms in Breast Cancer*. Boston: Kluwer, 1990.

Livingston-Wheeler, Virginia, et al. *The Conquest of Cancer: Vaccines and Diet*. New York: Franklin Watts Publishing, 1984.

Lloyd, G. E. R. *Hippocratic Writings*. London: Penguin Books, 1978.

Loewenstein, Werner R. *The Touchstone of Life*. New York: Oxford University Press Inc., 1999.

Longenecker, Gesina L., Ph.D. *How Drugs Work*. Emeryville, Calif.: Ziff-Davis Press, 1994.

Love, Susan M., M.D., et al. *Dr. Susan Love's Hormone Book*. New York: Random House, 1997.

Lyon, William S. *Encyclopedia of Native American Healing*. New York: W. W. Norton & Company, 1998.

Maines, Rachel P. *The Technology of Orgasm*. Baltimore, Md.: The John Hopkins University Press, 1999.

Malinowski, Bronislaw. *The Sexual Life of Savages in North-Western Melanesia*. Boston: Beacon Press, 1929.

Martin, Emily. *Flexible Bodies*. Boston: Beacon Press, 1994.

Martin, Raquel, et al. *The Estrogen Alternative*. Rochester, Vt.: Inner Traditions Intl. Ltd., 1997.

Mayr, Ernst. *What Evolution Is*. New York: Basic Books, 2001.

McLean, Adam. *The Triple Goddness*. Grand Rapids, Mich.: Phanes Press, 1989.

Mead, Margaret. *Blackberry Winter.* New York: Kodansha International Ltd., 1995.

———. *Male and Female*. New York: Quill/William Morrow, 1967.

Medina, John J. *The Clock of Ages*. Cambridge, England: Cambridge University Press, 1996.

Miller, K.R., et al. *Biology,* new ed. Needham, Mass.: Prentice Hall, 1993.

Millman, Marcia. *The Unkindest Cut: Life in the Backrooms of Medicine*. New York: William Morrow and Company, Inc., 1976.

Modrow, John, et al. *How to Become a Schizophrenic: The Case Against Biological Psychiatry*. Seattle, Wash.: Apollyon Press, 1992.

Moir, Anne, et al. *BrainSex*. London, England: Arrow Books, 1998.

Montagu, Ashley. *The Natural Superiority of Women*. New York: The Macmillan Company, 1968.

Moore, Keith L. *The Developing Human*. Philadelphia: W. B. Saunders Company, 1982.

Morgan, Elaine. *The Aquatic Ape Hypothesis*. London, England: Souvenir Press, 1997.

———. *The Descent of Woman*. London, England: Souvenir Press, 1972.

———. *The Scars of Evolution*. New York: Oxford University Press, 1994.

Morris, Simon Conway. *The Crucible of Creation*. New York: Oxford University Press, Inc., 1998.

Moss, Ralph W. *Questioning Chemotherapy*. Brooklyn, N.Y.: Equinox Press, 1995.

Neville, M.C., et al. *The Mammary Gland*. New York: Plenum, 1987.

Noble, Vicki. *Uncoiling the Snake*. New York: HarperCollins Publishing, 1993.

Nuland, Sherwin B. *How We Die*. New York: Vintage Books,1993.

Opie, Lionel H. *The Heart: Physiology, from Cell to Circulation*. New York: Lippincott-Raven Publishers, 1998.

Ortiz de Montellano, Bernard R. *Aztec Medicine, Health, and Nutrition*. New Brunswick, N.J.: Rutgers University Press, 1990.

Palmer, Gabrielle. *The Politics of Breast-feeding*. London, England: Pandora, 1988.

Patterson, J.T. *The Dread Disease*. Cambridge: Harvard University Press, 1987.

Paungger, Johanna, et al. *Moon Time*. Essex, England: Saffron Walden, 1995.

Pearsall, Paul. *The Heart's Code*. New York: Broadway Books, 1998.

Peat, F. David. *Who's Afraid of Schrodinger's Cat?* New York: Quill, 1997.

Perry, Michael C., et al. *The Chemotherapy Source Book*. Baltimore, Md.: Williams & Wilkins, 1997.

Pert, Candace B., et al. *Molecules of Emotion*. New York: Scribner, 1997.

Pinker, Steven. *How the Mind Works*. New York: W.W. Norton & Company Ltd., 1997.

Pollan, Michael. *The Botany of Desire*. New York: Random House, 2001.

Posner, Michael I. *Foundation of Cognitive Science*. Cambridge, Mass.: MIT Press, 1989.

Proctor, Robert N. *Cancer Wars*. New York: Basic Books, 1995.

Raine, Cedric S., et al. *Advances in Neuroimmunology*. New York: New York Academy of Sciences, 1988.

Rako, Susan. *The Hormone of Desire*. New York: Crown Publishing, 1996.

Ramet, Sabrina Petra. *Gender Reversals & Gender Cultures*. New York: Routledge, 1996.

Ratey, John J. *A User's Guide to the Brain*. New York: Vintage Books, 2001.

Raymo, Chet. *Skeptics and True Believers*. New York: Walker and Company, 1998.

Reed, Evelyn. *Women's Evolution: From Matriarchal Clan to Patriarchal Family*. New York: Pathfinder Press, Inc., 1975.

Reichman, Judith, M.D. *I'm Too Young to Get Old*. New York: Random House, 1996.

Richter, Curt Paul, Ph.D. *Biological Clocks in Medicine and Psychiatry*. Springfield, Ill.: Charles C. Thomas Publishers, 1965.

Riddle, John M. *Eve's Herbs*. Cambridge: Harvard University Press, 1997.

Ridley, Matt. *The Red Queen*. New York: Macmillan Publishing Company, 1993.

Rinzler, Carol Ann, et al. *Estrogen and Breast Cancer: A Warning to Women*. New York: Macmillan Publishing Company, 1993.

Rock, John, M.D. *The Time Has Come: A Catholic Doctor's Proposals to End the Battle Over Birth Control*. New York: Alfred A. Knopf, 1963.

Rodgers, Joann Ellison. *Sex: A Natural History*. New York: Times Books, 2001.

Rolling Stone Magazine, The Editors of. *The Rolling Stone Interviews. The 1980's*. New York: St. Martin's Press, 1989.

Romoff, Adam, M.D. *Estrogen: How and Why It Can Save Your Life*. New York: Golden Books, 1999.

Rosenberg, Charles E., et al. *Framing Disease*. New Brunswick, N.J.: Rutgers University Press, 1992.

Rosenthal, Sara M., et al. *The Thyroid Sourcebook for Women*. Los Angeles: Lowell House, 1999.

Rossi, Claudio, et al. *Tempos in Science and Nature: Structures, Relations, and Complexity*. New York: New York Academy of Sciences, 1999.

Rothman, David J., et al. *Medicine and Western Civilization*. New Brunswick, N.J.: Rutgers University Press, 1995.

Rowbotham, Sheila. *A Century of Women*. New York: Penguin Group, 1997.

Rubin, Emanuel, et al. *Essential Pathology*. Philadelphia: J. B. Lippincott Company, 1990.

Ruden, Ronald A., M.D., et al. *The Craving Brain*. New York: HarperCollins Publishers, 1997.

Sams, Jamie. *Earth Medicine*. New York: HarperCollins Publishers, 1994.

Sandblom, Philip, M.D. *Creativity and Disease*. New York: Marion Boyars, 1992.

Sayers, Janet. *Biological Politics: Feminist and Anti-Feminist Perspectives*. New York: Tavistock Publications, 1982.

Schwarzer, Alice. *After the Second Sex*. New York: Pantheon Books, 1984.

Seaman, Barbara. *Free and Female*. Greenwich, Conn.: Doubleday Book Club, 1972.

Seaman, Barbara, et al. *The Doctors' Case Against the Pill*. Alameda, Calif.: Hunter House Inc., Publishers, 1969.

———. *Women and the Crisis in Sex Hormones*. New York: Bantam Books, 1977.

Sears, Barry, Ph.D. *The Anti-Aging Zone*. New York: ReganBooks, 1999.

Sehgal, Pravinkumar B., et al. *Interleukin-6*. New York: New York Academy of Sciences, 1989.

Shandler, Nina. *Estrogen the Natural Way*. New York: Villard, 1997.

Sheehy, Gail. *The Silent Passage*. New York: Pocket Books, 1993.

Shilts, Randy. *And the Band Played On*. New York: Penguin Books, 1987.

Shimkin, M.B. *Contrary to Nature*. Bethesda, Md.: National Cancer Institute, 1979.

Sichel, Deborah, M.D., et al. *Women's Moods*. New York: William Morrow and Company, 1999.

Silva, Orlando E., et al. *Breast Cancer: A Guide for Fellows*. New York: Elsevier Science B.V., 1999.

Singer, Sydney Ross. *Dressed to Kill: The Link Between Breast Cancer and Bras*. New York: ISCD Press, March 2002.

Sipple, Horace L., et al. *Sugars in Nutrition*. New York: Academic Press, 1974.

Slevin, M.L., et al. *Randomized Trials in Cancer*. Philadelphia: Raven Press, 1986.

Small, Meredith F. *What's Love Got to Do with It?* New York: Anchor Books, 1995.

Squartini, F., et al. *Breast Cancer: From Biology to Therapy*. New York: Annals of the New York Academy of Sciences, 1993.

Stabiner, Karen. *To Dance Within the Devil*. New York: Delacorte Press, 1997.

Starr, Paul. *The Social Transformation of American Medicine*. New York: Basic Books, Inc., 1949.

Sternberg, Esther M. *The Balance Within*. New York: W.H. Freeman and Company, 2000.

Stryer, L. *Biochemistry*, 3d ed. New York: W. Freedman and Company, 1988.

Taylor, Timothy. *The Prehistory of Sex*. New York: Bantam Books, 1996.

Timiras, Paola S., et al. *Hormones and Aging*. New York: CRC Press, Inc., 1995.

Veggeberg, Scott K. *Medication of the Mind*. New York: Henry Holt and Company, 1996.

Walsh, Paul, et al. *Physicians' Desk Reference*, 55th ed., Montvale, N.J.: Medical Economics Company, 2001.

Weed, Susun S. *Menopausal Years: The Wise Woman Way*. Woodstock, N.Y.: Ash Tree Publishing, 1992.

West, Stanley, et al. *The Hysterectomy Hoax*. New York: Doubleday, 1994.

Wiley, T.S., et al. *Lights Out: Sleep, Sugar, and Survival*. New York: Pocket Books, 2000.

Wolpoff, Milford H. *Human Evolution*. New York: McGraw-Hill, 1996.

Wood, Lawrence C., M.D., et al. *Your Thyroid*. New York: Ballantine Books, 1985.

Yalom, Marilyn. *A History of the Breast*. New York: Alfred A. Knopf, 1997.

Yen, Samuel S.C., et al. *Reproductive Endocrinology*. Philadelphia: W.B Saunders Company, 1999.

Zuckerman, Solly. *Nuclear Illusion and Reality*. New York: Viking Press, 1982.

Index